Integrating Psychiatry and Primary Care

Series Editors

Dinesh Bhugra
Institute of Psychiatry
King's College London
London, United Kingdom

Michelle B. Riba
University of Michigan Rogel Cancer Center
Ann Arbor, Michigan, USA

This series of books will serve to provide models of clinical care; transfer research advances and evidence-based practices into practical applications for mental health providers and primary care providers; and increase knowledge about this field. Both editors are strongly associated with the World Psychiatry Association, one of the world's largest medical organizations, which together with its partners provides services to help bring new information and findings to clinicians in many disciplines, who are caring for patients and families. This series brings together well known editors and authors to develop important topics in primary care psychiatry.

More information about this series at http://www.springer.com/series/13818

Luigi Grassi • Michelle B. Riba • Thomas Wise
Editors

Person Centered Approach to Recovery in Medicine

Insights from Psychosomatic Medicine and Consultation-Liaison Psychiatry

Springer

WORLD PSYCHIATRIC ASSOCIATION

Editors
Luigi Grassi
Institute of Psychiatry, Department of Biomedical and Specialty Surgical Sciences
University of Ferrara
Ferrara
Italy

Michelle B. Riba
University of Michigan Rogel Cancer Center
Ann Arbor, MI
USA

Thomas Wise
Inova Fairfax Hospital
Johns Hopkins University Inova Fairfax Hospital
Falls Church, VA
USA

ISSN 2522-5693 ISSN 2522-5707 (electronic)
Integrating Psychiatry and Primary Care
ISBN 978-3-319-74735-4 ISBN 978-3-319-74736-1 (eBook)
https://doi.org/10.1007/978-3-319-74736-1

Library of Congress Control Number: 2018956338

This Springer imprint is published by the registered company Springer Nature Switzerland AG
The registered company address is: Gewerbestrasse 11, 6330 Cham, Switzerland

To my parents, my wife, and my daughter for their love and constant encouragement. To all my patients who have taught me the profound sense of being persons.

Luigi Grassi

Thank you to my family for their love and support. My sincere appreciation to my patients and their families for the privilege to participate in their care.

Michelle B. Riba

To Karen Wise who always supported my work and schedule

Thomas Wise

Preface

This volume offers an important compliment to the current texts about consultation-liaison psychiatry. Readers should understand that consultation-liaison is the clinical derivative of psychosomatic theory. The book discusses both and weaves into its chapters how the role of the individual with unique hopes and fears, with a biopsychosocial perspective, may collaborate with clinicians and family and others.

The book is divided into three parts. The first part starts with the historical roots of psychosomatic theory which are addressed with the current mandate to incorporate valid, efficient, and clinically useful screening methodologies to identify individuals in distress from common psychological maladies and how to follow them with clinimetric assessment.

The second part of this volume focuses on topics that are rarely covered in depth in other texts. It is essential to understand "who" the patient is as well as "what" symptoms or disease they present to their physician or what they think may be problematic. Cultural background understanding is essential to best organize the complaints with which a patient presents and how to organize such information. To conserve dignity in the seriously ill is essential for good care but is too often ignored. Topics about rehabilitation and prevention in psychosomatic medicine are discussed and remind the reader that psychosomatic concepts as well as psychiatric consultation interventions are important in public health constructs. The techniques of communication and establishing relationships are also highlighted.

The final part of this volume ends with the mandate for integrated care considering both psychiatric and psychological perspectives along with the medical biomedical approach. The unique specialty of psychosomatic medicine in German-speaking countries offers an insight into a different form of healthcare delivery from the traditional partition of psychiatry and internal medicine. The volume closes with an important contribution about training in consultation-liaison psychiatry in our field. The consultation psychiatrist is to be the true link between biomedicine and psychosocial interventions in offering patient-centered care, but all physicians and other healthcare professionals must know what is offered in this volume. This book will be of great value to all who understand this essential union.

Ferrara, Italy — Luigi Grassi
Ann Arbor, MI, USA — Michelle B. Riba
Falls Church, VA, USA — Thomas Wise

Contents

The Role of Patient-Centered and Recovery-Oriented Models in Medicine: An Introduction

1

Luigi Grassi, Thomas Wise, and Michelle B. Riba

Abstract

As medicine achieves new scientific findings regarding disease causation and treatment, a human element has receded in actual clinical practice. This has limited the importance of the doctor-patient relationship which has serious implications for medical care as both patient and health-care provider exist in a biopsychosocial matrix. Various international health organizations are now working together to better integrate person-centered and recovery-oriented approaches into general medical care. Such a comprehensive approach to clinical patient care as well as medical research is more than mere psychosomatic medicine but requires attention to issues of functionality in an autonomous manner as well as participation in social groups. Dignity conservation, reaffirmation, and spiritual needs are necessary elements of the doctor-patient relationship. This requires

L. Grassi (✉)
Institute of Psychiatry, Department of Biomedical and Specialty Surgical Sciences, University of Ferrara, Ferrara, Italy
e-mail: luigi.grassi@unife.it

T. Wise
Department of Psychiatry, Inova Fairfax Hospital, Falls Church, VA, USA

Johns Hopkins University, Baltimore, MD, USA

George Washington University, Washington, DC, USA

Virginia Commonwealth University, Richmond, VA, USA

M. B. Riba
Department of Psychiatry, University of Michigan, Ann Arbor, MI, USA

University of Michigan Comprehensive Depression Center and Psych Oncology Program, University of Michigan Comprehensive Cancer Center, Ann Arbor, MI, USA

L. Grassi et al. (eds.), *Person Centered Approach to Recovery in Medicine*, Integrating Psychiatry and Primary Care, https://doi.org/10.1007/978-3-319-74736-1_1

appropriate communication abilities which include such psychosocial information in addition to careful review of biologic systems in both health and disease. The psychosomatic legacy is only part of the journey toward a true patient-centered model. This volume attempts to provide a rationale for its importance and provides clinical and educational examples about how to achieve such goals.

1.1 Introduction

The World Health Organization (WHO) defines in its Constitution health as "a state of complete physical, mental and social well-being and not merely the absence of disease or infirmity" [1]. In turn, the WHO defines mental health as "[...] a state of well-being in which every individual realizes his or her own potential, can cope with the normal stresses of life, can work productively and fruitfully, and is able to make a contribution to her or his community" [2]. In this way, the WHO asserts that the aim of medicine is to help people to regain a state of physical, psychological, and social health—and we can add spiritual health [3]—that is far more complex than an absence of any disease. The WHO also states there is no universally accepted "definition" of well-being which should be interpreted within the sociocultural context of the individual. Thus there are different possible connotations for different individuals and groups (e.g., it could include the notion of happiness or contentment, or absence of disease, or economic prosperity), nevertheless well-being is part of what we need to purse in medicine. In fact, WHO also considers it mandatory to relate both well-being and mental health to a series of other concepts that have been the focus of attention of research related to clinical practice. These include resilience, as the capacity to cope with adversity and stressors; sense of coherence, which encapsulates factors that enable a person to use resources optimally; optimism; social engagement; satisfaction; autonomy; and achieving goals and expectations, all of which encompass the conceptualization of quality of life.

WHO indications are particularly important in the present time in which the increasing scientific reductionism and the focused attitude of medical practice upon technology have transformed the relationship of health-care professionals with their patients. This has resulted in dehumanized and exclusively disease-centered encounter with an individual that is ill that is, with a limited interest in the psychological, social, and spiritual well-being, as, in contrast the WHO strongly affirms. As chronic noncommunicable diseases such as diabetes, cancer, and cardiovascular and respiratory illnesses and severe mental disorders tend to become increasingly chronic burdens for the individual patient, new challenge for the medicine of the future will arise as patients' psychological and other elements of quality of life become more apparent and longer lasting. Currently and in the future, the personal experience and representations of the illness and the impact of these disorders on the individual patient life (i.e., the emotional, psychological, spiritual, and interpersonal levels of life) are an essential mission of what medicine must incorporate [4].

Finally, it has become clear, over the last 30 years of research, that every disease, whether somatic (e.g., cancer, diabetes) or mental (e.g., schizophrenia o bipolar spectrum disorders), is the result of multiple codeterminants and co-variables that are biological, psychological, spiritual, and social. All these variables together should be the target of prevention and treatment in all settings of medicine. Only then can medicine achieve its goals of reducing suffering and maximize both functioning and quality of life, in the biopsychosocial dimensions of the ill patient.

1.2 Person-Centered Medicine and Recovery-Oriented Approaches in Medicine

The above concepts are what both general medicine and psychiatry have proposed as central paradigms for promoting health and well-being of total individual, whether coping with a chronic disorder or terminally ill.

In general medicine, the person-centered approach has increased in the last years by the consideration of the reductionist limitations of current knowledge base of medical care and the urgency to reconquering the human side of medicine, which seems completely lost in the health system in all countries. As Cloninger states [5], the practice of person-centered medical care requires doctors to examine basic questions about the scope of medical responsibility, the nature of the therapeutic doctor-patient relationship, and the types of procedures that are appropriate in treatment and health promotion, when well-being is the goal to be reached. Thus a biopsychosocial framework for understanding both ill- and positive health, based on the need to promote the autonomy, values, and dignity of every person who consults a physician, as well as the diversity of patient populations, in their different sociocultural contexts is at the center of person-centered medicine [6].

In mental health and psychiatry, similar concepts have been expressed by the recovery-oriented movement, which strongly pursues an approach that should focus attention not to treat only the mental disease (or reduce the psychopathological symptoms) but to recover all the dimensions of the person, by seeing people beyond their problems—their abilities, possibilities, interests, and dreams—and by helping them to rehabilitate their social roles and relationships that give life value and meaning [7–9]. In this sense, recovery is affirmed in terms of existential constructs (e.g., sense of hope, empowerment, agency, as well as spiritual well-being). Furthermore functional actions (e.g., obtaining and maintaining valued societal roles and responsibilities), physical health (e.g., better health and a healthy lifestyle), and social engagements (e.g., enhanced and meaningful relationships and integration with family, friends, and the wider community) are issues to appreciate and improve [10].

A significant influence to both person-centered and recovery-oriented approaches has been given by positive psychology, which started in the 1990s by abandoning the exclusive disease model of illnesses and focusing attention on the need for people to live a meaningful life, to be oriented toward self-acceptance, autonomy, and purpose in life [11]. The scientific study of positive human functioning is flourishing on multiple levels that include the biological, personal, relational, institutional, cultural, and global dimensions of life [12], which are in fact coincident with what recovery proposes for mentally ill people and what person-centered medicine advocates in medicine in general [13, 14]. This has led positive psychiatry to emerge as the science and practice of psychiatry that seeks to understand and enhance well-being through assessments and interventions involving positive psychosocial characteristics in people with mental or physical illnesses [15].

Although the recovery-oriented approach in the context of patient-focused care was originally in mental health settings, general medicine has begun to utilize this positive approach. Initially focused on mental health, the World Psychiatric Association evolving collaboration with the World Association of Family Practice and the World Medical Association offers a larger vision for a medicine having the patient within as the center and goal of clinical care and health promotion, by articulating both a scientific and humanistic approach in order to optimize attention to both the objective factors of the disease in an ill person but also positive psychological and health aspects of the person [16, 17].

Therefore, in all the spheres of medicine and in all the medical specialties, the goals should not be restricted to merely curing one disease, or to symptom reduction when the disease is not curable, but to enhance patients' positive psychosocial characteristics is a way to reach and improve well-being when facing with disease (being it somatic or mental). This does not relegate the new scientific discoveries based on superb technology to a secondary position but implicates the shift from a sole disease-centered approach to personalized therapeutic intersubjective relationship of that particular health-care professional (as a person) with that particular patient (as, also, a unique person with spiritual and psychosocial needs) [18–20].

1.3 The Psychosomatic Legacy and the Person-Centered and Recovery-Oriented Approach

Many echoes of these approaches are evident in both the internal medicine and psychosomatic medicine of the last century. From the medical side, Francis W. Peabody was one of the many physicians who underscored the fact that the practice of medicine in its broadest sense should always include the whole relationship of the physician with his patient. In 1927, he said, *It is an art, based to an increasing extent on the medical sciences, but comprising much that still remains outside the realm of any science, since everyone, sick or well, is affected in one way or another, consciously or subconsciously, by the material and spiritual forces that bear on his life, and especially to the sick such forces may at as powerful stimulants or depressants* [21]. In 1950, Karl Jaspers, both a physician and philosopher, also underlined the dangerous change in medicine becoming too highly technological that could lead to negative consequences for the patient-doctor relationship. As he stated, *the patient enters the hospital as if he were entering a business concern, to be served in the best possible way by an impersonal apparatus. And the physician of modernity acts as if he were a collectivity, which cares for the patient without a physician's entering into the treatment in any personal way […]* [22]. In the same years, the Swiss physician Paul Tournier stated that the only possibility to speak of medicine is to consider it as a person-centered medicine, which has two pillars, science and faith, and thus it is a medicine of the whole person, including the biological, psychological, social, and spiritual aspects of health problems [23]. As he thought, the medicine of the person is not just another branch of medicine but a necessary approach toward health and disease, integrating the organic and the psychological. He urged this to be a basic attitude of the profound contact in patient care experience, which must be applicable in all areas of medicine. Tournier emphasizes the uniqueness and dignity of man, in his suffering, but also each person's resources and not just deficits, thus validating the individual's purposes in life and considering him as a whole individual in his community and society.

At least in part and albeit with several misunderstandings and ambiguities, the psychosomatic tradition has offered [24] the same line of clinical and research reasoning. In 1939, Franz Alexander suggested that acquiring a detailed knowledge of the relationship between emotional life and body processes extends the function of the physician by coordinating the physical and mental care of the patient into an integral whole of medical therapy [25]. The counterreformation against the mechanistic view of man and medicine has had its legacy in many other psychosomatic and psychiatry scholars, scientists, and clinicians, such as George L. Engel, Zbigniew J. Lipowski, Michael Balint, and others, stating that medicine should be actually reformulated as a biopsychosocial medicine [26–28], with its center and uniqueness in doctor-patient relationship as a therapeutic ingredient [29]. In this way the psychosomatic approach has to do with the inseparability and interdependence of psychosocial and biological (physiologic, somatic) aspects of humankind. Psychosomatic medicine should therefore be defined as the holistic dimension of medicine and the science aiming at (a) studying the correlations of psychologic and social phenomena with physiologic functions, normal or pathologic, and of the interplay of biologic and psychosocial factors in the development, course, and outcome of diseases and (b) advocacy of a holistic (or biopsychosocial) approach to patient care and application of methods derived from behavioral sciences to the prevention and treatment of human morbidity [30]. As Lipowski poignantly affirmed, *It is unfortunate that the word "holistic" has been appropriated recently by an anti-scientific and anti-intellectual so-called "holistic health movement" with resulting increment in semantic confusion and, in the eyes of many, loss of credibility for the misappropriated term. However, to retain it has merit as it is short, simple, and derived from the Greek—as were the very conceptions it has come to connote. Moreover, "holistic" has been part of the basic vocabulary of psychosomatic medicine from the beginning and conveys its core premises and purpose faithfully." Thus, the historic function of the psychosomatic movement has been to "vitalize the whole of medicine, psychiatry no less. . .. with the holistic and ecologic viewpoint* [31].

It is true that in some countries, such as the USA, psychosomatic medicine has been recognized as consultation-liaison (C-L) psychiatry, intended as a subspecialty of psychiatry focused on treating behavioral conditions in patients with medical and surgical problems, especially when patients have complex or long-term conditions [32–34].[1] And with respect to this, it involves psychiatrists to be specifically trained

[1] In November of 2017, The Academy of Psychosomatic Medicine (APM) voted to change its name to the Academy of Consultation-Liaison Psychiatry (ACLP). It followed a similar change in which the American Board of Medical Specialties voted to change the name of the field to Consultation-Liaison Psychiatry.

in the field and providing collaborative care, by bridging physical and mental health, as indicated by the consensus statement delineating the set of basic competencies and roles of a psychosomatic/C-L psychiatrists [35, 36]. On the other hand, C-L psychiatry has notably influenced in a profound way medicine, by allowing non-psychiatrists to understand through a continuous liaison with psychiatrists in the general hospital how to apply a biopsychosocial model and how to assess in clinical practice the concepts of psychosocial stress, psychophysiological response specificity, coping, adaptation, and social support [37–39].

However, in other countries, a number of networks and associations are proposing models that tend to consider psychosomatic medicine in a wider sense, by basically maintaining the original message from the old tradition of psychosomatic medicine as a scientific field of interest in the relationships among the psychological, biological, and social processes in human health and disease that cuts across all medical specialties and their basic sciences [40–42]. Therefore its clinical and educational message indicates that, besides specialists in psychiatry, all health-care teams, including physicians working in primary care and all the several medical specialties, psychologists, nurses, and other professionals, should have a "psychosomatic" training in order to practice a scientifically sound and rigorous biopsychosocial approach in their daily clinical activity [43, 44].

The need to advance and integrate the scientific study of biological, psychological, behavioral, and social factors in health and disease to be applied in clinical practice; to promote health as a state of physical, mental, sociocultural, and spiritual well-being; and to reduce disease, by acting on a mutual respect for the dignity and responsibility of each individual person (including the patient, the family and the health professional), is a common mission of these internationally recognized groups.[2] If, for example, we consider the specific aims of the several bodies interested into a medicine for the whole person, there are similarities if not almost complete overlapping of intents, with a wide space given to training students and health-care professionals (Table 1.1). The physicians who utilize the psychosomatic approach must understand that this is not a direct linear approach but a complex network of interacting biological, psychological, and social dimensions that continues to require significant research. It does not diminish to mandate never to forget the biopsychosocial approach for each patient in either the clinical experience or research arena.

[2] For more information, see the websites illustrating the aims and the mission of the associations and networks working in the area of psychosomatic medicine and person-centered medicine such as the International College of Psychosomatic Medicine (http://www.icpmonline.org/), the Academy of Consultation-Liaison Psychiatry (ACLP) (www.clpsychiatry.org//); the International College of Person-Centered Medicine (ICPM) (http://www.personcenteredmedicine.org); the European Association of Psychosomatic Medicine (EAPM) (http://eapm.org); the American Psychosomatic Society (APS) (http://www.psychosomatic.org/); the World Psychiatric Association section on Psychiatry, Medicine, and Primary Care (http://www.wpanet.org/detail.php?section_id=11&content_id=509); or the European Society for Person-Centered Healthcare (http://pchealthcare.org.uk), just to cite some.

Table 1.1 Conceptual bases and aims of professional associations and networks promoting new standard in a medicine for the whole person

International College of Psychosomatic Medicine	European Association of Psychosomatic Medicine	International College of Person-Centered Medicine
• To foster the development of psychosomatic medicine, i.e., the study, education, and application of knowledge and skills in biopsychosocial, brain-behavior-health-disease relationships • To foster cooperation and collaboration of researchers, educators, and practitioners of psychosomatic medicine throughout the world • To provide opportunities for communication and collegiality among persons and organizations that share and/or support the objectives of ICPM	• To promote an integrated psychosomatic (biopsychosocial) approach to health and disease • To promote the treatment and care of patients with psychiatric disorders and psychological problems in patients with or without physical disorders in general hospitals, medical clinics, other community outpatient clinics and primary care • To stimulate and support research in the areas of psychosomatic medicine, consultation-liaison psychiatry, and integrated care • To stimulate and support teaching and training and advanced professional education in the areas of psychosomatic medicine, consultation-liaison psychiatry, and integrated care • To foster interaction and collegiality among members of the association and provide opportunities for mutual support and assistance • To educate the patients, carers, and the general public regarding psychosomatic medicine • To provide a forum for the presentation, dissemination, and discussion of scientific problems in psychosomatic medicine, consultation-liaison psychiatry, and integrated care through the organization of meetings, conferences, workshops, and publications • To advise national and European organizations and to encourage and stimulate the formation of local, regional, and national organizations which further the goals of the association • To identify and reward outstanding achievement and/or service in psychosomatic medicine, consultation-liaison psychiatry, and integrated care	• Broad bio-psycho-socio-cultural-spiritual theoretical framework • Attention to positive health and ill-health as components of a broad concept of health • Enhancement of person-centered communication, diagnosis, treatment, prevention, and promotion of health • Respect for the autonomy, responsibility, and dignity of every person involved • Promotion of person-centered relationships and partnerships at all levels • Articulation of person-centered clinical medicine and people-centered public health

Therefore we need a medicine encompassing the conceptualizations derived from psychosomatic medicine, from person-centered and recovery-oriented approaches (i.e., humanistic-narrative individualized recovery-oriented care), and from what psychosomatic scientific literature has gathered in the last 40 years in terms of research (i.e., the relationship of psychosocial/spiritual individual dimensions with biological mechanisms at molecular and systemic levels, such as neuroendocrine-immune system, epigenetics, and so on) [45, 46].

1.4 Overview of Chapters

For all the abovementioned reasons, we have considered that it is time to move toward a unified conceptualization of a person-/family-centered and recovery-oriented approach in all fields of medicine, as the profession where care and cure are to be declared in a relational (the intersubjectivity between patients and health-care professionals) experience that has its background in a holistic approach, intended as a whole person-centered medicine that demands attention to the objective features of a disease but also the unique subjective elements of the person. These unique elements should include both strengths and limitations that help or hinder autonomous function in the physical and emotional spheres but also what factors limit or enhance integration into a group of the individual's choice.

In doing that, we decided not to take the challenge to go into the details of the single approach in the different specialty areas of medicine (e.g., cardiology, oncology, neurology, psychiatry), since many books are already available for this, and to try to cover the *deplorable gap between medicine and psychiatry* [30]. Instead, we tried to pursue the aim to give a framework about the need for a unified mission of medicine that can have for all people affected by any disorder and illness a whole biopsychosocial medical approach, basing the several steps of the clinical encounter (screening, assessment, intervention) according to evidence-based but also value-based principles, gaining the insights coming from psychosomatic and C-L psychiatry of the last 40 years. A second aim is to present innovative aspects and themes to have emerged from recent research and clinical experience, in terms of clinical practice, educational interventions, and organizational efforts to train students and health-care professionals to achieve such patient-centered care.

The book consists of three parts: (1) clinical concepts and methods in psychosomatic medicine, (2) clinical contexts of psychosomatic medicine, and (3) integrated intervention. Although this division is in part artificial and arbitrary, it gives the reader the opportunity to navigate within the methods, the practice of care, and the organizational issues related to proper person-centered and recovery-oriented approach in the several fields of medicine.

1.4.1 Part I: Clinical Concepts and Methods

In Part I, the general clinical concepts and methods in psychosomatic medicine are discussed in detail by experts in the field. Grassi and collaborators summarize in

Chap. 2 the old philosophical debate between the mind, as a subjective phenomenon that is linked to a sense of consciousness, and the body, as an objective phenomenon illustrating the role and importance of a biopsychosocial approach in all the spheres of medicine. The most recent data from biological, psychological, and social science are discussed according to the only possible approach, that is, the medicine of the whole person, as a way to contrast the still evident modern medicine reductionism.

In Chap. 3, Mezzich and Salloum summarize the most significant aspects related to psychosomatics within the framework of holistic theory and care, which happens to be one of the key concepts of person-centered medicine (PCM). The basic notions of person-centered medicine and the way this has evolved historically from ancient civilizations through modern medicine are also presented, from a systematic study organized by the International College of Person-Centered Medicine.

Mitchell in Chap. 4 focuses attention on the reliable assessment and measurement of psychological health as a key element of supportive care by examining the new evidence of screening of mood disorders, anxiety, distress, cognitive decline, and unmet needs in medicine and more specific assessment of the most frequent psychosocial/psychopathological conditions as a part of routine high quality of care that involves all health-care professionals.

Chapter 5 is dedicated to the clinimetric approach within a psychosomatic approach in medicine. Fava and Cosci illustrate how clinimetrics may help in expanding the narrow clinical approaches that minimize clinical trajectories or staging and focus too much on narrow state assessments or values in either the laboratory values or psychometric assessments. They point out the limited range of information that derives when only using the current traditional categorical nosography (i.e., the DSM-5). New approaches, such as the revised version of the Diagnostic Criteria for Psychosomatic Research (DCPR) that examine clinically significant dimensions in psychosocial medicine (e.g., the spectrum of maladaptive illness behavior, demoralization, irritable mood), are likely to improve outcomes both in clinical research and practice.

1.4.2 Part II: Clinical Contexts

Section II is dedicated to illustrate innovative issues in the clinical contexts of psychosomatic medicine. Chapter 6 by Grassi and collaborators explains the theory and practice of dignity-conserving care as a multifactorial construct taking into account illness-related concerns dignity-conserving perspectives and the social dimensions of dignity. In patients suffering from somatic or psychiatric disorders, loss of identity, shattering of self-image, discrimination or stigma, and having psychological, interpersonal, spiritual, and existential needs that are not being adequately addressed are all forms of loss of dignity. The delivery of dignity-conserving care and dignity-oriented intervention is illustrated as a way to achieve a holistic and healing approach in medicine to better allow the current focus upon technological strategies for disease treatment with the incorporation of our human needs that must be addressed.

In Chap. 7, Tarricone and collaborators belonging to the cross-cultural consultation-liaison psychiatry group of the European Association of Psychosomatic Medicine (EAPM) discuss the important and new emerging problems in medicine determined by the phenomenon of immigration in many countries worldwide. The role of culture on the symptom presentation, diagnostic process, and treatment strategies in these populations, as well as practical aspects of cultural competence, is discussed. The World Psychiatric Association (WPA) and the European Psychiatric Association (EPA) guidelines on mental health and mental health care for migrants and list a series of recommendations for policy makers, service providers, and clinicians are also presented as new needs in biopsychosocial medicine.

Chapter 8 by Fielding and Lam addresses the area of prevention in terms of the impacts of social, developmental, and environmental influences on the individual psychosomatic equilibrium in health and illness. The way in which political and economic contexts can exert a major influence on psychosomatic processes that affect health is also discussed with preventive options in addressing individual-level interventions presented and explored.

In Chap. 9 Kissane and collaborators examine the new insights from literature and clinical experience as far as effective communication in medicine is concerned. Two advanced communication training programs are presented, the first of which (i.e., the Comskil model) is relative to how to communicate distressing diagnostic and prognostic news to oncology patients and family and the second (the ComPsych model) focuses on schizophrenia and management approaches aligned to a recovery-orientated framework.

Stress and stress-related disorders from both physical and psychological viewpoints are the focus of Chap. 10, as presented by King. The author examines the long-lasting deleterious effects on mental and physical health caused by psychological trauma (e.g., childhood adversity and maltreatment, adult exposures to interpersonal violence, accidents and disasters, life-threatening medical events, such as myocardial infarcts or cancer). The consequences of post-traumatic stress disorder (PTSD) on the several psychobiological processes or “axes” (e.g., sympathetic autonomic system, the hypothalamic-pituitary-adrenal axis, and immune function and inflammatory processes) that lead to increased pathophysiological processes and disease risk are reviewed according to the most recent literature.

Javed and Carozza in Chap. 11 underline the role that psychiatric rehabilitation can have for medicine, as an example of helping individuals to develop skills and access resources needed to increase their capacity to be successful and satisfied in the living, working, learning, and social environments of their choice and how to incorporate principles of recovery and wellness, community support, person-centered care, and active involvement of individuals and families in the behavioral health system and services.

Chapter 12, by Linden, describes life span research in the development of individuals from conception to death, recognizing biological, psychological, and social factors. The problems of classification, assessment, and description of determinants of the course of illness, as well as treatment issues (i.e., when and how long to intervene; how to shift from a symptom/function approach to capacity limitations and impairment; how to evaluate treatment outcome), are also detailed.

Botbol and collaborators delineate in Chap. 13 the significant conceptualization related to the psychosomatic model starting from research in childhood and the role of the body in the interactions with the caring environment in terms of the modulation of both physiological and psychological mechanisms. Anorexia nervosa is taken as a specific example of alterations within family interpersonal relationships that foster misaligned meanings and intentions with a family system of mentalization (i.e., alexithymia, *operational thinking*, and *operational life*).

1.4.3 Part III: Integrated Intervention

Part III deals with the treatment implications in a person-centered and recovery-oriented approach in medicine. Biondi and collaborators, in Chap. 14, present the model of integrated interventions in a function-oriented rather than diagnosis-oriented approach and in the dimensional characterization of psychopathology. With respect to this, neuroendocrine concomitants (e.g., HPA) as well as personality aspects (e.g., resilience and coping styles) may be modulated by integrated (i.e., psychopharmacological and psychotherapeutic) intervention. Also, new data are presented on the telomere-telomerase-mitochondria system as a novel and relevant locus of interest in the interface between psychiatry and medicine and a possible common molecular mediator of both physical and psychiatric disturbances.

Chapter 15 by Boniolo deals with the field of ethical counselling as a special intervention centered on the needs and on the biographies of the patient when ethical problems intersect clinical decisions in medicine. This approach based on ethical counselling has the aims to improve the decision process concerning clinical option to be pursued and to increase the individual patient empowerment without reducing her autonomy.

Zipfel and collaborators, in Chap. 16, provide insights into the established German tradition of psychotherapy in medicine as an independent discipline within medicine and a model that both integrate psychosomatic medicine as a mandatory part of the curriculum in medicine and a specific specialty of psychosomatic medicine and psychotherapy. Examples of integrating multidisciplinary professionals (e.g., nurse, physician, psychologist, physiotherapist) in the intervention for patients with chronic pain, eating disorders, and somatoform/functional disorders are provided. Also the organization of Consultation-Liaison Psychosomatic Medicine (C-L PSM) services (e.g., departments of psychosomatic medicine, out- and inpatient services) with integration in several medical areas (e.g., psycho-cardiology, transplant C-L PSM, psycho-oncology, chronic pain) is illustrated.

In the last chapter, Chap. 17, Söllner and collaborators describe the role of training as a central issue in medicine, with particular reference to consultation-liaison

(C-L) psychiatry and psychosomatic medicine. As collaborative care becomes an increasing focus in the integration of psychiatry into medicine, the German model of training should be of interest to the current consultation-liaison curricula. The guidelines for training developed and agreed in the USA, Australia, New Zealand, and Europe are presented. The role of C-L psychiatrist and psychosomatic medical physicians in the education of medical students, general practitioners, residents and specialists of other medical specialties, and health-care professionals in general is delineated. Such training courses proved to be effective to improve communication with and treatment of patients with comorbid medical and mental health problems.

1.5 Discussion and Future Perspectives

The most significant challenge of medicine is to regain its role of science of human beings, that is, combining the progressive results and discoveries of science (in terms of physicalism and materialism) with the human side of the unique individual (humanistic medicine) [47]. At the same time, it is imperative to maintain the focus on both evidence-based- and value-based-oriented research (including quantitative and qualitative research) and to constantly work in daily clinical encounters according to the framework of a whole-centered medicine that takes into account the values of patients/families and health-care professional on their interpersonal relation (people-centered medicine) for the common aim not to get rid of the disease and/or symptoms but to orient all the interventions in improving the quality of life, that is, increasing the flourishing of the person (recovery-oriented medicine) [48]. In doing this it is necessary to avoid the risk that these concepts stay just as a rhetorical device or slogans in global health, without no investment in resources for a psychosomatic, person-centered and recovery-oriented education of health-care professionals and for the implementation of services really practicing what declared. And there is still a long road to go. In the recovery-oriented approach in psychiatry, connectedness, hope and optimism, identity, meaning and purpose, and empowerment, as part of the personal recovery journey [49], are not easily reached by the organization of current mental health services, still based on old models having traditional clinical outcome targets, rather than recovery in its specific meaning [50–52]. Furthermore, the site of clinical care is often siloed from general medical clinics which deprives both realistic integration of general medicine and psychiatric to patients but also limited educational experiences for both the mental health and general medical providers.

In general medicine, the difficulties and problems in integrating new technologies to a whole-person-centered approach are enormous. Current medicine is in fact powerfully supporting personalized medicine, which however has nothing to do with the person and in which "personalization" means again the reduction of the single individual and his family and clinical history to its genetic or molecular characterization for better targeting, in a purely biological way, the treatment and to prevent a disease. If it is extremely important and mandatory that medicine should improve its biological techniques and scientific methods, it cannot substitute scientific personalization for the humanistic art of medicine. It needs to be personal in the sense to responding to the needs of the people, who want and ask for personalized care, in terms of holistic approach, as a person-centered approach (or personalized care, as it has also been counter-defined) do [53–55]. In a sense, if there is no doubt that genomics, proteomics, pharmacogenomics, metabolomics, and epigenomics, are medical fields and expressions of extremely important conquests of science of and for the man, these should be tools to be used for and with the single specific individual with his own personality (e.g., personal history, resilience, coping, interpersonal relationships, values) and representation of health and disease, that is unique circumstances of the person—the "personome" (therefore, *personomics*) [56, 57]. The term "personalized" medicine is now being overtaken by labelling such molecular approaches as "precision" medicine. But to be "precise," it is essential to know "who" the patient as well as "what" disease they have and how biological interventions may help [58]. Thus *personomics* is a necessary aspect-component of modern medical care, from primary care to all the medical specialties [59].

With this in mind, the hope is that this book can give further and new insights in helping clinicians and researchers to constantly use a multidimensional approach when dealing with human suffering in medicine, by always applying, in all the several fields of medicine, a biopsychosocial attitude which can combine a whole-centered approach in the medical encounter by properly using the incredible discoveries that year after year science is giving us to better understand the human condition.

References

1. World Health Organization (WHO). Constitution of the World Health Organization. Geneva. http://apps.who.int/gb/bd/PDF/bd47/EN/constitution-en.pdf?ua=1.
2. World Health Organization (WHO). Promotion of mental health. Geneva: WHO. http://www.searo.who.int/entity/mental_health/promotion-of-mental-well-being/en/.
3. Milstein JM. Introducing spirituality in medical care: transition from hopelessness to wholeness. JAMA. 2008;299(20):2440–1.
4. Corbin J, Strauss AL. Accompaniments of chronic illness: changes in body, self, biography, and biographical time. Res Sociol Health Care. 1987;6:249–81.
5. Cloninger CR. Person-centred integrative care. J Eval Clin Pract. 2011;17:371–2.
6. Cox JL. Empathy, identity and engagement in person-centred medicine: the sociocultural context. J Eval Clin Pract. 2011;17(2):350–3.
7. Anthony W. Recovery from mental illness: the guiding vision of the mental health service systems in the 1990s. Psychosoc Rehabil J. 1993;16:11–23.
8. Slade M. Personal recovery and mental illness. Cambridge: Cambridge University Press; 2010.
9. Farkas M. The vision of recovery today: what it is and what it means for services. World Psychiatry. 2007;6:68–74.
10. Whitley R, Drake RE. Recovery: a dimensional approach. Psychiatr Serv. 2010;61(12):1248–50.
11. Resnick SG, Rosenheck R. Recovery and positive psychology: parallel themes and potential synergies. Psychiatr Serv. 2006;57:120–2.
12. Seligman MEP, Csikszentmihalyi M. Positive psychology: an introduction. Am Psychol. 2000;55(1):5–14.

13. Mezzich JE. Positive health: conceptual place, dimensions and implications. Psychopathology. 2005;38(4):177–9.
14. Cloninger CR. The science of well-being: an integrated approach to mental health and its disorders. World Psychiatry. 2006;5:71–6.
15. Jeste DV, Palmer BW, Rettew DC, Boardman S. Positive psychiatry: its time has come. J Clin Psychiatry. 2015;76(6):675–83.
16. Mezzich JE. World psychiatric association perspectives on person-centered psychiatry and medicine. Int J Integr Care. 2010;10:3–7.
17. Mezzich JE. Psychiatry for the person: articulating medicine's science and humanism. World Psychiatry. 2007;6:1–3.
18. Mezzich JE, Botbol M, Christodoulou GN, Cloninger CL, Salloum IM, editors. Person centered psychiatry. Berlin: Springer; 2016.
19. Miles A. On a *medicine of the whole person*: away from scientistic reductionism and towards the embrace of the complex in clinical practice. J Eval Clin Pract. 2009;15:941–9.
20. Miles A. Towards a medicine of the whole person--knowledge, practice and holism in the care of the sick. J Eval Clin Pract. 2009;15(6):887–90.
21. Peabody FW. The care of the patient. JAMA. 1927;9:877–82.
22. Jaspers K. Der Arzt im technischen Zeitalter. Universitas: Zeitschrift für Wissenschaft, Kunst und Literatur. 1959;14(4):337–54. (English translation by Grugan AA). The physician in the technological age. Theor Med Bioeth. 1989;10(3):251–67.
23. Tournier P. Médicine de la personne. Neuchatel: Delachaux et Niestlé; 1940. (English Tr. The Healing of Persons. Harper Collins Pub, 1965).
24. Jacob RG, Hugo JA, Dunbar-Jacob J. History of psychosomatic medicine and consultation-liaison psychiatry. In: Ackerman KD, Dimartini AF, editors. Psychosomatic medicine. New York: Oxford University Press; 2015.
25. Alexander F. Psychological aspects of medicine. Psychosom Med. 1939;1:7–18.
26. Engel GL. The need for a new medical model: a challenge for biomedicine. Science. 1977;196:129–36.
27. Lipowski ZJ. Review of consultation psychiatry and psychosomatic medicine. 3. Theoretical issues. Psychosom Med. 1968;30:395–422.
28. Lipowski ZJ. Review of consultation psychiatry and psychosomatic medicine. II. Clinical aspects. Psychosom Med. 1967;29(3):201–24.
29. Balint M. The doctor, his patient and the illness. London: Pitman Medical Publishing; 1957.
30. Lipowski ZJ. What does the word "psychosomatic" really mean? A historical and semantic inquiry. Psychosom Med. 1984;46(2):153–71.
31. Galdston I. Psychosomatic medicine. AMA Arch Neurol Psychiatry. 1955;74:441–50.
32. Gitlin DF, Levenson JL, Lyketsos CG. Psychosomatic medicine: a new psychiatric subspecialty. Acad Psychiatry. 2004;28(1):4–11.
33. Lipsitt DR. Psychosomatic medicine: history of a "new" specialty. In: Blumenfield M, Strain JJ, editors. Psychosomatic medicine. Philadelphia: Lippincott Williams & Wilkins; 2006. p. 3–20.
34. Boland RJ, Rundell J, Epstein S, Gitlin D.: Consultation-Liaison Psychiatry vs Psychosomatic Medicine: What's in a name? Psychosomatics. 2018;59(3):207–10.
35. Söllner W, Creed F, European Association of Consultation-Liaison Psychiatry and Psychosomatics Workgroup on Training in Consultation-Liaison. European guidelines for training in consultation-liaison psychiatry and psychosomatics: report of the EACLPP workgroup on training in consultation-liaison psychiatry and psychosomatics. J Psychosom Res. 2007;62(4):501–9.
36. Leentjens AF, Rundell JR, Diefenbacher A, Kathol R, Guthrie E. Psychosomatic medicine and consultation-liaison psychiatry: scope of practice, processes, and competencies for psychiatrists working in the field of CL psychiatry or psychosomatics. [corrected] a consensus statement of the European Association of Consultation-Liaison Psychiatry and Psychosomatics (EACLPP) and [corrected] the Academy of Psychosomatic Medicine (APM). Psychosomatics. 2011;52(1):19–25.

37. Lipowski ZJ. Psychosomatic medicine: past and present. Part II. Current state. Can J Psychiatr. 1986;31(1):8–13.
38. Lipowski ZJ. Psychosomatic medicine: past and present. Part III. Current research. Can J Psychiatr. 1986;31(1):14–21.
39. Lipowski ZJ. Consultation-liaison psychiatry at century's end. Psychosomatics. 1992;33(2):128–33.
40. Oken D. Current theoretical concepts in psychosomatic medicine. In: Kaplan HI, Sadock BJ, editors. Comprehensive textbook of psychiatry, vol. 2. 5th ed. Baltimore, MD: Williams & Wilkins; 1989. p. 1160–9.
41. Fava GA, Belaise C, Sonino N. Psychosomatic medicine is a comprehensive field, not a synonym for consultation liaison psychiatry. Curr Psychiatry Rep. 2010;12(3):215–21.
42. Deter HC. History, concepts and aims of internationally active societies in psychosomatic and behavioural medicine. Biopsychosoc Med. 2016;10:34. https://doi.org/10.1186/s13030-016-0085-1.eCollection.
43. Park EM, Sockalingam S, Ravindranath D, Aquino PR, Aggarwal R, Nemeroff SF, Gerkin JS, Gitlin DF, Academy of Psychosomatic Medicine's Early Career Psychiatrist Special Interest Group. Psychosomatic medicine training as a bridge to practice: training and professional practice patterns of early career psychosomatic medicine specialists. Psychosomatics. 2015;56(1):52–8.
44. Deter HC, Orth-Gomér K, Wasilewski B, Verissimo R. The European Network on Psychosomatic Medicine (ENPM)—history and future directions. Biopsychosoc Med. 2017;11:3. https://doi.org/10.1186/s13030-016-0086-0.eCollection2017.
45. Wise TN. Psychosomatics: past, present and future. Psychother Psychosom. 2014;83(2):65–9.
46. Wise TN, Balon R. Psychosomatic medicine in the 21st century: understanding mechanisms and barriers to utilization. In: Balon R, Wise T, editors. Clinical challenges in the biopsychosocial interface. Update on psychosomatics for the 21st century. Basel: Karger; 2015. p. 1–9.
47. Whatley SD. Borrowed philosophy: bedside physicalism and the need for a sui generis metaphysic of medicine. J Eval Clin Pract. 2014;20(6):961–4.
48. Martin CM, Félix-Bortolotti M. Person-centred health care: a critical assessment of current and emerging research approaches. J Eval Clin Pract. 2014;20(6):1056–64.
49. Leamy M, Bird V, Le Boutillier C, et al. A conceptual framework for personal recovery in mental health: systematic review and narrative synthesis. Br J Psychiatry. 2011;199:445–52.
50. Davidson L, O'Connell MJ, Tondora J, et al. Recovery in serious mental illness: a new wine or just a new bottle? Prof Psychol Res Pr. 2005;36(5):480–7.
51. Slade M, Amering M, Farkas M, et al. Uses and abuses of recovery: implementing recovery-oriented practices in mental health systems. World Psychiatry. 2014;13(1):12–20.
52. Drake RE, Whitley R. Recovery and severe mental illness: description and analysis. Can J Psychiatr. 2014;59(5):236–42.
53. Vogt H, Ulvestad E, Eriksen TE, Getz L. Getting personal: can systems medicine integrate scientific and humanistic conceptions of the patient? J Eval Clin Pract. 2014;20(6):942–52.
54. El-Alti L, Sandman L, Munthe C. Person centered care and personalized medicine: irreconcilable opposites or potential companions? Health Care Anal. 2017. p. 1–15. https://doi.org/10.1007/s10728-017-0347-5. [Epub ahead of print].
55. Cornetta K, Brown CG. Balancing personalized medicine and personalized care. Acad Med. 2013;88(3):309–13.
56. Ziegelstein RC. Personomics. JAMA Intern Med. 2015;175(6):888–9.
57. Ziegelstein RC. Personomics: the missing link in the evolution from precision medicine to personalized medicine. J Pers Med. 2017;7-11:1–5.
58. Ziegelstein RC. Personomics and precision medicine trans. Am Clin Climatol Assoc. 2017;128:160–8.
59. Ziegelstein RC. Perspectives in primary care: knowing the patient as a person in the precision medicine era. Ann Fam Med. 2018;16(1):4–5.

Part I

Clinical Concepts and Methods in Psychosomatic Medicine

Psychosomatic and Biopsychosocial Medicine: Body-Mind Relationship, Its Roots, and Current Challenges

2

Luigi Grassi, Thomas Wise, David Cockburn, Rosangela Caruso, and Michelle B. Riba

We have at present no conception of what an explanation of the physical nature of a mental phenomenon would be. Without consciousness the mind-body problem would be much less interesting. With consciousness it seems hopeless. The most important and characteristic feature of conscious mental phenomena is very poorly understood.

(Nagel, 1974; page 436) [1]

L. Grassi (✉)
Institute of Psychiatry, Department of Biomedical and Specialty Surgical Sciences, University of Ferrara, Ferrara, Italy
e-mail: luigi.grassi@unife.it

T. Wise
Department of Psychiatry, Inova Fairfax Hospital, Falls Church, VA, USA

Johns Hopkins University, Baltimore, MD, USA

George Washington University, Washington, DC, USA

Virginia Commonwealth University, Richmond, VA, USA

D. Cockburn
Department of Philosophy, University of Wales Trinity Saint David, Lampeter, UK

R. Caruso
Department of Biomedical and Specialty Surgical Sciences, Institute of Psychiatry, University of Ferrara, Ferrara, Italy

University Hospital Psychiatry Unit, Integrated Department of Mental Health and Addictive Behavior, S. Anna University Hospital and Health Authorities, Ferrara, Italy

M. B. Riba
Department of Psychiatry, University of Michigan, Ann Arbor, MI, USA

University of Michigan Comprehensive Depression Center and Psych Oncology Program, University of Michigan Comprehensive Cancer Center, Ann Arbor, MI, USA

L. Grassi et al. (eds.), *Person Centered Approach to Recovery in Medicine*, Integrating Psychiatry and Primary Care, https://doi.org/10.1007/978-3-319-74736-1_2

Abstract
The basis of psychosomatic medicine is a fundamental philosophical debate between mind (a subjective phenomenon that is linked to a sense of consciousness) and body (which is empirically demonstrable). Starting from the Greek tradition to the Cartesian *res cogitans-res extensa* dichotomy, the chapter illustrates the role and importance of a biopsychosocial approach in all the spheres of medicine as a way to contrast the still evident modern medicine reductionism. The evidence coming from biological, psychological, and social science, merging in biopsychosocial (or psychosomatic) integrated view in medicine, is also discussed. Although the term psychosomatic can be misleading, since, as Alexander underlined in the first issue of the journal Psychosomatic Medicine in 1939, *it may imply dichotomy between psyche and body (soma). If however we understand psychic phenomena as nothing but the subjective aspect of certain bodily (brain)* processes, this dichotomy disappears, becoming medicine of the whole person, away from scientistic reductionism and toward the embrace of the complex in clinical practice.

2.1 Historical Antecedents

The basis of psychosomatic medicine is a fundamental philosophical debate between mind (a subjective phenomenon that is linked to a sense of consciousness) and body (which is empirically demonstrable). As one of the most debated issues in the history of humanity, the relationship between the mind and the body is based in various theories, particularly in the Western world that fundamentally attempted to unify two contrasting elements, body and soul [2], to arrive at either a dualistic or a monistic position.

The conceptualization of a spiritual soul with respect to a concrete body has always been discussed within a framework of dialectic constructs, such as life and death, mortality and immortality, materiality and immateriality, divine and human, heavenly and earthly, and purity and impurity. A final synthesis of such opposing ideas has yet to be constructed.

The psychological-somatic partition can be already traced in the Homeric tradition, where the psychosoma paradigm was stringently related to death and life. The word σῶμα (*soma*) denoted the dead body, while ψυχή (*psyche*) was the last breath when dying and the ghost of the person wandered in the afterlife of ᾞδης (Hades). This school of thought localized the "psychological" (belonging to ψυχή) aspects of existence within the physical body by labelling them θυμός (*thymos*), φρήν (*phren*), and νοῦς (*nous*) as the expressions of emotional life, the mind, and intelligence, respectively.

A more structured dualistic position, in the following centuries, is traceable in the Orphic religion that considered the soul to be of divine origin (δαίμων)[1] (and

[1] It is interesting that the Greek word has different roots, deriving from both δαίμων (daemon = deity) and δαήμων (daemon = knowing or wise) but also from the word δαίω (to divide, to distribute destinies, to allot).

therefore immortal), immaterial and incorporeal, while the body, as a material and mortal element, holds the soul in bondage, coercing it to live for a period of time. The idea of transmigration of the soul after death, in other bodies in order to purify the spirit from sins committed during the life (μετεμψύχωσις), is also part of this vision, with a dialectic contrast between purity versus impurity, heaven versus earth, and freedom versus coercion. These concepts were initially shared by the Pythagorean schools of philosophy and, subsequently, by Socrates and then the Platonic schools—who clearly stated that the soul is the factor animating the body as a living being and that, at the same time, possesses a body which metaphorically imprisons the soul (the similarity between the words σῶμα (*soma* = body) and σημα (*sema* = prison, tomb), demonstrates this association). Platonic beliefs best summarized in *Phaedo* concluded that the soul inhabits the body temporarily and otherwise exists in the infinite metaphysical sphere as rational knowledge. Plato presents the soul as the seat of the reason, whereas the functions of the less rational elements, appetite and spirit, are localized in the animate body. In *Republic*, Plato re-conceptualizes the soul as consisting of three parts, conventionally translated as λογιστικόν (*logistikon*, the logical reason, attached to knowledge and truth), the θυμοειδές (*thymoeides*, or spirit, that in the just soul, aligns with the *logistikon*) and the ἐπιθυμητικόν (*epithymetikon*, the appetitive part which ignores the *logistikon* and expresses the desires as eating and libido).

Subsequently Aristotle in his essay *On the Soul* (Περὶ Ψυχῆς Latin *De Anima*) considered the soul consisting of two parts, rational and irrational, the latter subdivided into vegetative and sensitive (also present in plants and animals) and the former subdivided in a passive nous (the passive intellect destined to die with the body) and an active nous, divine, immortal, and detached from the body. For Aristotle the mind is a faculty of the soul, and when the body perishes, so does the soul.

2.2 The Cartesian Approach and Psychosomatics

The debates about the interaction of "mind" and "body" continued over the centuries but became more evident when Descartes (1596–1650) published his ideas. Descartes abandoned the traditional Scholastic Aristotelian philosophy and constructed a new mechanistic science. He formulated a modern version of the mind-body problem by contrasting two different dimensions, *res cogitans* and *res extensa*, the first immaterial and the second material. Over a period of 10 years, Descartes in his published works especially *Discours de la méthode (Discourse on the Method) (1637), Meditationes de prima philosophia (Meditations on First Philosophy) (1641),* and *Les passions de l'âme (Passions of the soul) (1649)* expanded the debate on the body-mind relationships of the following questions: ontological (are mental states and physical states entirely distinct, one class a subclass of the other, are all mental states physical, or vice versa?); causal (do physical states influence mental states or vice versa? In which way?); questions related to consciousness, intentionality, and the self (how can we define these concepts? How are they related to the brain and the body?); and finally the embodiment question (is the mind housed in a body and in which way? What is it for a body to belong to a particular subject?).

2.2.1 Descartes and the Problem of Body-Mind Dualism/Triadism

In Descartes, the basis for a psychosomatic explanation of the human being has two essential components: the doctrine of mind-body dualism (i.e., a clear distinction between the mind as a thinking, non-divisible, non-extended phenomenon and the body as a nonthinking, divisible, extended object) and the doctrine of the body-machine (i.e., a mechanization of the human body that, according to him, can be compared to a statue or a machine like an artificial fountain). In this analogy, the nerves are like pipes, the muscles like springs and levers, and the brain cavities like storage tanks, while the soul is the fountain-keeper. The human soul, however, has the important role to give the human a sense of uniqueness. Descartes defines the different aspects of the thought (soul) in terms of actions of the soul, mainly volition and passions which are our perceptions of objects that stimulate the nerves or are due to other less common causes, such as fantasies of the imagination that stir the soul, the temperament, or the intellectual emotions ("all the sort cases of perceptions and knowledge").

In spite of the fact that the two substances, body and soul, share nothing in common, Descartes holds that there is a union unique to humans established by nature and constituted by their mutual dependence and interaction that he localizes in the pineal gland, as the seat of the soul (*siège de l'àme*) [3].

Descartes theorized that the pineal gland displays properties that place it as a third object somewhere between the soul and the body. Descartes suggests the idea of the union between mind and body a "third primitive notion," which is basic and unanalyzable. Union is not essential to either mind or body, since either can exist without the other, but, unless united to a soul, a body is not a human body, suggesting that the "human body," body and soul together, can be considered as a unity, a thing, a substance, in its own right, a substance created from the union of body and soul. If the relationship between the soul and the body is something more than the sum of its two parts, some scholars [4, 5] propose the notion of "triadism" when discussing the Cartesian theories, suggesting a "quality," which is specifically represented by the interaction between the two substances that make up human beings, as an experience of unity. In the need to try to solve the separation between the mind and the body, Descartes, according to Machamer and McGuire [6], created an epistemological shift where a sense of wholeness starts to prevail on a firm dualism. The relation between the soul and the body is redefined, with the soul, although without extension, size, shape, or position, cohered in something akin to the totality of the body. The body in this view seems to be reinterpreted not as an accumulation of discrete and separate parts but as an organizational whole, in the totality of which a soul is present. Descartes' last writings in a sense introduce a sort of "corporealization" (materialization) of the soul and at the same time of a sort "mentalization" (indivisibility) of the body, where memory, imagination, and sense perception are faculties rooted in corporeal-material processes, while thought, corresponding to myself, is linked to the soul [5].

2.2.2 Descartes' "Guilt" and the Need for Holistic Vision

In spite of these attempts to rehabilitate and give more light to Descartes' last writings where the "human" itself seems to be conceived as a being in itself, an individuated whole or unity greater than just the combination of soul and body [7], many critiques have been raised. Descartes has been and continues to be considered responsible of the Western dichotomy ever made both from the ontological (mind and body) and the epistemological point of view (subject and object). Binswanger also, as an existential psychiatrist, was convinced that the Cartesian dichotomy is *the cancer of all psychology and psychiatry up to now [...] It is a question of attempting to understand and to explain the human being in the totality of his/her existence. But that is possible only from the perspective of our total existence: in other words, only when we reflect on and articulate our total existence, the "essence" and "form" of being human* [8].

In a totally different way, years later, Damasio a contemporary behavioral neurologist [9] also criticizes Descartes pointing out that the separation of mental activity from the structure of the brain and its inner workings, as conceptualized by Descartes, is an error since the brain and the rest of the organism form an inseparable entity consisting of numerous neuronal and biochemical channels that relate the subject to its surroundings, and mental activity is a result of this interaction. One of the mechanisms enabling feelings of emotion to emerge is the activation of neural "as if body loops." These simulation mechanisms, bypassing the body proper through the internal activation of sensory body maps, create a representation of emotion-driven body-related changes. The activation of these "as if body loops" can likely be not only internally driven but also triggered by the observation of other individuals. Thus, any consensus about Descartes' vision of the human being is still debatable [10].

2.3 Psychosomatic as Biopsychosocial

From the perspective of psychoanalysis, the interest in the body-mind question was, in contrast, an extremely intriguing field. Freud himself changed several times his conviction about the interpretation of the body-mind relationship, being initially as a dualist, and evolving into an epiphenomenalist, and eventually a parallelist [11].

In spite of that, a number of scholars within the psychoanalytical movement, such as Ferenczi, Groddeck, Dunbar, Alexander, Mirsky in the 1950s, and later Bahnson [12], used a psychoanalytical paradigm to try to understand the "mysterious leap" from mind to body [13]. The paradigm, however, was for most part linked to ascertain how mental phenomena could influence the body to foster vulnerabilities for causing medical disorders [14, 15].

Lipowski corrected the psychoanalytic mistake of reducing psychosomatic to psychogenic by viewing the individual in a holistic manner within a framework that values all the dimensions of the human being. Lipowski [16, 17] profoundly restated the constitution of psychosomatic medicine, advising physicians to avoid the trap of etiological and causal relationships between mind and body and considering psychosomatic medicine in a more integrated framework as a discipline:

> The task of psychosomatic medicine is to attempt to integrate the 3 modes of abstraction, viz., biological, psychological, and social. [...] Psychosomatic" does not imply a value judgment that psychic events are more important than somatic or vice versa. Nor does it connote the assumption of specific causal relationships, i.e., psychic events causing somatic ones and somatic causing psychic. The use of terms "psychosomatic" and "somatopsychic" does give the impression of implied causal sequences, but this is only a problem of semantics and not of causality. [...] Psychosomatic medicine is more than a set of techniques, more than an approach; it is also a science. (page 397)

Thus a science, *since one which studies the relationships between psychological and biological phenomena in humans, as they occur in and are influenced by the human and nonhuman environment, in both health and disease,* and, at the same time, an approach since the *hallmark of the psychosomatic approach is the insistence that psychosocial as well as biological factors be considered in the diagnosis, treatment, and prevention of all disease* [14, 15].

Engel popularized the term "biopsychosocial" from a different perspective as a way to contrast the dogma of a medicine only based on a reductivist biomedical approach [18].

> What is being and can be done to neutralize the dogmatism of biomedicine and all the undesirable social and scientific consequences that flow therefrom? How can a proper balance be established between the fractional-analytic and the natural history approaches, both so integral for the work of the physician and the medical scientist? How can the clinician be helped to understand the extent to which his scientific approach to patients represents a distinctly "human science"[...]? (page 135)

It was possible in his opinion by starting from and using a multifactorial frame of reference as in von Bertalanffy's general system theory [19]. He underlined the impossibility to separate the biological, psychological, behavioral, and social aspects of our being in the world, since health and illness (whatever illness, be it a somatic or a psychiatric disease) are codetermined by a series of interacting variables, from the cellular to the social. In his model, both understanding the determinants of disease and determining at rational treatments and patterns of health care, the patient, the social context in which he lives, and the complementary system devised by society to deal with the disruptive effects of illness should be taken contemporarily always into account.

Engel was however aware of the formidable resistances of the biomedical system (both as science and as dogma) to a different approach, including the power of vested interests, social, political, and economic, where the delivery of health care is a major industry, the professionalization of biomedicine which has engendered a caste system among health-care personnel, and a peck order concerning what constitutes appropriate areas for medical concern and care.

Thus, not only biological factors, but the personal experience of the disease, what it means to him/her and how this meaning may influence his/her behavior, the role of the environment, and the interaction with others are components to be studied in an integrated way to understand both health and illness, as a total human response. It is up to the physician, taking into consideration these interactions through a biopsychosocial lens in order to promote the healing of patients' illnesses, as opposed to narrow efforts to diagnose and cure diseases [20, 21].

Forty years later, these basic concepts and the related problems that Engel raised regarding the biomedical approach still reverberate in medicine. However, biopsychosocial or psychosomatic medicine remains an important attempt to reduce the level of extremism of biologically oriented theories and approaches, on one side, and psychological-oriented theories and approaches, on the other side, by integrating what has emerged from biological, psychological, and social studies [22–24]. An essential task of psychosomatic research is to carefully consider biological and psychosocial variables.

2.3.1 Biological Issues

A series of data have accumulated regarding psychosomatic medicine in terms of psychoneurobiology, over the last years [25, 26]. Data exist relative to the genetic influences on brain structure and functions, including the genetically determined differences in receptor morphology and density or in transporter function in regulatory systems as co-responsible for individual variation in personality, stress reactivity, and potential for somatic reactions to stress. Studies on the functional neuroanatomic bases of mental states have shown that the vast majority of mental life takes place outside of conscious awareness and that bottom-up processing of subcortical and bodily emotional information is associated with subsequent top-down inhibition or modulation of those structures that generate emotional responses. The role of neurotransmitter systems is clearer and allows to understand the individual variation in regulatory systems as contributors of the differences in personality, temperament, and emotional reactivity. The existence of interactions between the central nervous system, the autonomic nervous system, the endocrine system, and the immune system, including conditioning of immune responses, immune effects of brain lesions or stimulation, stress effects, and brain changes during immune reactions, has been demonstrated [27, 28], as well as the role of genetics in modulating the immune response to stress [29], which is extremely important in the view of the immune system as a sixth sense to perceive and interpret the world [30].

These information are important in how we approach medical disorders, such as cardiovascular disorders, cancer, neurological disorders, and medical disease in general, which, according to Lane et al. [31], should follow an A (mind, behavior), B (brain), C (information transfer system, i.e., autonomic, neuroendocrine, immune), and D (end organ, e.g., heart) model. The “Cartesian” pineal gland has also been taken into account modulator of the stress-immune response [32].

Major advances have been done with regard to neurosciences and the biological concomitants of psychological disorders. In psychiatry, it has been repeatedly indicated that depression is a systemic disease, involving the brain, the hormonal, the immune system (IS), and the autonomic nervous (AN) system [33]. Some interesting data regards the fact that chronic inflammation and oxidative stress have been implicated in the pathophysiology of depression and, since similar mechanisms have been reported in a number of chronic medical conditions. Psychological and physical stressors have been considered possible cofactors in systemic diseases, and conversely, systemic diseases have been considered to facilitate the development of depression [34]. This hypothesis is in agreement with data showing that chronic inflammation is implicated in the pathophysiology of immune suppression in the context of chronic illnesses, such as cancer, while markers of impaired cellular immunity (e.g., decreased natural killer cell cytotoxicity) and inflammation (e.g., elevated IL-6, TNFα, and CRP) are associated with depression [35], suggesting that immune dysregulation may be a central feature common to both depression and medical comorbidities. Regarding chronobiology and stress, alterations in the circadian axis have been proposed, for example, as a possible biological concomitant of physical symptoms in cancer patients, with psycho-neuroendocrine-immune stress-related pathways possibly influencing circadian disruption and negative implications for cancer prognosis [36, 37].

2.3.2 Psychological Issues

Increasing research has focused attention to psychological aspects of medical disorders, both in terms of the onset of psychological disorders secondary to a diagnosis of medical illness of the role of psychological factors in the adjustment to the stressors caused by the illness and of a possible modulation of the progression of the disorder itself, especially if chronic [38]. Use of valid psychometric assessment approaches has further improved the reliability of the psychosocial dimension of psychosomatic research.

Attachment theory has been applied in a series of studies regarding medical illness, with data indicating that attachment is a factor influencing the individual responses to stress (as a psychobiological phenomenon) via psycho-neuro-endocrino-immunological pathways [39]. Thus, health and disease states can be interpreted as psychobiological entities that are at least in part socially constituted, through the role of attachment and attachment styles among individuals [40]. In a psychosomatic sense, the sequences of attunement, misattunement, and reattunement, between the dialogic/dyadic child-mother relationship, that mediate the regulation of emotions, wherein the mother (primary caregiver) co-regulates the infant's postnatal development, are also considered important for the development of the structural right brain neurobiological systems involved in processing of emotion and self-regulation [41]. In summary, the individual's attachment styles can be understood as a the result of an internal working model accompanying the human being and mold our disposition toward certain perceptions of others and of the self, as well as certain preferred strategies to deal with the existence and life events. All these aspects have significant implications in terms of intervention and treatment [42].

Major advances have been done in terms of psychological diagnostic issues, with new criteria specifically developed for psychosomatic medicine, showing the importance of a wide vision catching the several dimensions of suffering, not only the classical psychopathological symptoms for a nosologically-oriented psychiatric diagnosis. The Diagnostic Criteria for Psychosomatic Research (DCPR) originally formulated in 1995 [43] and recently revised [44] have been applied in patients affected by different medical illnesses [45], as also illustrated in Chap. 5 in this book.

Relevant scientific data have been also collected in the area of psychological well-being. Concepts like hedonic (subjective) (e.g., positive affect, life satisfaction, happiness) and eudaimonic well-being (e.g., personal growth, purpose in life, autonomy, self-acceptance, positive relationships, meaning, self-realization) [46–48] have been indicated to be extremely important in contributing to individuals' health through functional salutogenic brain mechanisms [49]. In line with the idea that well-being is not just the absence of distress and that positive emotions are not merely the opposite of negative emotions [50], a number of authors have found that intervention centered on the aforesaid aspects can promote psychological well-being [51].

2.3.3 Social and Interpersonal Issues

The environment in which we live in is both a source for support and stress. Stressful life events have been one of the first areas of studies regarding the impact of stress on individuals and the implications in terms of vulnerability to develop medical or psychiatric diseases [52, 53]. Both major life events and chronic daily hassles and minor events may determine a decrease of the defense natural mechanisms, although eustress (i.e., the "right" quantity of stress in terms of allostasis) is beneficial for the organism [54]. Data have shown that stressors in the environment can have long-lasting effects on development, depending upon the stage of life at which they are experienced, and that adverse childhood experiences can alter the later capacity of individuals to respond normally to adverse situations in adulthood [55]. However, under the right circumstances, the brain can reenter plastic states, and negative outcomes may be mitigated, even later in life [55]. These circumstances are frequently represented by positive and effective social relationships. In fact, a number of studies over the last 20 years have on the other hand provided evidence of the importance of the support (e.g., emotional, practical, informational) deriving from interpersonal ties in improving coping abilities against stressful events [56]. Both close (e.g., family, friends) and diffuse social support (e.g., social network) are important in this respect [57]. It has been demonstrated that social relationships, as instruments for integration and care, are related to the maintenance of health behavior (e.g., diet, physical activity, adherence to treatment) that are important both in disease prevention and in adjustment to the disease [58]. Resilience (as the ability to recover from or adjust easily to a stressful event) [59] has been also related to social support, which connoted as a buffering hypothesis works as an external coping mechanism favoring the activation of internal coping [60, 61] and the psychobiological capacity of the organism to react [62–64].

2.3.3.1 Interpersonal Support and Doctor-Patient Relationship

A special area of support in interpersonal relationship regards doctor-patient communication and the importance of health-care professionals' use of empathy in facilitating patients' adjustment to their illness. This is the territory where both cure and care integrate each other, and only within the space created between a dyadic clinical relationship, a mutual, holistic existence of two beings is created in terms of "physicianship" [65]. Such a healing space can be described, in Buber's and Levinas' conceptualization [66, 67], as an authentic encounter with true subjectivity being formed with and through the other [68].

The scientific literature on these issues is extremely vast, ranging from the identification of the skills and the key competences doctors and health-care professionals should have to the association between empathy and patient outcomes, the role of cultural background in communication, and the impact of education and training in changing doctors' communication behavior and attitudes and in improving the relationship with their patients, in different medical fields [69–71].

As a psychosomatic implication, it has been demonstrated that the mirror neuron system has been not only implicated in action but also in communication, language, and social interaction, with a possible extension to emotions, sensations, and thoughts [72–74]. In other words, this matching mechanism might be related to the way in which human beings access and understand the minds of others (theory of mind, mentalization), facilitating social behavior and social competence [75, 76] and making intentionality and intersubjectivity possible [77]. Although this explains only a part of a more complex neural network involving subcortical and neurohormonal mechanisms associated with affective communication, parental care, and social attachment processes [78, 79], a series of data now exist trying to relate the mirror neuron system to interpersonal and behavioral problems in psychiatric disorders [80] and to understand compassion and empathic communication, as a mirroring-based interpersonal morality [81] in medical settings [82].

Because of the essential mutuality in the doctor-patient relationship, a bulk of data are available on the emotional implication of curing and caring in health-care settings. The overidentification with suffering, the overwhelming sense of compassion (compassion fatigue) up to vicarious traumatization, and the erosion in values, dignity, and will among health-care professionals are all part of this scenario [83].

However, compassion is an integral part for a humanistic approach in a doctor-patient relationship. According to several scholars [84], compassion seems to reside between objective and affective understanding oriented to another (empathy) and subjective responses oriented to the self, rooted in pity toward another (sympathy) [85].

2.4 Challenges to Biopsychosocial Medicine

There are however some problems to be taken into account and discussed. The first is related to the fact that the biomedical reductionism has determined at least an apparent partial crisis of evidence-based medicine and the onset of a bulk of paradigms (e.g., holistic, humanistic, narrative and narrative evidence-based medicine, medical cosmology) [86–89]. This has sometimes determined the loss of a scientific approach, making again evident a powerful dualism and the impossibility of a constructive dialogue between the bio and the mental. In this sense, the risk that a nonscientific approach can become equally reductionist and damaging was noted by Engel himself with what he described as possible "counter dogmas," such as those of "holistic" and "humanistic" medicine, if based on faith, superstitions, and obscure belief systems [90]. However, the principles underlying humanistic medicine include aspects (e.g., open communication, mutual respect, and emotional connection between physicians and their patients) which indicate that care is the key element of these principles. But this does not imply that care cannot be part of observation (outer viewing), introspection (inner viewing), and dialogue (interviewing), as Engel proposed as the basic methodological triad for clinical scientific study of medical diseases [91]. This triad was demonstrated in Engel and Reichsman's long-term case study investigating an infant with a gastro-tracheal fistula. Monica carefully identified various affective states that allow reliable correlation between the interviewer (whether verbally and facially empathic or stoic) and the biological variable of gastric acid levels [92]. Although some suggest that subjectivity was apparently less considered by Engel [93], the role of working on a scientific framework "biopsychosocial factor" (and not the static concept of "model") has been and can be a stimulus for a psychosomatic broad vision of health care [94, 95].

A paradoxical and opposite aspect is that, in spite of the psychosomatic/biopsychosocial lesson, medicine tends to maintain its biological-/technical-oriented framework that, in contrast with all the complaints about rehumanizing the health-care system, strongly molds the personalization (and uniqueness) of the individual in a very objective materialistic way. Therefore, the meaning of modern personalized medicine has to do with the individual genomic profile, bringing per se to the opposite result of a depersonalized medicine [96, 97], with no attention to the psychosocial inner dimensions (profile) of the person, according to a true person-centered approach [98].

A further problem has been raised by some scholars, such as McLaren [99] that criticizes Engel's biopsychosocial approach in that he suggests that *to be science, the theory itself must be more than a mere metaphysical claim; its propositions must be cast in a form which permits empirical testing, which is where the model comes into its own.* And for McLaren, the biopsychosocial model/theory (that in fact should be considered as completely different concepts) should be contextualized in the time in which it was developed and did not solve the problem that psychiatry lacks—and continues to lack—a well-formulated, theoretical basis and logically derived models with true predictive power.

From a different philosophical perspective, Van Oudenhove and Cuypers [100] point out the need to restructure the biopsychosocial theory considering that different metaphysical views on the "mind-body problem" may have important implications for the conceptual foundations of psychosomatic medicine, in terms of integration between biomedical (including neuroscience), psychological, and social sciences. In particular they consider that a simplistic biopsychosocial approach should be analyzed in a more sophisticated way taking into account the contribution of philosophical approaches such as reductive physicalism (i.e., mental states are both nothing over and above physical states and reducible to physical states) and supervenience physicalism (i.e., every mental phenomenon must be grounded in, or anchored to, but not reduced to an underlying physical-neural state).

From another perspective, Ghaemi [101] considers the need to rescue other approaches—such as Jaspers' non-dogmatic, non-eclectic approach to be defined as method-based medicine (including psychiatry)—in order to maintain a true interdisciplinary way of working in medicine in terms of both humanism (e.g., the holistic consideration of the patient) and science (e.g., the need for the assessment of psychosocial factors through a scientific approach) [102]. In a sense, as Ghaemi [103] says, an art based on science, not simply a science but also not merely an art, is a concept that Engel explicitly rejected, arguing that it denigrated psychosocial factors into idiosyncratic interpersonal skills.

It was in fact Jaspers who, in his essay on *The Physician in the Technological Age* [104], two decades before Engel and with words that are still extremely modern, admonished about the risk that the physician's identity was weakened by the use of high technical-diagnostic instrumentation and the relationship between physician and patient might progressively be deprived of its ethical value in terms of meeting, listening, and treating subjects.

> We call to mind three harmful tendencies in the modem physician, which at the moment are shadows of great things. First, the intensification of the technological presuppositions of medical ability through the organization of the physician has, as a side-effect, ruinous influence on the reality of the idea of the physician. Second, the advance of scientific knowledge has, as a side-effect, a medicine which, if it does not see its limits, does violence through theories to therapy and to the patient, and restricts the spirit and the soul. Third, the substance of the philosophical idea of the physician at those limits has, as a side-effect, the disorder of non-philosophy. (page 265)

Jaspers strongly recommended the need to reinstate the ancient model of the physician-philosopher, as proposed by Hippocrates, so as to counteract the regressive aspects of a medical practice which has already been completely integrated within the increasingly "technically enhanced" domain of natural sciences. Thus the answer for Jaspers is to readmit philosophy into the mainstream of medicine, since philosophy does not mean abstract, a vacuum, or an airless space wherein the voice does not carry, as it has often believed. As Jaspers writes:

> The answer to that would have been: space is not airless, but is in fact like pure air; seemingly nothing, yet is the air in which we must breathe in order to exist; the air of reason, without which we suffocate in the mere intellect. It becomes the life's breath of existenz. Only through it does reality speak out of a deeper origin. [...] (page 265) science without philosophy—despite its having correct knowledge of many particulars—becomes on the whole uncritical, and in the inner constitution of its supports becomes a dark reserve. (page 264)

However, the problem with these critics is that complicated theories do not practically help physicians in understanding the way in which they can recuperate their own sense of being doctors in a human relationship with their patients. In this sense, the most urgent aspect of mind-body dualism is of a practical, not theoretical, nature and should be based on something understandable and transferrable in clinical practice, yet scientific based [105].

Conclusions

The biopsychosocial approach in medicine, with an evolution in the psychosomatic literature proposing the multivariant nature of this phenomenon over the last 30 years, seems to maintain its utility, if we speak, in an evidence-based but at the same time, ethically speaking, value-based way, of our being in the world as biological, social, psychological, and spiritual entities. Thus, human life should be viewed as a wholeness, requiring and deserving both the tough-mindedness of the scientist (evidence-based medicine) and the compassion of the physician (person-centered medicine) [106, 107], integrating the cure and the care as inseparable parts of the medical approach.

What Alexander wrote, in the first inaugural issue of the "new" journal *Psychosomatic Medicine*, as a "new" chapter of medicine [108] in 1939, could maintain its validity if we continue to integrate the discoveries and results of different disciplines working together for a better and more comprehensive approach in medicine:

> The fundamental philosophical postulate of modern medicine is that the body and its function can be understood in terms of physical chemistry, that living organisms are physico-chemical machines and the ideal of the physician is to become an engineer of the body. The recognition of psychological forces, a psychological approach to the problems of life and disease, appears as a relapse back to the ignorance of the dark ages in which disease was considered as the work of the evil spirit and therapy was exorcism, the expelling of the demon from the diseased body. [...] (pages 7–8)
>
> The totality that is a human being has been divided for study into parts and systems; one cannot decry the method but one is not obliged to remain satisfied with its results alone. [...] The need for more knowledge here is of an excruciating obviousness. Contributions from other fields are to seek from psychology, cultural anthropology, sociology and philosophy as well as from chemistry and physics and internal medicine to resolve the dichotomy of mind and body left us by Descartes. (page 9)

Descartes' legacy is in fact still challenging. It is true that despite increasingly detailed knowledge of neural processes on one hand and psychological functioning on the other, we seem no closer to the actual transition of one to the other, the identity of mind and body [109]. Furthermore it is true that, if we are in a world that is indeterminant and ambiguous, where no event is certain and the entire outcome of anything is a probability, speaking about body-mind relation is an extremely hard challenge [110]. However, as Fava et al. suggest [111, 112], psychosomatic medicine has demonstrated to allow science to have a complex and not reductionist view of the person and remains a name to be kept and may be defined as a comprehensive interdisciplinary framework. It maintains also its mission with specific aims:

1. The scientific investigations on the role of psychosocial factors affecting individual vulnerability, course, and outcome of any type of medical disease
2. The personalized and holistic approach to the patient, adding psychosocial assessment to the standard medical examination
3. The integration of psychological and psychiatric therapies in the prevention, treatment, and rehabilitation of medical disease
4. The multidisciplinary organization of health care that overcomes the artificial boundaries of traditional medical specialties

It is true, as Alexander himself thought, that the term psychosomatic can be misleading: the word *"psychosomatic medicine maybe is not most fortunate because it may imply dichotomy between psyche and body (soma). If however we understand psychic phenomena as nothing but the subjective aspect of certain bodily (brain) processes this dichotomy disappears"* (page 14). Becoming de facto a medicine of the whole person: away from scientistic reductionism and towards the embrace of the complex in clinical practice [113].

References

1. Nagel T. What is it like to be a bat? Philos Rev. 1974;83:435–50.
2. Porter R. The flesh in the age of reason. The modern foundation of body and soul. New York: W.W. Norton; 2003.
3. Descartes R. Discourse on method and mediations of first philosophy (translated by Donald A. Cress), 4th ed. Cambridge: Hackett Publishing Company, Inc; 1998.
4. Alanen L. Reconsidering descartes's notion of the mind-body union. Synthese. 1996;106:3–20.
5. Bassiri N. Material translations in the cartesian brain. Stud His Philos Biol Biomed Sci. 2012;43:244–55.
6. Machamer P, McGuire JE. Descartes's changing mind. Stud Hist Phil Sci. 2006;37:398–419.
7. Hoffman P. The unity of descartes' man. Philos Rev. 1986;95(3):339–70.
8. Binswanger L. Grundformen und erkenntnis menschlichen daseins, 1942 (Basic forms and the realization of human "Being-in-the-World") Zurich (3rd édition, Munich/Basle; 1962).
9. Damasio A. Descartes' error: emotion, reason, and the human brain. New York: Putnam; 1994.

10. Kirkebøen G. Descartes' embodied psychology: descartes' or damasio's error? J Hist Neurosci. 2001;10(2):173–91.
11. Smith DL. Freud's philosophy of the unconscious. Dordrecht: Kluwer Academic; 1999a.
12. Bahnson CB. Epistemological perspectives of physical disease from the psychodynamic point of view. Am J Public Health. 1974;64(11):1034–40.
13. Deutsch F, editor. On the mysterious leap from the mind to the body. New York: International Universities Press; 1959.
14. Wise TN. Psychosomatics: past, present and future. Psychother Psychosom. 2014;83(2):65–9.
15. Lipsitt DR. Consultation-liaison psychiatry and psychosomatic medicine: the company they keep. Psychosom Med. 2001;63:896–909.
16. Lipowski ZJ. Review of consultation psychiatry and psychosomatic medicine. 3. Theoretical issues. Psychosom Med. 1968;30:395–422.
17. Lipowski ZJ. Psychosomatic medicine: past and present. Part I. Historical background. Can J Psychiatr. 1986;31:2–7.
18. Engel GL. The need for a new medical model: a challenge for biomedicine. Science. 1977;196:129–36.
19. von Bertalanffy L. General system theory. New York: George Braziller; 1968.
20. Engel GL. The clinical application of the biopsychosocial model. Am J Psychiatry. 1980;137:535–44.
21. Novack DH, Cameron O, Epel E, Ader R, Waldstein SR, Levenstein S, Antoni MH, Wainer AR. Psychosomatic medicine: the scientific foundation of the biopsychosocial model. Acad Psychiatry. 2007;31(5):388–401.
22. Adler RH. Engel's biopsychosocial model is still relevant today. J Psychosom Res. 2009;67(6):607–11.
23. Karl SR, Holland JC. The roots of psychosomatic medicine II: George L. Engel. Psychosomatics. 2015;56(6):630–3.
24. Fava GA, Sonino N. From the lesson of George engel to current knowledge: the biopsychosocial model 40 years later. Psychother Psychosom. 2017;86(5):257–9.
25. Lane RD, Waldstein SR, Chesney MA, Jennings JR, Lovallo WR, Kozel PJ, Rose RM, Drossman DA, Schneiderman N, Thayer JF, Cameron OG. The rebirth of neuroscience in psychosomatic medicine, part I: historical context, methods, and relevant basic science. Psychosom Med. 2009;71(2):117–3.
26. McEwen BS. Epigenetic interactions and the brain-body communication. Psychother Psychosom. 2017;86:1–4.
27. Quan N, Banks WA. Brain-immune communication pathways. Brain Behav Immun. 2007;21(6):727–35.
28. Kemeny ME, Schedlowski M. Understanding the interaction between psychosocial stress and immune-related diseases: a stepwise progression. Brain Behav Immun. 2007;21:1009–18.
29. Mathews HL, Janusek LW. Epigenetics and psychoneuroimmunology: mechanisms and models. Brain Behav Immun. 2011;25:25–39.
30. Blalock JE, Smith EM. Conceptual development of the immune system as a sixth sense. Brain Behav Immun. 2007;21:23–33.
31. Lane RD, Waldstein SR, Critchley HD, Derbyshire SW, Drossman DA, Wager TD, Schneiderman N, Chesney MA, Jennings JR, Lovallo WR, Rose RM, Thayer JF, Cameron OG. The rebirth of neuroscience in psychosomatic medicine, part II: clinical applications and implications for research. Psychosom Med. 2009;71(2):135–51.
32. Couto-Moraes R, Palermo-Neto J, Markus RP. The immune-pineal axis: stress as a modulator of pineal gland function. Ann N Y Acad Sci. 2009;1153:193–202.
33. Gold PW, Charney DS. Diseases of the mind and brain: depression: a disease of the mind, brain, and body. Am J Psychiatry. 2002;159:1826.
34. Iwata M, Ota KT, Duman RS. The inflammasome: pathways linking psychological stress, depression, and systemic illnesses. Brain Behav Immun. 2013;31:105–14.
35. Rawdin BS, Mellon SH, Dhabhar FS, Epel ES, Puterman E, Su Y, Burke HM, Reus VI, Rosser R, Hamilton SP, Nelson JC, Wolkowitz OM. Dysregulated relationship of inflammation and oxidative stress in major depression. Brain Behav Immun. 2013;31:143–52.

36. Sephton S, Spiegel D. Circadian disruption in cancer: a neuroendocrine-immune pathway from stress to disease? Brain Behav Immun. 2003;17:321–8.
37. Eismann EA, Lush E, Sephton SE. Circadian effects in cancer-relevant psychoneuroendocrine and immune pathways. Psychoneuroendocrinology. 2010;35:963–76.
38. de Ridder D, Geenen R, Kuijer R, van Middendorp H. Psychological adjustment to chronic disease. Lancet. 2008;372(9634):246–55.
39. Maunder RG, Hunter JJ. Attachment and psychosomatic medicine: developmental contributions to stress and disease. Psychos Med. 2001;63:556–67.
40. Wilce JM. Social and cultural lives of immune systems. London: Routledge; 2003.
41. Schore AN. The seventh annual John Bowlby Memorial Lecture, Minds in the making: attachment, the self-organizing brain, and developmentally-oriented psychoanalytic psychotherapy. Br J Psychother. 2001;17:299–328.
42. Hunter J, Maunder R, editors. Improving patient treatment with attachment theory a guide for primary care practitioners and specialists. Berlin: Springer; 2016.
43. Fava GA, Freyberger HJ, Bech P, Christodoulou G, Sensky T, Theorell T, Wise TN. Diagnostic criteria for use in psychosomatic research. Psychother Psychosom. 1995;63:1–8.
44. Fava GA, Cosci F, Sonino N. Current psychosomatic practice. Psychother Psychosom. 2017;86(1):13–30.
45. Porcelli P, Rafanelli C. Criteria for psychosomatic research (DCPR) in the medical setting. Curr Psychiatry Rep. 2010;12:246–54.
46. Seligman MEP, Steen TA, Park N, Peterson C. Positive psychology progress: empirical validation of interventions. Am Psychol. 2005;60:410–21.
47. Ryan RM, Deci EL. On happiness and human potential: a review of research on hedonic and eudaimonic well-being. Annu Rev Psychol. 2001;52:141–66.
48. Ryff CD, Singer BH. Know thyself and become what you are: a eudaimonic approach to psychological well-being. J Happiness Stud. 2008;9:13–39.
49. Smith DF. Functional salutogenic mechanisms of the brain. Perspect Biol Med. 2002;45:319–28.
50. Kobau R, Seligman ME, Peterson C, Diener E, Zack MM, Chapman D, Thompson W. Mental health promotion in public health: perspectives and strategies from positive psychology. Am J Public Health. 2011;101(8):e1–9.
51. Sin NL, Lyubomirsky S. Enhancing well-being and alleviating depressive symptoms with positive psychology interventions: a practice-friendly meta-analysis. J Clin Psychol. 2009;65:467–87.
52. Ellis BJ, Del Giudice M. Beyond allostatic load: rethinking the role of stress in regulating human development. Dev Psychopathol. 2013;26:1–20.
53. Jaremka LM, Lindgren ME, Kiecolt-Glaser JK. Synergistic relationships among stress, depression, and troubled relationships: insights from psychoneuroimmunology. Depress Anxiety. 2013;30:288–96.
54. McEwen BS, Gianaros PJ. Stress- and allostasis-induced brain plasticity. Annu Rev Med. 2011;62:431–45.
55. Karatsoreos IN, McEwen BS. Annual research review: the neurobiology and physiology of resilience and adaptation across the life course. J Child Psychol Psychiatry. 2013;54(4):337–47.
56. Seeman TE. Social ties and health: the benefits of social integration. Ann Epidemiol. 1996;6:442–51.
57. Uchino BN. Social support and physical health: understanding the health consequences of relationships. New Haven: Yale University Press; 2004.
58. Tay L, Tan K, Diener E, Gonzalez E. Social relations, health behaviors, and health outcomes: a survey and synthesis. Appl Psychol Health Well Being. 2013;5:28–78.
59. Aburn G, Gott M, Hoare K. What is resilience? An integrative review of the empirical literature. J Adv Nurs. 2016;72(5):980–1000.
60. Schetter CD, Dolbier C. Resilience in the context of chronic stress and health in adults. Soc Personal Psychol Compass. 2011;5(9):634–52.

61. Stewart DE, Yuen T. A systematic review of resilience in the physically ill. Psychosomatics. 2011;52:199–209.
62. Kalisch R, Müller MB, Tüscher O. A conceptual framework for the neurobiological study of resilience. Behav Brain Sci. 2015;38:e92.
63. Ménard C, Pfau ML, Hodes GE, Russo SJ. Immune and neuroendocrine mechanisms of stress vulnerability and resilience. Neuropsychopharmacology. 2017;42(1):62–80.
64. Karatsoreos IN, McEwen BS. Psychobiological allostasis: resistance, resilience and vulnerability. Trends Cogn Sci. 2011;15:576–84.
65. Fuks A, Brawer J, Boudreau JD. The foundation of physicianship. Perspect Biol Med. 2012;55:114–26.
66. Buber M. I and thou. Edinburgh: T. & T. Clarke; 1944.
67. Levinas E. Totality and infinity: an essay on exteriority. Pittsburgh, PA: Duquesne University Press; 1969.
68. Clifton-Soderstrom M. Levinas and the patient as other: the ethical foundation of medicine. J Med Philos. 2003;28:447–60.
69. Grassi L, Caruso R, Costantini A. Communication with patients suffering from serious physical illness. Adv Psychosom Med. 2015;34:10–2.
70. Mitchell AJ. Reluctance to disclose difficult diagnoses: a narrative review comparing communication by psychiatrists and oncologists. Support Care Cancer. 2007;15(7):819–28.
71. Papageorgiou A, Loke YK, Fromage M. Communication skills training for mental health professionals working with people with severe mental illness. Cochrane Database Syst Rev. 2017;6:CD010006.
72. Rizzolatti G, Sinigaglia C. Mirrors in the brain: how our minds share actions and emotions. Oxford: Oxford University Press; 2008.
73. Keysers C, Fadiga L. The mirror neuron system: new frontiers. Soc Neurosci. 2008;3(3-4):193–8.
74. Gallese V. The 'shared manifold' hypothesis. From mirror neurons to empathy. J Conscious Stud. 2001;8:33–50.
75. Kaplan JT, Iacoboni M. Getting a grip on other minds: mirror neurons, intention understanding, and cognitive empathy. Soc Neurosci. 2006;1(3-4):175–83.
76. Iacoboni M. Imitation, empathy, and mirror neurons. Annu Rev Psychol. 2009;60:653–70.
77. Fusar-Poli P, Broome M, Stanghellini G. From Brentano to mirror neurons: bridging phenomenology and clinical neuroscience. Psychiatry Res. 2010;183:245–6.
78. Decety J. The neuroevolution of empathy. Ann N Y Acad Sci. 2011;1231:35–45.
79. Decety J, Norman GJ, Berntson GG, Cacioppo JT. A neurobehavioral evolutionary perspective on the mechanisms underlying empathy. Prog Neurobiol. 2012;98:38–48.
80. Buccino G, Amore M. Mirror neurons and the understanding of behavioural symptoms in psychiatric disorders. Curr Opin Psychiatry. 2008;21:281–5.
81. Reich TW. From ancient consolation and negative care to modern empathy and the neurosciences. Theor Med Bioeth. 2012;33:25–32.
82. Riess H. Empathy in medicine—a neurobiological perspective. JAMA. 2010;304:1604–5.
83. Cole TR, Carlin N. The suffering of physicians. Lancet. 2009;374:1414–5.
84. Goetz JL, Keltner D, Simon-Thomas E. Compassion: an evolutionary analysis and empirical review. Psychol Bull. 2010;136(3):351–74.
85. Sinclair S, Norris JM, McConnell SJ, Chochinov HM, Hack TF, Hagen NA, McClement S, Bouchal SR. Compassion: a scoping review of the healthcare literature. BMC Palliat Care. 2016;15:6. (2-16).
86. Charon R. The patient-physician relationship. Narrative medicine: a model for empathy, reflection, profession, and trust. JAMA. 2001;286:1897–902.
87. Gordon J. Medical humanities: to cure sometimes, to relieve often, to comfort always. Med J Aust. 2005;182:5–8.
88. Laine C, Davidoff F. Patient-centered medicine. A professional evolution. JAMA. 1996;275:152–6.
89. Greaves D. Reflections on a new medical cosmology. J Med Ethics. 2002;28:81–5.

90. Smith GC, Strain JJ. George Engel's contribution to clinical psychiatry. Aust N Z J Psychiatry. 2002;36:458–66.
91. Engel GL. From biomedical to biopsychosocial. Being scientific in the human domain. Psychosomatics. 1997;38(6):521–8.
92. Engel GL, Reichsman F, Segal HL. A study of an infant with a gastric fistula I. Behavior and the rate of total hydrochloric acid secretion. Psychosom Med. 1956;18(5):374–98.
93. Benning TB. Limitations of the biopsychosocial model in psychiatry. Adv Med Educ Pract. 2015;6:347–52.
94. Wise TN. Psychosomatic medicine: an approach needed now more than ever. Int J Clin Pract. 2010;64(8):999–1001.
95. Fava GA, Ruini C, Tomba E, Wise TN. The biopsychosocial factor. Psychother Psychosom. 2012;81(1):1–4.
96. Horwitz RI, Cullen MR, Abell J, Christian JB. (De)personalized medicine. Science. 2012;339:1155–6.
97. Horwitz RI, Hayes-Conroy A, Singer BH. Biology, social environment, and personalized medicine. Psychother Psychosom. 2017;86:5–10.
98. Martin CM, Félix-Bortolotti M. Person-centred health care: a critical assessment of current and emerging research approaches. J Eval Clin Pract. 2014;20(6):1056–64.
99. McLaren N. A critical review of the biopsychosocial model. Aust N Z J Psychiatry. 1998;32:86–2.
100. Van Oudenhove L, Cuypers S. The relevance of the philosophical 'mind-body problem' for the status of psychosomatic medicine: a conceptual analysis of the biopsychosocial model. Med Health Care Philos. 2014;17(2):201–13.
101. Ghaemi SN. Paradigms of psychiatry: eclecticism and its discontents. Curr Opin Psychiatry. 2006;19(6):619–24.
102. Pilgrim D. The biopsychosocial model in Anglo-American psychiatry: past, present and future. J Ment Health. 2002;11:585–94.
103. Ghaemi SN. The rise and fall of the biopsychosocial model. Br J Psychiatry. 2009;195(1):3–4.
104. Jaspers K. Der Arzt im technischen Zeitalter. Universitas: Zeitschrift für Wissenschaft, Kunst und Literatur 1959;14(4):337–54. English translation by Arthur A. Grugan. The physician in the technological age. Theor Med Bioeth. 1989;10(3):251–67.
105. Shelton W. A new look at medicine and the mind-body problem: can Dewey's pragmatism help medicine connect with its mission? Perspect Biol Med. 2013;56(3):422–41.
106. Price AI, Djulbegovic B, Biswas R, Chatterjee P. Evidence-based medicine meets person-centred care: a collaborative perspective on the relationship. J Eval Clin Pract. 2015;21(6):1047–51.
107. Weaver RR. Reconciling evidence-based medicine and patient-centred care: defining evidence-based inputs to patient-centred decisions. J Eval Clin Pract. 2015;21(6):1076–80.
108. Alexander F. Psychological aspects of medicine. Psychos Med. 1939;1:7–18.
109. Albuquerque J, Deshauer D, Grof P. Descartes' passions of the soul—seeds of psychiatry? J Affect Disord. 2003;76:285–91.
110. Clarke PGH. Neuroscience, quantum indeterminism and the Cartesian soul. Brain Cogn. 2014;84:109–17.
111. Fava GA, Belaise C, Sonino N. Psychosomatic medicine is a comprehensive field, not a synonym for consultation liaison psychiatry. Curr Psychiatry Rep. 2010;12(3):215–21.
112. Fava GA, Sonino N. Psychosomatic medicine: a name to keep. Psychother Psychosom. 2010;79(1):1–3.
113. Miles A. On a medicine of the whole person: away from scientistic reductionism and towards the embrace of the complex in clinical practice. J Eval Clin Pract. 2009;15(6):941–9.

Psychosomatic and Person-Centered Medicine

3

Juan E. Mezzich and Ihsan M. Salloum

Abstract

Psychosomatics involves an important approach to medical care that is connected to a holistic theoretical perspective as well as a practical guide to clinical work. To this effect, this paper briefly reviews psychosomatics within the framework of holistic theory and care, which happens to be one of the key concepts of person-centered medicine (PCM). Next, the paper considers the basic notions of person-centered medicine and the way this has evolved historically from ancient civilizations through modern medicine. The conceptualization of PCM is further approached from a systematic study organized by the International College of Person Centered Medicine. After that, the paper focuses on person-centered psychiatry in general and then more specifically on person-centered diagnosis both as a theoretical model and as a practical guide.

J. E. Mezzich (✉)
Icahn School of Medicine at Mount Sinai, New York, NY, USA

Section on Classification, Diagnostic Assessment and Nomenclature,
World Psychiatric Association, New York, NY, USA

I. M. Salloum
Section on Classification, Diagnostic Assessment and Nomenclature,
World Psychiatric Association, Miami, FL, USA

University of Miami Miller School of Medicine, Miami, FL, USA

L. Grassi et al. (eds.), *Person Centered Approach to Recovery in Medicine*,
Integrating Psychiatry and Primary Care, https://doi.org/10.1007/978-3-319-74736-1_3

3.1 Introduction

It is said that person-centered medicine (PCM) is definitionally aimed at placing the whole person at the center of health [1] and as the goal of health care [2]. Cassell [3] has articulated well the key importance of the person and personhood in medicine. Also the key in the definition of PCM is the concepts of wholeness and health, i.e., an important component of its basic conceptualization. This holistic framework extends the concept of psychosomatic medicine by adding to the somatic and the psychological the dimensions of the social, the cultural, and the spiritual.

After articulating the relationship of psychosomatics and PCM, this paper reviews in some detail the general concepts of the latter perspective from its historical roots to its notions in modern medicine. This is followed by the presentation of a study to appraise systematically the conceptualization of PCM and explore its measurement. Finally, the manuscript deals with the more specific field of person-centered psychiatry, both in general and concerning person-centered diagnosis, theoretically and practically.

3.2 Psychosomatics and Wholeness in Health

Psychosomatics or the psychosomatic approach to health deals basically with the integration of the somatic and the psychic in medicine and health [4]. This is the principal focus of the present book. The holistic approach or the wholeness in health extends the scope of psychosomatics to also include the social, the cultural, and the spiritual. As such, this extension speaks to the articulation of psychosomatics and person-centered medicine.

The importance of wholeness in health may be illustrated through an etymological review. According to the Oxford Dictionaries [5], *health* comes from *Old* English *hal* of Germanic origin meaning wholeness. Wholeness in health is often discussed with regard to a multi-perspective framework, e.g., biological, psychological, and social [6], which can also encompass the cultural and the spiritual. Wholeness in health may also refer to contextualization. Its value is usually posited with regard to being aware of and responsive to social and environmental circumstances, including cultural ones [7]. The significance of contextualization is even deeper when, with high pertinence to the person and PCM, one considers the perspectives and dictum of Ortega y Gasset, "Yo soy yo y mi circunstancia, y si no la salvo a ella no me salvo yo" ("I am I and my circumstance, and if I do not take care of it I do not take care of myself") [8].

It can be argued, respecting natural complexity, that the scope of wholeness, contextualization, and circumstance in health should not be restricted to the multi-perspective and the cross-sectional but that it should also encompass a longitudinal and historical dimension. A number of aspects of this longitudinal dimension of relevance to health and health care may be identified, as follows.

One of these aspects is usually termed life history. This refers to the unfolding of life from birth to death. It may be also called life course, and as such it has been prominently discussed in PCM [9]. Another conceptual aspect of the longitudinal dimension of wholeness in health refers to the life cycle, often framed in terms of life stages. This concern is so well established in health care that specific professional specialties are organized for such stages, such as pediatrics and geriatric medicine. Person-centered approaches to them have been cogently articulated for these two medical specialties [10, 11].

Also of interest is personal development, pointedly helpful to understand personhood and health. Thus, as one could expect, this human development aspect has been specifically addressed concerning person-centered care [12] and person-centered education [13].

Furthermore, the longitudinal aspect of wholeness in health has been engaged in reference to major medical pathology. This has taken place particularly concerning multi-morbidity [14, 15] and chronic diseases. The latter represents the greatest current epidemic [16], and it is clear that to address it effectively we need to engage the involved patients and their sense of responsibility to adopt required lifestyle changes [17]. In other words, we need for clinical and public health efforts to succeed with these challenging and enduring conditions a person- and people-centered approach [18].

3.3 Person-Centered Medicine

3.3.1 General Concepts

The term **person** (from the Latin *personare*, i.e., resonance), in Greek *prosopon* (resonance mask), refers to a mask that the actors and actresses worn in Greco-Roman theaters to amplify their voices. When the actor or actress appeared with the mask, the audience exclaimed, "here comes the person." The term *person* has evolved to absorb notions of complexity, autonomy, dignity, and rights [19].

Historical roots of a medicine focused on the person can be found in the most ancient civilizations. A holistic theoretical framework and a personalized approach in dealing with health problems were prevalent in these civilizations. Among the oldest correspond to Chinese and Ayurvedic medicine, which are still practiced today as traditional medicines [20]. The same, mutatis mutandis, is true for the ancient cultures of Africa (e.g., from Ubuntu: "I am because you are and you are because we are") [21] and of America [22]. These cultures focus more on the overall health of the patient than just on disease [23]. They tend to articulate a comprehensive and harmonious framework of health and life and to promote a highly personalized approach for the treatment of specific diseases and the promotion of life quality [24].

Analyzing the ancient Greek culture as the cradle of Western civilization, one finds that holistic medicine had been strongly argued by Hellenic philosophers and physicians. Socrates and Plato discussed that "if the whole is not well, it is impossible that a part be well" [4]. This position was enriched by Aristotle, philosopher and naturalist *par excellence*, who analyzed the method of medicine and its relationship to ethics and treatment focused on the person [25]. For his part, Hippocrates articulated theory, emotion, and individuality in the practice of medicine [26].

Closer antecedents can be encountered in the pioneering work of Paul Tournier [27] and Carl Rogers [28], as well as in the World Medical Association's International Code for Medical Ethics [29] and Ethical Principles for Medical Research [30], the founding of family medicine [31], and the establishment of the World Psychiatric Association as an attempt to articulate science and humanism [32] from which emerged more recently an Institutional Program on Psychiatry for the Person [33]. Likewise, the World Health Organization (WHO) through the 2008 World Health Report [34] and the 2009 World Health Assembly resolutions [35] has been seeking to upgrade public health by engaging people-centered care as a key pivot.

Crucial in the conceptual, operational, and institutional development of person-centered medicine have been the Geneva Conferences annually celebrated around this perspective since 2008. This maturational process took place in collaboration with the World Health Organization, the World Medical Association, the Council for International Organizations of Medical Science, the International Council of Nurses, the International Federation of Social Workers, and the International Pharmaceutical Federation, with the support of the Geneva University Hospital and Medical School and the Paul Tournier Society, all headquartered in Geneva or surrounding cities, as well as with other global entities such as the World Organization of Family Doctors, the International Alliance of Patients' Organizations, and a growing number of universities from across the world.

The Geneva Conferences [2, 36–38] led to the emergence of the International Network (more recently named College) of Person Centered Medicine (INPCM, ICPCM) [39–41]. They are established and headquartered as a nonprofit organization in New York. The College provides a key focus of fellowship for the cultivation and sharing of ideas, experiences, and educational and research projects in an intercultural and multi-professional setting. The College has extended the impact of the Geneva Conferences through the Geneva Declarations and their accompanying academic papers, as illustrated by the early ones focused on person-centered health research [42, 43] and person- and people-centered integrated health care for all [44, 45]. A major institutional achievement has been the establishment of the International Journal of Person Centered Medicine in collaboration with the University of Buckingham Press [46]. Through its quarterly issues, it is promoting research and scholarship on person-centered medicine in many countries and world regions and across them [17]. A major book on person-centered psychiatry has been published by Springer Verlag [47].

It has also been emphasized that PCM seeks fundamentally to articulate science and humanism in medicine and health care and to refocus these on the whole person [2]. Furthermore, it has been posited that person-centered medicine is dedicated to the promotion of health as a state of physical, mental, sociocultural, and spiritual well-being, as well as to the reduction of disease, and founded on mutual respect for the dignity and responsibility of each individual person [48].

The purposes of person-centered medicine have been also summarized as promoting a medicine *of the person* (of the totality of the person's health, including its ill and positive aspects), *for the person* (promoting the fulfillment of the person's life project), *by the person* (with clinicians extending themselves as full human beings with high ethical aspirations), and *with the person* (working respectfully, in collaboration and in an empowering manner) [33, 38].

3.3.2 Systematic Conceptualization of Person-Centered Medicine

While the definitional notes listed above have been well received and used frequently, a need has been pointedly recognized to conceptualize systematically person-centered medicine especially in terms of person- and people-centered care and to develop measures to assess progress in these directions.

A study was organized by the International College of Person Centered Medicine with support of the World Health Organization aimed at elucidating the core concepts of person-centered medicine and health care, and on the basis of these, designing a prototype measuring instrument and appraising its metric structure, instrumental prospects, acceptability, reliability, and validity [49].

3.3.2.1 Elucidating Key Concepts

The domains elucidated from a literature review were organized into a form to facilitate its presentation to and handling by a Broad Consultation Group. The responses received from the Broad Consultation Group members were tabulated. The majority (but not all) of the domains received a predominantly high importance rating for person centeredness. There were 20 additional domains identified by 1 or more Broad Consultation Group members.

Through this sequential and iterative process, the following key concepts of person-centered medicine and people-centered health care were delineated: (1) ethical commitment, (2) cultural sensitivity, (3) holistic scope, (4) relational focus, (5) individualized care, (6) common ground for collaborative diagnosis and care, (7) people-centered systems of care, and (8) person-centered education and research. Furthermore, a number of sub-concepts were identified under each broad concept, which amounted to a total of 33 sub-concepts.

3.3.2.2 Design of a Person-Centered Care Index (PCI)

On the basis of the abovementioned interactions with the international consultation groups, work toward the design of a metrically suitable person-centered care index prototype was initiated. This involved first the formulation of the eight broad items of person-centered medicine and health care as well as of the 33 subitems referred to above, nested under the eight broad items.

Second, a four-point rating scale was agreed to. Initially, this was based on the *degree of presence* (None, Moderate, Substantial, High) of the corresponding items and subitems in a given health service. Later, the anchor points of the scale were reformulated in terms of *frequency of presence* of the corresponding items, as follows: Never, Occasionally, Frequently, and Always.

Then, on the basis of consultations with the involved international panels and the whole group of investigators co-authoring the present paper, the wording of the broad items and subitems was refined. Rating guidelines were established, as well as guidelines for computing a global average score by adding the partial scores and dividing the result by the number of items actually rated. Additionally, space was agreed to at the end of the scale in order to encourage and accommodate narrative evaluative comments.

Table 3.1 displays the person-centered care index (PCI), with all the featured content (8 broad items and 33 subitems), four-point rating scale, completion guidelines, and all other aspects of the PCI mentioned above.

Table 3.1 Person-centered care index (PCI)

No	Indicators	Never	Occasionally	Frequently	Always
1.	*Ethical commitment*				
1.1	The dignity of every person involved (patients, family, clinicians) is honored	1	2	3	4
1.2	Patient's rights are respected	1	2	3	4
1.3	Patient's autonomy is supported	1	2	3	4
1.4	Patient's empowerment is advanced	1	2	3	4
1.5	The fulfillment of the patient's life project (purpose in life) is enabled and encouraged	1	2	3	4
1.6	The patient's personal values, choices, and needs are understood and respected	1	2	3	4
2.	*Cultural sensitivity*				
2.1	The patient's ethnic identity and cultural values are recognized	1	2	3	4
2.2	The patient's language and communication needs and preferences are actively considered	1	2	3	4
2.3	The patient's gender and sexual preferences are acknowledged and respected	1	2	3	4
2.4	The patient's spiritual needs are factored in	1	2	3	4
3.	*Holistic scope*				
3.1	The biological, psychological, social, cultural, and spiritual factors of health inform understanding and care	1	2	3	4
3.2	Both ill health (health problems, disabilities) and positive health or well-being (functioning, resilience, strengths, resources, and quality of life) are the focus of attention	1	2	3	4
4.	*Relational focus*				
4.1	Clinicians, patients, and families work in partnership	1	2	3	4
4.2	Empathy in clinical communication is emphasized	1	2	3	4
4.3	Interpersonal trust is fostered throughout the care process	1	2	3	4
5.	*Individualized care*				
5.1	The patient's individuality and unique qualities inform care	1	2	3	4
5.2	The patient's historical and social context are factored in	1	2	3	4
5.3	The patient's personal growth and development are promoted	1	2	3	4
6.	*Common ground for diagnosis and care*				
6.1	Diagnosis of health status, experience, and contributory factors involve shared understanding	1	2	3	4
6.2	Diagnosis is worked out taking into account the whole person	1	2	3	4
6.3	Care plan decisions are made collaboratively	1	2	3	4
7.	*People-centered systems of care*				
7.1	The health and rights of all people in the community are advocated and promoted	1	2	3	4
7.2	The community participates in the planning of health services	1	2	3	4

Table 3.1 (continued)

No	Indicators	Never	Occasionally	Frequently	Always
7.3	Collaboration across disciplines and programs is promoted at all levels of service organization	1	2	3	4
7.4	Personalized services are aimed at attaining high quality and excellence	1	2	3	4
7.5	Health services are responsive to specific community needs and expectations	1	2	3	4
7.6	Health services are integrated and coordinated around patients' needs	1	2	3	4
7.7	Services emphasize people-centered primary care	1	2	3	4
7.8	Services ensure continuity of care	1	2	3	4
7.9	Services are informed by person-centered international perspectives and developments	1	2	3	4
8.	*Person-centered education and research*				
8.1	The health system promotes person-centered public education	1	2	3	4
8.2	The health system promotes person-centered health professional training	1	2	3	4
8.3	The health system promotes person-centered clinical research	1	2	3	4
Global average score					

Please rate the following person-centered care indicators in terms of the frequency of their presence in a given health service. The term "patient" here refers to a person who experiences health problems and/or uses health services, whose personhood transcends these roles and circumstances. To obtain a global average PCI score, please add the partial scores, and divide this by the number of items actually rated

Additional evaluative comments: Copyrighted by the International College of Person Centered Medicine. 2016

3.4 Person-Centered Psychiatry

A brief discussion of person-centered psychiatry and the place and role of mental health in person-centered medicine need to touch on two domains. The first one relates to the various activities and manners through which mental health has contributed to the conceptualization and experience of person-centered medicine. The second corresponds to the development of person-centered psychiatry within the framework of person-centered medicine.

3.4.1 Mental Health Perspectives Toward Person-Centered Medicine

At the 54th World Health Assembly, Gro Brundlandt, former Prime Minister of Norway and then WHO Director General, proclaimed "There is no development without health, and no health without mental health" [50]. This summarizes the growing perception of the cruciality of mental health to achieve general health and well-being. The following sections illustrate why this is so, from various angles, particularly with attention to person-centered health and person-centered medicine.

3.4.1.1 The Importance of Behavioral Factors for Addressing Chronic Diseases

Chronic noncommunicable diseases such as diabetes, cancer, and cardiovascular and respiratory illnesses are responsible for over 70% of morbidity and mortality across the world. Their prominence as a global epidemic has attracted the urgent attention of the United Nations and the World Health Organization [16].

Addressing chronic disease is particularly pertinent for the International College of Person Centered Medicine given that effective care for such conditions requires indispensably the engagement of persons and their sense of responsibility to undertake actively and creatively required adjustments in lifestyle [51, 52]. Consequently, the International College dedicated its 5th Geneva Conference to *Person Centered Care for Chronic Diseases* and issued its first Geneva Declaration, which was dedicated to this topic [18]. Among its recommendations are to monitor risk and protective factors (intrinsic and extrinsic; biological, psychological, and social), as well as outcomes for positive health (vitality and resilience despite exposure and adversity).

The World Health Alliance (World Medical Association, International Council of Nurses, International Dental Federation, and International Pharmaceutical Federation) has recently identified through a Health Improvement Card [53] a number of factors to prevent chronic diseases. The majority of such factors have to do with behavior and lifestyle. Among these are diet, exercise, avoidance of alcohol and other hazardous drugs, stress control, adequate rest and sleep, and participation in social and creative activities.

3.4.1.2 Psychological Elements in Adaptive Systems for the Promotion of Well-Being

Keyes and Ryff's research [54] has shown the overlap of physical, mental, and social well-being, as well as the inadequacy of focusing only on the presence of physical and mental disorders in assessing health. Flourishing involves dynamic interactions between healthy functioning, contributions to health, and the experience of health. As argued by Herrman et al. [55], in order to develop well-being, people must be aware of the causes of both their distress and disability as well as of the paths open to them to develop in health and happiness with community support as well as personal effort.

Cloninger et al. [56] have endeavored to explain the dynamic origins of well-being. The causes of well-being and ill-being appear to involve a complex adaptive network of components and processes that are being gradually specified, measured, and treated according to the principles of person-centered medicine. Some of the key factors promoting well-being seem to be the development of self-awareness, cooperation, and self-transcendence [57].

3.4.1.3 The Importance of Subjectivity and Intersubjectivity in Person-Centered Care

As noted by Botbol [58], person-centered medicine should not be reduced to individualization of care or respect for patients' rights, as it has wider aspirations. These include the recognition of the individual subjectivity of the whole person of the patient beyond what characterizes his or her illness or the status or role of patient. What is of interest here is dealing with the inner world of a patient in his particular situation of suffering and dependence caused by illness, as proposed in Aristotle's *Nicomachean Ethics*: "Cure of a unique person (not of a generalized nosological case), in a specific situation, within a specific, unrepeatable period of one's life" [59]. What becomes crucial here is the commitment of the mental health professional to approach the patient's subjectivity in such singular vital situation.

In addition to the attention paid to the medico-biological aspects of the person's health status, a person-centered assessment needs to give enough consideration to the patient's subjective feelings [60]. Whether or not one suspects a psychic or psychosomatic causality to the disorder that a patient brings to the clinic, it is essential to keep in perspective the factors involved in the patient's health situation. Beyond reasserting this principle, one needs to utterly enhance the methodology for accessing these subjective dimensions among different partners involved in the diagnostic process and the therapeutic relationship. For health professionals, the only way to access these subjective dimensions is through what the patient (and or his/her carers) says in words or shows in acting, as long as these words or acts can trigger in the professionals enough empathy to approach the patient's subjective feelings to which these expressions are related.

Working on a person-centered diagnostic approach has become an important element to meet this methodological goal. This diagnostic model includes, besides the objective elements about the patient and his or her context, the subjective elements reported by the idiographic formulations of the person who is being cared for, their carers, and assisting professionals.

This approach appears to lead to a closer examination of the role of the professional's empathy in the methodology to access the subjectivity of the patient, trying to go beyond the general assertions on the importance of this concept in therapeutic relationships and care activities [60].

At first seen as the professional's ability to listen sympathetically to the comments of the patient and to consider his wishes and needs, the notion of empathy has gradually widened to include representations that the physician (or other health professional) makes of the clinical situation in which the person in need of care is involved. In short, these are representations that the professional makes of the health situation of the person suffering through his/her (the professional) own empathy, triggered by the words and the acts of the patients and of their carers. This mechanism is well described by the concept of "metaphorizing-empathy" proposed by Lebovici [61] from his work with babies and their mothers. It is also close to the notion of "narrative empathy" proposed by Jacques Hochmann [62] based on his work with autistic children and on the philosophical ideas brought by Paul Ricoeur in his book "Time and Narrative" [63]. It is also consistent with Kleinman's assumptions [64] on illness narratives. This important development in person-centered medicine marks the full recognition of the role of the physician's subjectivity as a diagnostic and treatment tool within the framework of the physician-patient relationship.

3.4.1.4 Recovery Orientation in Mental Health and Its Relations to Person-Centered Medicine

Recovery-oriented concepts emerged from a coalescence of efforts from both service users and professional groups in the mental health field. On one hand, individuals who suffered and recovered from mental illnesses formed a recovery movement and a national and international community of activists. For example, Chamberlin [65] and Deegan [66], expressed their criticism against negatively experienced psychiatric treatment and demanded to be considered active protagonists and partners rather than passive recipients of care. On the other hand, well-known experts in the field of psychosocial rehabilitation, such as Anthony [67] welcomed the statements of service users and the need to attend to their subjective experiences, speaking against improving just functioning and adaptation and not also promoting the flourishing of the individual human being. At least since the beginning of the 1990s, many professionals in rehabilitation and other fields and various service user groups have started substantial collaboration through joint publications and conferences. Recently, reflecting progress in this regard, Mary Barber [68] has considered recovery as "the new medical model for psychiatry."

Recovery orientation engages multidisciplinary cooperation, where professionals aim at helping not only to reduce symptoms, disease, and disability but also to assist individuals to have a home again, to return to work, and to have friends. The key here is to cultivate a partnership attitude in which the individual can contribute actively based on his/her former illness experience and include family members and friends who know well the patient's needs. Furthermore, peer support (a recovery-oriented development) is becoming frequently complementary to standard treatment in the United States, the United Kingdom, and Australia [69].

Patients' participation in treatment planning is being increasingly advocated in mental health [70]. "Shared decision-making" was an early contribution of the recovery movement to clinical care and is becoming gradually a valued tool in person-centered medicine. It is considered a promising method of engaging patients in medical decisions and improving health-related outcomes [71, 72]. The concept of "shared decision-making" serves as a clinical tool toward enhancing communication and optimizing treatment planning as well as implementing respect for the autonomy, responsibility, and dignity of every person involved. It is now a core concept applied in both recovery orientation as well as person-centered care, especially useful for chronic patients. The patient or client, an expert by experience, and the practitioner, an expert by training, are now expected to contribute from their own perspectives and determine collaboratively a course of treatment.

A comparison of the essentials of recovery orientation and person-centered care identified unique characteristics for each approach as well as substantial elements of convergence. Recovery orientation is primarily centered within the mental health and psychosocial fields, while the person-centered approach covers general medicine and health care at large. Their points of convergence encompass a holistic theoretical perspective, an emphasis on contextualization and establishing a common ground for understanding an action, development of person-centered procedures for clinical care and health promotion, and, last but not least, an ethical commitment [73].

3.4.2 From Psychiatry for the Person to Person-Centered Medicine

The organized and institutional development of person-centered care in the psychiatry and mental health field has been unfolding in two phases. The first one from 2005 to 2008 took place in the form of an Institutional Program on Psychiatry for the Person within the World Psychiatric Association. The second one, since 2008 to date, evolved from the first one by extending its domain from psychiatry to medicine at large and progressing institutionally through collaboration with a large number of top global institutions in medicine and health.

3.4.2.1 WPA Institutional Program on Psychiatry for the Person

The Institutional Program on Psychiatry for the Person (IPPP), established by the 2005 General Assembly of the World Psychiatric Association (WPA), involved an organization-wide initiative affirming the *whole person of the patient within his context* as the center and goal of clinical care and health promotion, at both individual and community levels. This was set to involve the articulation of science and humanism to optimize attention to the ill and positive health aspects of the person. As care is basically a partnership experience, the program involved the integration of all relevant health and social services. Furthermore, the program also involved advancing appropriate public health policies.

Historians Garrabe and Hoff [32] have noted that the principles behind psychiatry for the person could be already detected at the very beginnings of the WPA. As a conceptual introduction to the whole Institutional Program, two editorials were published by the first author of the present paper, then WPA president, one broadly focusing on articulating medicine's science and humanism [74] and another on the dialogic basis of the profession [75].

The work of the Institutional Program was organized in four components: conceptual bases, clinical diagnosis, clinical care, and public health. These are summarized next.

Conceptual Bases

This component dealt with analyses and delineations of the conceptual bases of psychiatry for the person. It produced an editorial and a regular article in international journals presenting the objectives of this component [76, 77].

Additionally, a monographic set on the conceptual bases of psychiatry for the person was prepared and eventually published with the following table of contents: Introduction [77], Historical perspectives [32], Philosophy of science perspectives

[78], Ethics perspectives [79], Biological perspectives [80], Psychological perspectives [12], Social perspectives [81], Cultural perspectives [82], Spiritual perspectives [83], Users perspectives [84], and Literature and art perspectives [85].

Clinical Diagnosis

There were two work objectives in this component. The first one involved collaborating with the WHO toward the development of ICD-11. There was a preliminary background phase in this process during the first half of the preceding decade involving principally the WPA Classification Section and the WHO Classification Office and leading to two monographs [86, 87]. A full development of the ICD-11 Mental Disorders Chapter started in early 2007 under the direction of the WHO Mental Health Department.

The second and main work objective of the IPPP clinical diagnosis component was the development of a person-centered integrative diagnosis (PID) model. At its heart was a concept of diagnosis defined as the description of the positive and negative aspects of health, interactively, within the person's life context. The PID would include the best possible classification of mental and general health disorders (expectedly the ICD-11 classification of diseases and its national and regional adaptations) as well as the description of other health-related problems and positive aspects of health (adaptive functioning, protective factors, quality of life, etc.), attending to the totality of the person (including his/her dignity, values, and aspirations). The approach would employ categorical, dimensional, and narrative approaches as needed, to be applied interactively by clinicians, patients, and families. A starting point for the development of the PID was the schema combining standardized multiaxial and personalized idiographic formulations at the core of the WPA International Guidelines for Diagnostic Assessment (IGDA) [88].

As an introduction to this IPPP component's work, a broad-ranging volume on *Psychiatric Diagnosis: Challenges and Prospects* [89] was prepared. A paper on "Towards innovative international classification and diagnostic systems: ICD-11 and person-centered integrative diagnosis" was published by Mezzich and Salloum as an invited editorial in *Acta Psychiatrica Scandinavica* [90]. Other papers pertinent to this developmental work included an editorial on clinical complexity and person-centered integrative diagnosis [91] and on person-centered integrative diagnosis [92].

Clinical Care

The thrust of the work of this component encompassed educational efforts toward achieving person-centered care. The two main developments which were outlined were an approach to person-centered clinical care and a curriculum to carry out training on the abovementioned approach.

It was noted that the teaching of medicine and that of psychiatry in particular has experienced many changes. There was a time when the core curriculum in psychiatry, written by the WPA together with the World Federation for Medical Education, became a landmark because it did not only define the competencies in psychiatry that every physician should be taught but mainly because it called attention to prevention of illness and promotion of health.

Public Health

Public health in modern times has a broad scope as the organized global and local effort to promote and protect the health of populations and reduce health inequities. This ranged from the control of communicable diseases to the leadership of intersectoral efforts in health [93]. It was noted that evidence is growing for the value of integrating mental health in general health and public health practice [94, 95]. Despite this, public health programs in many countries around the world have yet to recognize and include mental health and mental illness as areas of relevant action.

Psychiatry for the person is a basis for advocacy that emphasizes the value and dignity of the person as essential starting points for public health action. This includes development of policies and services and research and evaluation supporting these. Failure to recognize the humanity and dignity of citizens living with mental illness as well as the value of mental health to the individual and community has resulted in abuse and neglect of the former and lost opportunities to improve mental health through population-based and person-based initiatives. The neglect of individual needs and the fragmentation and inadequacies of health and social services undermine policy development [96, 97]. Public health actions to promote mental health prevent illness and provide effective and humane services that benefit from and contribute to the development of psychiatry for the person.

3.4.2.2 Events of the Institutional Program of Psychiatry for the Person

1. *London Conference on Person-centered Integrative Diagnosis and Psychiatry for the Person:* It was organized on October 26–28, 2007, by both the WPA IPPP and the Health Department of the United Kingdom. It represented a path-opening opportunity for synergism between person-centered care and Britain's Shared Vision Project.
2. *Paris Conference on Psychiatry for the Person:* This was organized on February 6–8, 2008, by the WPA IPPP, the French Member Societies of WPA, and the five WPA European Zonal Representatives. The city and the professional community that served 58 years earlier as the cradle of WPA offered a special type of conference, focused and interactive, without commercial accompaniments.
3. *Philippe Pinel Prize on Psychiatry for the Person: Articulating Medicine's Science and Humanism.* In 2007, the WPA Executive Committee established this Prize to honor Philippe Pinel, a pioneer in the systematization of clinical psychiatry and an inspiring humanist who broke the chains of his hospital's mental patients. The awardee was Prof. Yrjo Alanen of Turku, Finland, world acclaimed for his innovative work on *Need Adaptive Assessment and Treatment* integrating scientifically valid therapeutic techniques with attention to the experience and views of patients with psychotic disorders.

3.4.3 Development of Person-Centered Psychiatry Within Person-Centered Medicine

Around 2008, contacts between the leaders of WPA and those of other important organizations such as the World Medical Association, the World Federation of Neurology, the World Organization of Family Doctors (Wonca), the International Council of Nurses, and the international Alliance of Patients' Organizations, among others, revealed wide interest for placing the person at the center of general medicine and health care. This led to the collaborative organization of the first Geneva Conference on Person Centered Medicine at Geneva University Hospital. This started a process of annual Geneva Conferences. Of note, the World Health Organization joined in formally cosponsoring the Conferences since its third edition in 2010 to date. From this process emerged the International Network, now International College, of Person Centered Medicine [40].

Within the framework of this broader conceptual scope and wide inter-institutional collaboration, work on person-centered psychiatry has continued with greater vigor and reach. Illustrative of these efforts are the following projects.

3.4.3.1 Development of the Person-Centered Integrative Diagnosis (PID) Model and Practical Guides

This work has involved the publication of a consolidated structural model for person-centered integrative diagnosis (PID), following up on the work on person-centered clinical diagnosis initiated during the period of the Institutional Program on Psychiatry for the Person mentioned above. Thus, most immediately, this is a model for person-centered psychiatric diagnosis but potentially extensible to medicine at large.

The PID model [98] articulates science and humanism to obtain a diagnosis *of* the person (of the totality of the person's health, both its ill and positive aspects), *by* the person (with clinicians extending themselves as full human beings, scientifically competent and with high ethical aspirations), *for* the person (assisting the fulfillment of the person's health aspirations and life project), and *with* the person (in respectful and empowering relationship with the person who presents for evaluation and care). This notion of diagnosis goes beyond the more restricted concepts of nosological and differential diagnoses.

The person-centered integrative diagnostic model is defined by three key features: (a) broad informational domains, covering both ill health and positive health along three levels, health status, contributors to health, and health experience and values, (b) pluralistic descriptive procedures (categories, dimensions, and narratives), and (c) evaluation partnerships among clinicians, patients, and families. Evolving research on the PID includes a conceptual validation of its basic elements [99].

The Latin American Psychiatric Association Section on Diagnosis and Classification has prepared and published the Latin American Guide for Psychiatric Diagnosis, Revised Version (GLADP-VR) [100]. It was built starting with the original GLADP [101] and largely incorporating the basic elements of the person-centered integrative diagnosis (PID) model [99]. For coding disorders, it uses the categories and codes of WHO's International Classification of Diseases.

The GLADP-VR is being increasingly used throughout the various Latin American countries. It is the official guide from the Latin American Psychiatric Association.

There are also plans to develop under the auspices of the International College of Person Centered Medicine a PID practical guide intended for use in general medicine.

3.4.3.2 Person-Centered Psychiatry Book

The purpose of this book is to present authoritatively the emerging field of person-centered psychiatry. It is organized under the aegis of the International College of Person Centered Medicine. The World Psychiatric Association (WPA) is officially cosponsoring it. Eighteen WPA Scientific Sections are engaged in its authorship. It has been published by Springer Switzerland.

Its editors are JE Mezzich, M. Botbol, G. Christodoulou, CR Cloninger, and I. Salloum. It has 90 chapter authors. It includes 40 chapters organized into the following five sections: Principles, Diagnosis and Assessment, Person-Centered Care Approaches, Person-Centered Care for Specific Mental Conditions, and Special Topics.

3.5 Colophon

As the present century unfolds in the field of health, a programmatic movement on person-centered medicine has emerged. It shares with the psychosomatic approach a holistic framework to understand and deal with ill health and positive health. The reaffirmation of medicine's central mission, recognizing the person as a fundamental center and goal rather than just as a carrier of disease, is informed by the wisdom of major ancient civilizations as well as contemporary insights from the clinical and public health arenas. Person-centered medicine values emerging biological, psychological, and sociocultural scientific advances and incorporates them within a whole person framework. Improving on reductionistic epistemological formulations, it proposes a medicine informed by evidence, experience, and values and oriented to the service and promotion of the totality of the person.

Acknowledgments and Disclosures The authors do not have any conflicts of interest to report.

References

1. Mezzich JE, Snaedal J, van Weel C, Botbol M, Salloum IM. Introduction to person-centered medicine: from concepts to practice. J Eval Clin Pract. 2011;17:330–2.
2. Mezzich JE, Snaedal J, van Weel C, Heath I. Toward person-centered medicine: from disease to patient to person. Mt Sinai J Med. 2010;77:304–6.
3. Cassell E. The person in medicine. Int J Integr Care. 2010;10(Supplement):50–1.
4. Christodoulou GN, editor. Psychosomatic medicine. New York: Plenum Press; 1987.

5. Oxford University Press. Oxford dictionaries. Oxford: Oxford University Press; 2016.
6. Engel G. The need for a new medical model: a challenge for biomedicine. Science. 1977;196:129–36.
7. Kirmayer LJ, Bennegadi R, Kastrup MC. Cultural awareness and responsiveness. In: Mezzich JE, Botbol M, Christodoulou GN, Cloninger CR, Salloum IM, editors. Person centered psychiatry. Heidelberg: Springer; in press.
8. Ortega y Gasset J. Meditaciones del Quijote. Obras Completas de José Ortega y Gasset. vol 1. Madrid: Editorial Santillana; 1914, 2004. p. 745–825.
9. Appleyard J. Person-centered and integrated care across the life-cycle. Int J Pers Cent Med. 2015;5(1):15–20.
10. Appleyard J. Child-centered medical care. Int J Pers Cent Med. 2011;1:460–2.
11. Snaedal J. Person centered medicine for the old with specific reference to dementia. Int J Pers Cent Med. 2011;1:53–5.
12. Botbol M, Alanen YO, Schmolke M. Psychological perspectives on psychiatry for the person. Int J Pers Cent Med. 2011;1:134–6.
13. Tischler V, Chopra A, Nixon N, McCormack L. Loss and tomorrow's doctors: how the humanities can contribute to person and professional development. Int J Pers Cent Med. 2011;1:547–52.
14. Millar HL. The burden of multimorbidity: physical health in the severely mentally ill population. Die Psychiatrie. 2012;3:137–42.
15. Salloum IM, Mezzich JE, Cordoba SE. Conceptual and methodological considerations in comorbidity. In: Salloum IM, Mezzich JE, editors. Psychiatric diagnosis: challenges and prospects. Oxford: Wiley-Blackwell; 2009.
16. World Health Organization. Global health status report on non-communicable diseases. Geneva: World Health Organization; 2012.
17. Mezzich JE, Appleyard J. Continuing development of person centered medicine and addressing chronic disease. Int J Pers Cent Med. 2013;3:1–4.
18. International College of Person-centered Medicine. Geneva declaration on person-centered care for chronic diseases. Int J Pers Cent Med. 2012;2:153–4.
19. Lalande A. Vocabulario Técnico y Crítico de la Filosofia. In: Alfonso TL, Quintero V, editors. Sociedad Francesa de Filosofía. Buenos Aires: Librería El Ateneo; 1953.
20. Patwardhan B, Warude D, Pushpangadan P, Bhatt N. Ayurveda and traditional Chinese medicine: a comparative overview. Evid Based Complement Alternat Med. 2005;2:465–73.
21. Ramose MB. The philosophy of the Ubuntu and Ubuntu as a philosophy. In: Coetzee PH, Roux APJ, editors. The African philosophy reader. 2nd ed. NewYork: Routledge; 2003. p. 230–8.
22. Montiel E. El humanismo americano. Filosofía de una comunidad de naciones. Asunción: Fondo de Cultura Económica; 2000.
23. Wolf E. Pueblos y Culturas de Mesoamérica. Mexico: Ediciones Era; 1967.
24. Anzures, Bolaños MC. Medicinas tradicionales y antropología. Anales de Antropología (México). 1978;15:151. I.I.A./U.N.A.M.
25. Ierodiakonou CS. Medicine as a model for Aristotle's ethics and his person-centered approach. Int J Pers Cent Med. 2014;4:31–4.
26. Jouanna J. Hippocrates. Translated by M.B. Debevoise. Baltimore: Johns Hopkins University Press; 1999.
27. Tournier P. Médecine de la Personne. Neuchatel: Delachaux et Niestle; 1940.
28. Rogers CR. On becoming a person: a therapist's view of psychotherapy. Boston: Houghton Mifflin; 1961.
29. WMA Declaration of Geneva 1948. World medical association international code of medical ethics. Pilanesberg, South Africa; 2006. www.wma.net.
30. WMA Declaration of Helsinki. Ethical principles for medical research. http://www.wma.net/en/30publications/10policies/index.html.
31. McWhinney IR. Family medicine: a textbook. Oxford: Oxford University Press; 1989.

32. Garrabe J, Hoff P. Historical views on psychiatry for the person. Int J Pers Cent Med. 2011;1:125–7.
33. Mezzich JE. Psychiatry for the person: articulating medicine's science and humanism. World Psychiatry. 2007;6:65–7.
34. World Health Organization. World health report. Geneva: World Health Organization; 2008.
35. World Health Organization. World health assembly resolutions on primary health care, including health system strengthening, WHA 62.12, 22 May 2009; 2009.
36. Mezzich JE, Snaedal J, van Weel C, Heath I. Conceptual explorations on person-centered medicine. Int J Integr Care. 2010;10(Suppl):e002.
37. Mezzich JE, Snaedal J, van Weel C, Botbol M, Salloum I. Introduction to person-centred medicine: from concepts to practice. J Eval Clin Pract. 2011;17(2):330–2.
38. Mezzich JE, Snaedal J, Van weel C, Botbol M, Salloum I, Van Lerberghe W. Articulating person-centered medicine and people-centered public health: a report from the fourth Geneva conference on person-centered medicine. World Med J. 2011;57:171–4.
39. Mezzich JE. The Geneva conferences and the emergence of the international network of person-centered medicine. J Eval Clin Pract. 2011;17:333–6.
40. Mezzich JE, Snaedal J, van Weel C, Heath I. The international network for person-centered medicine: background and first steps. World Med J. 2009;55:104–7.
41. Mezzich JE. The construction of person-centered medicine and the launching of an international college. Int J Pers Cent Med. 2012;2:6–10.
42. International College of Person Centered Medicine. Geneva declaration on person centered health research. Int J Pers Cent Med. 2013;3:106–7.
43. Salvador L, Cloninger CR, Thornicroft A, Mezzich JE, et al. Geneva declaration on person centered health research. Int J Pers Cent Med. 2013;3:109–13.
44. International College of Person Centered Medicine. 2014 Geneva declaration on person- and people-centered integrated health care for all. Int J Pers Cent Med. 2014;4:66–8.
45. Cloninger CR, Salvador-Carulla L, Kirmayer LJ, Schwartz MA, Appleyard J, Goodwin N, Groves J, Hermans MHM, Mezzich JE, van Staden CW, Rawaf S. A time for action on health inequities: foundations of the 2014 Geneva declaration on person- and people-centered integrated health care for all. Int J Pers Cent Med. 2014;4:69–89.
46. Miles A, Mezzich JE. Advancing the global communication of scholarship and research for personalized healthcare: the international journal of person centered medicine. Int J Pers Cent Med. 2011;1:1–5.
47. Mezzich JE, Botbol M, Christodoulou GN, Cloninger CR, Salloum IM, editors. Person centered psychiatry. Heidelberg: Springer; 2016.
48. Cloninger CR, Salloum IM, Mezzich JE. The dynamic origins of positive health and well being. Int J Pers Cent Med. 2012;2:179–87.
49. Mezzich JE, Kirisci L, Salloum IM, Trivedi JK, Kar SK, Adams N, Wallcraft J. Systematic conceptualization of person centered medicine and development and validation of a person-centered care index. Int J Pers Cent Med. 2016;6:219–47.
50. Brundtland G. Preface to mental health: a call for action by world health ministers. Ministerial rounds at the 54th world health assembly. Geneva: World Health Organization; 2001.
51. Greenhalg T. Patient and public involvement in chronic illness: beyond the expert patient. Br Med J. 2009;338:49.
52. Cloninger CR. What makes makes people healthy, happy, and fulfilled in the face of current world challenges? Mens Sana Monogr. 2013;11:16–24.
53. Seyer J. Development of the health improvement card developed by the world health professions alliance. In: Paper presented at the 5th Geneva conference on person-centered medicine. International College of Person Centered Medicine, May 2012; 2012.
54. Keyes CL, Shmotkin D, Ryff CD. Optimizing well-being: the empirical encounter of two traditions. J Pers Soc Psychol. 2002;82(6):1007–22.
55. Herrman H, Stewart DE, Diaz-Granados N, Berger EL, Jackson B, Yuen T. What is resilience? Can J Psychiatr. 2011;56(5):258–65.

56. Cloninger CR, Salloum IM, Mezzich JE. The dynamic origins of positive health and wellbeing. Int J Pers Cent Med. 2012;2(2):1–9.
57. Cloninger CR. Feeling good: the science of well-being. New York: Oxford University Press; 2004. p. 374.
58. Botbol M. Du manifeste au subjectif: ce qu'est la médecine de la personne [from objectivity to subjectivity : what is person centered medicine]. In: Kipman SD, editor. Manifeste pour la médecine de la personne [Manifesto for person centered medicine]. Paris: Dion; 2012.
59. Warne C. Aristotle's nicomachean ethics: reader's guide. London: Continuum; 2007.
60. Botbol M, Lecic-Tosevski D. Person-centered medicine and subjectivity. In: Cornelius-White JHD, Motschnig- Pitrik R, Lux M, editors. Interdisciplinary applications of the person-centered approach. New York: Springer; 2013. p. 73–82.
61. Lebovici S. L'arbre de vie—éléments de la psychopathologie du bébé [the tree of life—principles of infant psychopathology]. Toulouse: Eres; 1999.
62. Hochmann J. Une histoire de l'empathie [a history of empathy]. Paris: Odile Jacob; 2012.
63. Ricoeur P. Temps et récit [Time and narrative]. Paris: Le Seuil; 1983.
64. Kleinman A. The illness narratives. New York: Basic Books; 1988.
65. Chamberlin J. On our own: patient-controlled alternatives to the mental health system. New York: McGraw-Hill; 1979.
66. Deegan P. The independent living movement and people with psychiatric disabilities: taking back control over our own lives. Psychosoc Rehabil J. 1992;15:3–19.
67. Anthony W. Recovery from mental illness. The guiding vision of the mental health service system in the 1990s. Psychosoc Rehabil J. 1993;16:11–23.
68. Barber ME. Recovery as the new medical model for psychiatry. Psychiatr Serv. 2012;63(3):277–9.
69. Davidson L, Chinman M, Sells D, et al. Peer support among adults with serious mental illness: a report from the field. Schizophr Bull. 2006;32(3):443–50.
70. Deegan PE, Drake RE. Shared decision making and medication management in the recovery process. Psychiatr Serv. 2006;57(11):1636–9.
71. Stevenson FA, Barry CA, Britten N, Barber N, Bradley CP. Doctor–patient communication about drugs: the evidence for shared decision making. Soc Sci Med. 2000;50(6):829–40.
72. Hamann J, et al. Shared decision making for in-patients with schizophrenia. Acta Psychiatr Scand. 2006;114:265–73.
73. Schmolke MM, Mezzich JE. Contrasting the essentials of recovery orientation and person-centered care. Int J Pers Cent Med. 2013;3:31–5.
74. Mezzich JE. Psychiatry for the person: articulating medicine's science and humanism. World Psychiatry. 2007;6:1–3.
75. Mezzich JE. The dialogal basis of our profession: psychiatry with the person. World Psychiatry. 2007;6:129–30.
76. Christodoulou G, Fulford B, Mezzich JE. Psychiatry for the person and its conceptual bases. Int Psychiatry. 2008;5:1–3.
77. Mezzich JE, Christodoulou G, Fulford KWM. Introduction to the conceptual bases of psychiatry for the person. Int J Pers Cent Med. 2011;1:121–4.
78. Thornton T, Schaffner KF. Philosophy of science perspectives on psychiatry for the person. Int J Pers Cent Med. 2011;1:128–30.
79. Fulford KWM, Christodoulou G, Stein DJ. Values and ethics: perspectives on psychiatry for the person. Int J Pers Cent Med. 2011;1:131–3.
80. Cloninger CR, Abou-Saleh MT, Mrazek DA, Möller H-J. Biological perspectives on psychiatry for the person. Int J Pers Cent Med. 2011;1:137–9.
81. Rutz W, Fernandez M, Trivedi J. Social perspectives on psychiatry for the person. Int J Pers Cent Med. 2011;1:140–2.
82. Fabrega H Jr, Wintrob R. Ethnomedical and cultural foundations of psychiatry for the person. Int J Pers Cent Med. 2011;1:143–5.
83. Cox J, Verhagen PJ. Spirituality, religion and psychopathology: towards an integrative psychiatry. Int J Pers Cent Med. 2011;1:146–8.

84. Sukhanova E, Thomashoff H-O, Thoret Y. Literature and arts perspectives on psychiatry for the person. Int J Pers Cent Med. 2011;1:149–51.
85. Wallcraft J, Steffen S, Amering M. Service user and family perspectives on psychiatry for the person. Int J Pers Cent Med. 2011;1:152–4.
86. Mezzich JE, Ustun TB. International classification and diagnosis: critical experience and future directions. Psychopathology. 2002;35(2–3):59–201.
87. CEM B, Mezzich JE, Berganza CE. Philosophical and methodological foundations of psychiatric diagnosis. Psychopathology. 2005;38(4):155–230.
88. World Psychiatric Association (WPA). Essentials of the world psychiatric association's international guidelines for diagnostic assessment (IGDA). Br J Psychiatry. 2003;182(Suppl. 45):37–66.
89. Salloum IM, Mezzich JE, editors. Psychiatric diagnosis: challenges and prospects. Chichester: Wiley-Blackwell; 2009.
90. Mezzich JE, Salloum IM. Towards innovative international classification and diagnostic systems: ICD-11 and person-centered integrative diagnosis. Acta Psychiatr Scand. 2007;116:1–5.
91. Mezzich JE, Salloum IM. Clinical complexity and person-centered integrative diagnosis. World Psychiatry. 2008;7:1–2.
92. Mezzich JE, Salloum IM. On person-centered integrative diagnosis. Die Psychiatrie. 2007;4:262–5.
93. Beaglehole R, editor. Global public health: a new era. Oxford: Oxford University Press; 2003.
94. Herrman H, Saxena S, Moodie R. Promoting mental health: concepts, emerging evidence, practice. Geneva: WHO; 2005.
95. Rutz W. Social psychiatry and public mental health: present situation and future objectives. Time for rethinking and renaissance? Acta Psychiatr Scand. 2006;429(Suppl):95–100.
96. Strauss JS. The person—key to understanding mental illness: towards a new dynamic psychiatry, III. Br J Psychiatry. 1992;161(18):19–26.
97. WHO. The world health report 2001: mental health: new understanding, new hope. Geneva: World Health Organization; 2001.
98. Mezzich JE, Salloum IM, Cloninger CR, Salvador-Carulla L, Kirmayer L, Banzato CE, Wallcraft J, Botbol M. Person-centered integrative diagnosis: conceptual bases and structural model. Can J Psychiatr. 2010;55:701–8.
99. Salloum IM, Mezzich JE. Conceptual appraisal of the person-centered integrative diagnosis model. Int J Pers Cent Med. 2011;1:39–42.
100. Asociación Psiquiátrica de América Latina, Sección de Diagnóstico y Clasificación. Guía Latinoamericana de Diagnóstico Psiquiátrico, Version revisada (GLADP-VR). Lima: Asociación Psiquiátrica de América Latina; 2012.
101. Asociación Psiquiátrica de América Latina, Sección de Diagnóstico y Clasificación. Guía Latinoamericana de Diagnóstico Psiquiátrico. Guadalajara: Asociación Psiquiátrica de América Latina; 2004.

Screening for Psychosocial Distress and Psychiatric Disorders in Medicine: From Concepts to Evidence

4

Alex J. Mitchell

Abstract

A key element of supportive care is the reliable assessment and measurement of psychological health. This includes detection of frank psychiatric disorders as well as broader psychological symptoms and generalized distress. Many organizations have made recommendations for assessment of psychiatric disorders and psychological distress, but despite the potential benefits, uptake of screening has been slow, and evidence that patient outcomes improve is mixed. New evidence supports multidomain-/algorithm-based screening as well on screening online and in new smartphone apps. Psychosocial assessment can be pragmatically divided into screening, clinical assessment (case finding) and severity measurement. Screening is designed to quickly ascertain which individuals in a large population need further assessment and where necessary additional care. The target of screening may be mood disorders, anxiety, distress, cognitive decline, unmet needs or any combination (multidomain approach). For patients with complex needs, a multidimensional approach may be preferable, and a multidimensional tool can be valuable as it can serve as a roadmap to a more effective way of addressing patient concerns in a timely way with appropriate referral to the right professional. Yet some forms of screening can be an additional burden to patients and clinicians unless conducted at home, online or in the waiting room. Screening for distress and/or psychological assessment should not be considered a one-off exercise but part of routine high quality of care that involves all healthcare professionals.

A. J. Mitchell
Department of Cancer Studies and Molecular Medicine,
University of Leicester, Leicester, UK
e-mail: ajm80@le.ac.uk

L. Grassi et al. (eds.), *Person Centered Approach to Recovery in Medicine*,
Integrating Psychiatry and Primary Care, https://doi.org/10.1007/978-3-319-74736-1_4

4.1 Introduction

In the last 10 years, there has been raised awareness of the importance of mental health in both primary care and secondary (hospital) care. A large body of evidence suggests that the quality of mental healthcare is lower than expected in these settings [1]. Further specific mental health mood and anxiety disorders adversely influence mortality following myocardial infarction [2], heart disease [3], COPD [4], stroke [5] and haemodialysis [6, 7]. The same observation applies for severe mental illnesses such as schizophrenia, bipolar disorder and dementia [8, 9]. Ultimately these deficits in care contribute to a large mortality gap of approximately 5–10 years for patients with mild-to-moderate mental illness and 10–20 years for patients' severe mental illness [8, 10]. However, it is not only mortality that is a concern. Comorbid mental health problems have a greater effect on quality of life than physical comorbidities [11]. Distress itself is associated with reduced health-related quality of life and poor satisfaction with medical care [12]. Comorbid anxiety results in greater disability and lower quality of life after controlling for confounding variables [13]. Given these concerns several organizations have promoted the concept of parity of esteem, namely, valuing mental health as much as physical health. Several recent guidelines outline how to reduce these inequalities in diagnosis, treatment, follow-up and attitudes [14–16].

Perhaps the first step in reducing inequalities in mental health in medical settings is appropriate diagnosis and screening. There is no doubt that there is significant under-diagnosis of every mental health condition studied in primary and secondary care [17]. Further psychiatric illnesses are more often overlooked when they occur in patients with pre-existing physical comorbidity. Over half of all cases of depression in the general hospital setting go unrecognized by physicians and nursing staff, and there are similar problems with detection in primary care [18, 19]. This may be in part because clinicians have little training in this area, have low awareness of mental illness and in these settings do not have the time to use assessment tools preferring instead to rely upon their own clinical judgement [20]. As a result emotional issues are often not emphasized during clinical consultations [21, 22]. To address this, many organizations have recommended screening for depression, delirium or dementia (or mental illness as a whole) in primary care and in hospital settings.

4.2 Concepts of Diagnosis, Case Finding and Screening

Clinical diagnosis is a process, whereby a clinician or trained researcher establishes the most likely condition based on the evidence available. That evidence may simply be symptoms in the history or signs elicited in the medical examination, or it may be psychometric scores from assessment scales. To date no reliable biomedical tests have contributed significantly to clinical psychiatric diagnosis outside of dementia and cognitive impairment. Once symptoms, signs and/or test results have been elicited there must be pattern recognition ideally against standardized criteria achieved by either clinical judgement or computer matching/artificial intelligence. The ideal is to correctly identify all cases as well as correctly identifying all non-cases. Sensitivity is the proportion of true positives out of all with the condition (cases), and specificity is the proportion of true negatives out of all those without the condition (non-cases). Although these are the most popular metrics, both sensitivity and specificity are abstract concepts for clinicians and are really only useful when they approach 100%. A more useful metric is the ability to identify true positives (cases) as a proportion of all positive screening attempts which is known as the *positive predictive value* (PPV). PPV is essentially a measure of case-finding ability. The ability to spot (true) non-cases as a proportion of all negative test results is the *negative predictive value* (NPV) and is a measure of screening acumen (see Box 4.1). In an epidemiological sense, *screening studies* are those where a test is applied to those at low or modest risk of a condition or in a population where the prevalence is low. The aim in most screening studies is to initially exclude a large number of clear non-cases. In this application, a first-stage screener may not have perfect PPV, but it should have high NPV because those ruled-out are unlikely to receive a second examination and false negatives should be avoided. Conversely *case-finding studies* are usually applied in high-prevalence settings such as hospitalized care where a final confirmation is needed of caseness and false positives should be avoided.

Box 4.1 Pragmatic Definitions of Case-Identification

Screening

The application of a diagnostic test or clinical assessment in order to optimally rule-out those without the disorder with minimal false negatives (missed cases).

Screening is often performed as a broad population strategy as a first step.

Case-Finding

The application of a diagnostic test or clinical assessment in order to optimally identify those with the disorder with minimal false positives.

Case finding is often performed in a selected population at high risk the condition.

Recently newer metrics have attempted to improve upon sensitivity and specificity when evaluating screening and diagnostic studies. Sensitivity and specificity are essentially measures of occurrence. Contrastingly, PPV and NPV are measures of discrimination. Clinically relevant rule in accuracy would be product of the PPV and sensitivity. This is called the positive clinical utility index (CUI+ = sensitivity × PPV) [23]. Similarly clinically relevant rule out accuracy would be product of the NPV and specificity. This is called the negative clinical utility index (CUI− = specificity × NPV). The utility index can be considered a measure of the clinical value of a diagnostic test (see www.clinicalutility.co.uk for further information).

4.3 Implementation of Screening

There are three major types of studies. Psychometric studies examine various characteristics of the instrument such as reliability and consistency. Diagnostic validity studies examine accuracy against a known standard. Implementation studies examine how well does screening work in practice [24]. This might involve examination of the uptake of the tool, acceptability of the tool, change in referral patterns, influence on patient care and ultimately effect of patient well-being. Phases in the development and testing of a screening tool have been reported [25]. Once a screening tool has been developed and tested for potential accuracy against an accepted "gold standard", it can be evaluated in a clinical setting. This is the implementation phase. The implementation can be non-comparative or observational. For example, the effect of screening on quality of care (process measures) or patient-reported outcomes can be monitored using current or historical data. Observational studies will reveal how well screening is working, but will not reveal how much better screening is over usual care. For this, interventional screening studies are required. These can be randomized or non-randomized. In the randomized study, two equal groups of clinicians, or in the case of cluster randomization two centres, are randomized to have either access to screening or no access to screening. A variant on this design is to randomize two groups to have either access to results of screening or screening, but no feedback of the results of screening. In effect it is feedback of results that are randomized not screening. Theoretically this may help distinguish which effects are related to application of the screener and which are related to the receipt of screening results.

The aim of screening is fundamentally to facilitate effective and efficient treatment by focussing on people who would most benefit from a proven intervention. However, to justify the time and effort required, screening must be more worthwhile than not screening (treatment-as-usual). Usually this is assessed using patient-reported outcome measures (PROMs) but may also include clinician behaviour (e.g. number of accurate diagnoses recorded, doctor-patient communication, referrals made to specialist services and psychosocial help given by clinicians). These quality of care markers, sometimes called process measures can influence PROMs. For example, Carlson et al. [26] found that the best predictor of decreased anxiety and depression was receipt of referral to psychosocial services. If screening studies show benefits in quality of care or clinician behaviour but not patient well-being, then this suggests that there are significant barriers to care downstream of the screening process. An important measure in all studies is acceptability of the screening programme to patients and clinicians. This can be measured by satisfaction scores or by proxy measures such as uptake and participation. Thought needs to be given to the location of the screen, the method of application (e.g. pencil and paper or computer or touch tablet) and the timing and number of applications. Screening may be conducted systematically on every qualifying patient or targeted on the basis of clinician decision. Systematic screening (i.e. screen everyone within a service) has the advantage of not missing low-risk individuals who might nevertheless be in need of help but is more resource intensive.

4.4 Screening for Depression

Depression comorbidity has been extensively studied in virtually all medical areas and in primary care. Depression is seen in approximately 15% of primary care patients, and about half of those who consult their general practitioner are incorrectly diagnosed [27]. The same error rate is seen in hospital settings for those who do not receive a specialist assessment by a mental health professional [28]. Prevalence rates vary according to the tool used, duration after diagnosis and background risk factors. As a rule of thumb depressive symptoms are more common than mild-moderate clinical depression which is more common in turn than severe clinical depression. The most commonly applied criteria are those for major depression set out in *Diagnostic and Statistical Manual of Mental Disorders, 5th Edition* (DSM5) [29] which requires five of nine qualifying symptoms, together with a minimum duration of 2 weeks and clinical significance defined by concomitant distress or impaired daily function. Other forms of depression include minor depression, dysthymia and adjustment disorder with predominant depression. Depression is very often comorbid with other mental health conditions as well as a wide range of medical conditions (multi-morbidity). Rates of depression are threefold higher for patients with two or more medical conditions compared with those with no comorbidity [30]. Rates of depression are broadly similar in well-designed studies conducted in patients with stroke, multiple sclerosis, Parkinson's disease, epilepsy, diabetes, myocardial infarction, heart failure, cancer, rheumatological disease and lung disease [31]. About 50% of patients have symptoms of depression and 20% have major depression early after a medical diagnosis a prevalence rate which is approximately 50% higher than rate seen in the general population [32]. In longitudinal studies persistent depression increases the risk of later dementia, diabetes, heart disease and cancer [33]. Compared to hospitalized inpatients without depression, those discharged with depressive symptoms are more likely to be readmitted (20.4% vs 13.7%) and more likely to die within 30 days (2.8% vs 1.5%) [34]. Depression also increases the risk of adverse outcomes (mortality and morbidity) among those who already have established medical conditions [35, 36]. This may be because depression influences receipt of medical care, quality of medical care and participation in medical treatment [37–39].

Over the last decade, numerous depression screening studies and depression screening guidelines have been published. The UK National Institute for Health and Care Excellence (NICE) [40, 41] states:

> *Be alert to possible depression (particularly in people with a past history of depression, possible somatic symptoms of depression or a chronic physical health problem with associated functional impairment) and consider asking people who may have depression two questions, specifically: During the last month, have you often been bothered by feeling down, depressed or hopeless? During the last month, have you often been bothered by having little interest or pleasure in doing things?*

In 2016 the US Preventive Services Task Force (USPSTF) updated its recommendation on the screening of depression in the general adult population (aged 18 years or older including pregnant women and postpartum women) as follows [42].

> *The USPSTF concludes with at least moderate certainty that there is a moderate net benefit to screening for depression in adults, including older adults, who receive care in clinical practices that have adequate systems in place to ensure accurate diagnosis, effective treatment, and appropriate follow-up after screening.*

It is important to note that routine screening is not always successful and is not without risks of false positives and false negatives and, in addition, requires adequate follow-up with good-quality evidence-based treatments. Where treatments are not given, screening alone is unlikely to be beneficial, and this has been strongly asserted by several groups [43]. Further the evidence from randomized controlled trials that screening improves quality of care is currently modest. There is a small but statistically significant evidence base in primary care and in cancer care but with an absence of evidence in other settings. This has led the Canadian Task Force on Preventive Health Care (CTFPHC) to downgrade its original 2005 recommendation to "not routinely screen adults with no apparent symptoms of depression" but nevertheless "that clinicians be alert to the clinical symptoms of depression, especially in individuals with characteristics that may increase their risk for depression" [44].

Regarding choice of individual tools, numerous tools have been developed, tested and validated with item counts varying from 1 to 90 items or more [45]. Most are self-report, but there are also brief structured verbal questions and computerized questionnaires [46]. USPSTF suggests screening with the Patient Health Questionnaire (PHQ), the Hospital Anxiety and Depression Scales (HADS) in adults, the Geriatric Depression Scale (GDS) in older adults and the Edinburgh Postnatal Depression Scale (EPDS) in postpartum and pregnant women [42]. No scale is perfect, and each should be judged on accuracy, reliability and acceptability [47]. Scales are more likely to be successful in screening (ruling out) than case finding when assessing a low prevalence condition such as depression. For example, recent reviews found that the HADS could not be recommended as a case-finding (diagnostic) instrument but it may be suitable as an initial screening tool, length permitting [48, 49]. Other tools including the Beck Depression Inventory (BDI) [50], the Edinburgh Postnatal Depression Scale (EPDS) [51] and the Centers for Epidemiological Studies-Depression Scale (CES-D) tend to be too lengthy for non-specialists [52, 53]. Currently the most popular strategy is to use the Patient Health questionnaire (PHQ-2 and PHQ-9) [54]. Best estimates of sensitivity and specificity were 81.3% and 85.3% (95% CI 81.0–89.1) and 89.3% and 75.9% for the PHQ-9-linear and PHQ-2, respectively [54]. For case finding (confirming a diagnosis) no self-report tool is entirely satisfactory, but for screening (ruling out non-cases) almost any validated tool can be used with the exception of a single verbal item which is inaccurate [55, 56]. That said, an increasingly favoured strategy is to routinely screen with a short one- or two-item questionnaire (e.g. PHQ-2) and then apply a longer scale in screen positive patients (e.g. PHQ9).

4.5 Screening for Anxiety Disorders

Anxiety and related disorders are the most prevalent mental disorders in the general population, and there is a strong bidirectional association with general medical conditions [57]. Anxiety disorders include several subtypes including generalized anxiety disorder (GAD), panic disorder, phobias, obsessive compulsive disorder and post-traumatic stress disorder. PTSD, for example, is seen in about 10–20% patients after coronary heart disease or cancer and influences quality of life outcomes, adherence to treatments and likelihood of readmission [58]. About 20% of primary care patients have one or more anxiety disorders, and recognition may be as low as 24%. Further 5 year treatment uptake may be as low as 60% even after diagnosis [59, 60].

Anxiety is the most common patient-reported emotional complication of most medical disorders including cardiovascular disease, most neurological conditions and cancer [17, 61]. Conversely the most common medical comorbidities in hospital patients with anxiety appear to be hypertension, asthma, cataract and ischaemic heart disease [62]. If one controls for physical comorbidities (i.e. number of physical conditions), anxiety disorder remains significantly associated with gastrointestinal conditions and chronic pain [63]. Self-reported anxiety is typically found in more than 40% of patients in the early stages of treatment, but unlike depression anxiety is usually more persistent with time especially in cancer survivors [64]. Anxiety is underestimated by clinicians, and it is under-represented by semi-structured interviews [17]. Anxiety and depression are frequently comorbid, and both are independently associated with poorer QoL [65].

Clinicians rarely use formal instruments when assessing anxiety but typically rely on verbal and nonverbal cues [66]. Recognition of anxiety appears to be significantly worse than recognition of depression. Simple clinically relevant screening tools are likely to improve recognition rates. A single verbal item ("How anxious have you felt this week?") and single-item Anxiety Thermometer (from www.emotionthermometers.com) offer a rapid screen for anxiety that can be quickly adopted into routine care but may lack specificity [67, 68]. A number of brief generic self-report questionnaires have been studied in several medical settings and in primary care. These include the anxiety subscale of the HADS, the STAI, the Beck Anxiety Inventory, the Pen State Worry Questionnaire and the GAD7. Several organizations have authored anxiety screening guidelines and many recommend the GAD7 which has a modest evidence base but importantly does not accurately follow DSM5 algorithm for GAD [69]. Our group proposed a new questionnaire GAD-DSM which is compliant. Regarding anxiety screening NICE states [70]:

> *Be alert to possible anxiety disorders (particularly in people with a past history of an anxiety disorder, possible somatic symptoms of an anxiety disorder or in those who have experienced a recent traumatic event). Consider asking the person about their feelings of anxiety and their ability to stop or control worry, using the 2-item Generalized Anxiety Disorder scale (GAD-2). If the person scores less than three on the GAD-2 scale, but you are still concerned they may have an anxiety disorder, ask the following: 'Do you find yourself avoiding places or activities and does this cause you problems?'. If the person answers 'yes' to this question consider an anxiety disorder and follow the recommendations for assessment (see section 1.3.2).*

Unfortunately the criteria for GAD may be too restrictive for medical settings, as they require "excessive anxiety" for at least 6 months. In addition there is low agreement between ICD10 and DSM-IV criteria for GAD [71]. Further, screening standards for non-GAD anxiety disorders remains a problem. For example, NICE states regarding panic disorder "there is insufficient evidence on which to recommend a well-validated, self-reporting screening instrument to use in the diagnostic process, and so consultation skills should be relied upon to elicit all necessary information" [72].

4.6 Screening for Distress

Emotional distress is common to most mental health conditions and therefore may represent a valid screening target in itself. In addition "distress" is a patient-friendly term which is usually easily understood in most cultures. A definition of distress is "the experience of significant emotional upset arising from any physical or psychiatric condition" [73, 74]. Distress is not a specific category in DSM5 nor ICD10 (International Classification of Diseases, 10th Edition) but rather a qualifying clinical significance criteria. Accumulating evidence suggests that the presence of distress is associated with reduced health-related quality of life [75], poor satisfaction with medical care [76] and possibly reduced survival [77]. Unfortunately, interventions for distress and related emotional disorders have failed to show any benefit on survival as a whole implying distress is linked with mortality through confounding factors [78, 79]. In 1998 the NCCN released a one-item, visual-analogue scale (VAS) known as the Distress Thermometer (DT) [80, 81]. This is a simple one-item visual-analogue thermometer with good sensitivity and modest specificity [82, 83]. NICE recognizes distress as an important symptoms and states:

> *For people with significant language or communication difficulties, for example people with sensory impairments or a learning disability, consider using the DT and/or asking a family member or carer about the person's symptoms to identify a possible common mental health disorder. If a significant level of distress is identified, offer further assessment or seek the advice of a specialist.*

Despite the popularity of the DT, more sophisticated distress measures are available, and several have been widely studied in primary care including the General Health Questionnaire (GHQ). Indeed several promising variants of the thermometer format have been developed [84, 85]. Recently, Mitchell et al. developed a five-item Emotion Thermometer designed to measure multidomain emotional complications with better accuracy and yet no appreciably drop in acceptability compared with the original DT [68].

4.7 Screening for Bipolar Disorder and Severe Mental Illness

Screening for bipolar disorder is a relatively new area that has long been overlooked in hospital settings and in primary care. However detection is not always straightforward because patients with bipolar disorder may have infrequent or very brief manic/hypomanic symptoms and patients may not recall past manic symptoms at all [86]. Several screening tests and self-completed questionnaires have been developed to facilitate the early detection of bipolar disorder including the Mood Disorders Questionnaire (MDQ) and the Bipolar Spectrum Disorders Scale [87]. The MDQ is a single-page screener for a lifetime history of manic or hypomanic symptoms using 13 yes/no items [88]. In a review of studies with mixed unipolar and bipolar patients, the MDQ was found to have modest accuracy (sensitivity 76% and specificity 81%), but sensitivity was only 37%, and specificity was 88% when undiagnosed patients were considered [89]. Given a concern over high false-positive rates, several authors propose that screening for bipolar is confined to those with current depression, focussing on the longitudinal history of bipolar disorder [90]. Indeed screening for bipolar disorder is not a common practice outside of specialist settings, and guidelines are rare. In the UK, NICE states [91]:

> *Do not use questionnaires in primary care to identify bipolar disorder in adults.*

4.8 Screening for Dementia

Dementia is an increasing problem in society due to increasing longevity. In the UK recent national campaigns have called attention to dementia and encouraged early help seeking [92, 93]. Sixty to seventy percent of all people with dementia are not formally diagnosed [94]. Around 6–10% of inpatients in general hospital have dementia roughly 10 times the rate in the community [95, 96]. Typically only one in three hospital cases of dementia were previously known before admission, therefore many incident cases come to light in hospital.

The needs of patients with dementia are often overlooked, and such patients are also susceptible to environmental change and may find it difficult to communicate their needs in busy environments. General hospitals are not a good environment to manage dementia. GPs (primary care physicians) are usually the first source of contact for individuals and their families worried about their memory [97]. GPs often competently manage patients with cognitive impairment without referral to hospital specialists [98]. Yet clinicians are understandably hesitant about using the term “dementia” prematurely and are generally cautious about disclosing this diagnosis [99, 100]. This concern over false-positive errors might reduce rates of inappropriate treatment but, equally, might favour omission or delay in making a correct diagnosis. Studies show that documentation of dementia is often poor [101], and the typical time taken to reach a diagnosis of dementia or Alzheimer’s disease after first symptoms are noted by patient or family ranges from 10 months in Germany to 32 months in the UK [96, 102]. Dementia is a feared diagnosis, and people under investigation should be asked if they wish to know the diagnosis, and with whom this should be shared. Several surveys suggest that GPs may not be confident in making a diagnosis of dementia and are often unsure about which tests or tools to use [103, 104]. Only a quarter use standardized criteria such as those provided by DSM-IV, ICD10 and DSM5 [105, 106]. Most non-specialists rely on their clinical judgement, occasionally enriched with a basic cognitive screening tool such as the Mini-Mental State Examination (MMSE) [107, 108]. Official criteria for dementia require prolonged impairment in short- and long-term memory, deficits in other areas of cognition and functional impairment, but not all criteria agree precisely [109]. Ngo (2014) summarized current clinical guidelines for dementia [110]. From 12 recent guidelines, 8 addressed cognitive testing, and there was agreement that a cognitive assessment should be performed using a validated, standardized tool. However the specific tools recommended are not very accurate in cases of mild dementia. Short cognitive tests include the MMSE, abbreviated mental test score (AMTS), and six-item cognitive impairment test (6CIT) and GPCOG. The Montreal Cognitive Assessment (MOCA), Addenbrooke's Cognitive Assessment-Revised (ACE-R) and CAMCOG are probably more appropriate in cases of early dementia; indeed six guidelines recommended performing neuropsychological testing as an adjunct to the standard tools. Self-assessment tools such as TYM (Test Your Memory) often performed online are currently under development. Extensive in-depth cognitive testing can be conducted by trained staff such as neuropsychologists, neuropsychiatrists or occupational therapists. Diagnosis is part of a process including history taking, cognitive and mental state examination, physical examination and biomedical investigations. NICE states that primary healthcare staff should consider referring people who show signs of mild cognitive impairment (MCI) for assessment by memory assessment services to aid early identification of dementia [111]. NICE also states [112]:

> *1.4.1.3 Clinical cognitive assessment in those with suspected dementia should include examination of attention and concentration, orientation, short and long-term memory, praxis, language and executive function. As part of this assessment, formal cognitive testing should be undertaken using a standardised instrument. The Mini Mental State Examination (MMSE) has been frequently used for this purpose, but a number of alternatives are now available, such as the 6-item Cognitive Impairment Test (6-CIT), the General Practitioner Assessment of Cognition (GPCOG) and the 7-Minute Screen. Those interpreting the scores of such tests should take full account of other factors known to affect performance, including educational level, skills, prior level of functioning and attainment, language, and any sensory impairments, psychiatric illness or physical/neurological problems.*

4.9 Screening for Delirium

Delirium is an important cognitive disorder with the hallmark of disturbed attention and/or awareness which normally develops rapidly. Delirium is very common in general medical settings with rates of between 15 and 20% of older medical patients and 25–70% after high-risk post-operative surgery, in palliative care units and in critical care, depending on the patient population and assessment methods [113]. However, delirium is frequently overlooked or misdiagnosed due to fluctuating symptoms and signs, overlap with dementia and due to infrequent use of routine cognitive screening [114, 115]. Delirium and dementia differ in their course and cognitive items attention and vigilance [116]. Delirium is costly, causing functional impairment, increased falls, increased healthcare costs, prolonged hospitalization with an increased risk of placement in long-term care at discharge and increased risk of mortality [117]. It worsens pre-existing dementia and increases the risk for future dementia [118]. Delirium also causes significant psychological distress for patients, families and healthcare providers [119].

Detection rates for mental health conditions among older patients are typically very low. For example, one study found that delirium was missed in up to two-thirds of cases [120]. Even when problems are identified, the treatment provided by clinical staff in acute hospitals is sometimes suboptimal despite availability of effective pharmacological and non-pharmacological treatments [121]. Many of the complications of delirium could be prevented with better risk assessment and early prophylactic treatment according to some studies [122].

Many screening tools have been developed and validated for delirium. One review of 31 studies describing 21 delirium screening tools across a broad range of inpatient settings [123]. However there is a lack of evidence that screening implementation positively influencing patient outcomes. Nevertheless some organizations have recommend screening all patients or screening of specific patients considered at risk for delirium. The British Geriatrics Society guidelines include a recommendation to identify all patients over 65 years with cognitive impairment on admission [124]. Risk factors for delirium include dementia, recent surgery, untreated biochemical change, old age and visual and hearing impairment. Serial assessments are sometimes recommended but are not often conducted in practice. The Australian clinical practice guideline on management of delirium recommends establishment of a structured process for screening and diagnosis of delirium in all healthcare settings [125]. Clinical practice guidelines from the American College of Critical Care Medicine of the Society of Critical Care Medicine recommend routine assessment for the presence of delirium, including ICU patients [126]. The NICE guideline on diagnosis, prevention and management of delirium recommends assessment of risk factors for delirium in all patients when they first present as follows:

> *If indicators of delirium are identified, carry out a clinical assessment based on the Diagnostic and Statistical Manual of Mental Disorders (DSM-IV) criteria or short Confusion Assessment Method (short CAM) to confirm the diagnosis. In critical care or in the recovery room after surgery, CAM-ICU should be used. A healthcare professional who is trained and competent in the diagnosis of delirium should carry out the assessment. If there is difficulty distinguishing between the diagnoses of delirium, dementia or delirium superimposed on dementia, treat for delirium first* [127, 128].

The Confusion Assessment Method is the most commonly employed custom tool to identify delirium [123, 129], but others include Delirium Rating Scale and Memorial Delirium Assessment Scale. However, the MMSE is also very widely used despite numerous limitations [130, 131]. All scales show significant limitations in accuracy and can be challenging to use in patients with very severe symptoms.

4.10 Screening for Alcohol Problems

Alcohol problems are a significant public health problem [132, 133]. Alcohol consumption has been estimated to cause about 4–5% of all deaths and all disability [134]. Alcohol problems include alcohol use disorder (AUD), alcohol dependence and acute intoxication. Alcohol use disorders include a spectrum of excessive drinking often described using the terms alcohol abuse (DSM-IV), hazardous drinking (WHO) or harmful drinking (ICD10). In the general population, hazardous drinking is seen in 30–40% [135] and alcohol dependence in 10% [136]. In primary care and hospital settings, approximately 7–30% have an AUD [137] and approximately 4–10% have alcohol dependence [138]. In spite of these concerns, it seems that only a minority of patients with alcohol problems are detected and treated. Studies conducted in the USA, Australia, the UK and Finland indicate that clinicians frequently do not screen for AUD and fail to address the problem in at least one-third to one-half of cases even when the diagnosis is known. About a third of individuals with alcohol problems are detected by their general practitioner (GP), and screening for alcohol problems is not a routine in primary care [139–141] or in specialist settings. In most cases diagnosis is made by clinical judgement without the use of scales, blood tests or reference to diagnostic criteria [139, 140]. Similarly, only about a third of clinicians use alcohol screening questions and 15% cite use of biochemical markers [142, 143]. Patient surveys suggest that only 30–40% receive any enquiry about their alcohol habits [144–146] and a small percentage of those with alcohol problems report receiving advice to cut-down [147]. Screening followed by brief alcohol intervention results in significant reductions in consumption after discharge from hospital [148].

Many factors have been cited as barriers to appropriate and prompt recognition. These include clinician confidence as to what constitutes alcohol misuse [149], inadequate training [150], contractual incentives [151], lack of time [152], fear of labelling due to the stigma associated with substance abuse [153] and a belief that patients will not honestly disclose their drinking practices [154, 155].

In response to these concerns, the Institute of Medicine, the National Institute on Alcohol Abuse and Alcoholism (NIAAA), the American Medical Association and the American Society of Addiction Medicine have all recommended that clinicians *routinely* ask patients about alcohol use [156–158]. However the Scottish Intercollegiate Guidelines Network advocates clinical assessment with judicious use of questionnaires only where there is suspicion of alcohol problems [159]. The NIAAA and the US Preventive Services Task Force (USPSTF) recommend population screening to identify problem drinking, that is, clinicians should ask all attendees whether they drink and assess the specific quantity, frequency and pattern of consumption, but they do not recommend a specific tool [160]. The NIAAA also recommended targeted screening in that all patients who drink alcohol should be screened with the CAGE questions [161]. To date, variations of the AUDIT (Alcohol Use Disorder Identification Test), CAGE and MAST (Michigan Alcohol Screening Test) have been the most common questionnaires for alcohol problems, but these tools are difficult to use in a primary care practice [141, 157].

4.11 Mixed Psychiatric Multidomain Screening

Screening for several psychiatric disorders at one time is potentially efficient but difficult to achieve in practice. Probably the best method is an algorithm starting with simple broad questions proceeding to more in-depth questions depending on response. A number of multidomain tools have been developed which encompass several biopsychosocial domains. For example, in cancer settings the Edmonton Symptom Assessment System (ESAS) has been extensively used and it includes six physical symptoms (pain, tiredness, nausea, depression, anxiety, drowsiness, appetite, well-being, shortness of breath) and three psychosocial symptoms (well-being, depression, anxiety). The tool has been applied to nearly a million cancer patients in Canadian cancer hospitals [162]. Mitchell and colleagues proposed a multidomain extension to the distress thermometer called the Emotion thermometers (see www.emotion thermometers.com) incorporating distress, depression, anxiety and anger. Preliminary validation in early- and late-stage cancers and also in cardiology and neurology settings suggests the ET improves upon the accuracy of the DT [163]. Other multidomain tools such as the 27-item My Mood Monitor (M-3) have been developed and tested in mental health and primary care settings [164]. Houston et al. (2011) developed a 17-item instrument for differential diagnosis of GAD, MDE, past/present mania and ADHD [165]. The Health of the Nation Outcome Scale (HoNOS) is a 12-item scale and was developed by the Royal College of Psychiatrists' measuring behaviour, impairment, symptoms and social functioning (Wing et al., 1996) [166]. HoNOS has been widely used in the NHS mostly in mental health trusts and fairly extensively field tested [167]. Another commonly used scale is the Clinical Outcomes in Routine Evaluation (CORE) [168] which is a widely used patient self-report measure across service settings particularly those delivering psychological treatments.

4.12 Conclusion: Judging the Effectiveness of Screening for Psychiatric Disorders

Screening is fundamentally designed to improve patient outcomes, but positive benefits are not invariable [169–171]. Large-scale studies comparing care before and after screening (sequential cohort) or in groups randomized to screening are not common. There is much interest in what determines whether screening leads to an effective psychological assessment. Evidence suggests screening can benefit communication and clinician referral patterns, but it has a weaker effect on the ability of clinicians to correctly identify cases. When mandated as clinical routine, screening can be widely disseminated, and therefore acceptability to both clinicians and patients is key. Acceptability can be enhanced by using a brief tool (possibly an algorithm or multidimensional design), with simple scoring, ideally one that generates meaningful results and one that does not duplicate work. Staff who are involved in tool development and dissemination tend to be more invested in the screening programme itself. To be effective screening must be allied with appropriate follow-up and effective treatment. Screening should be used in combination with good quality of care because good-quality screening cannot compensate for poor-quality care in other areas. An alternative to systematic screening is targeted screening of preselected high-risk groups, such as those with troubling physical complication or those people whose family members ask for help.

Following on from screening, a key question is what happens to patients who screen positive and those who screen negative. Generally, an evidence-based management plan is important to ensure that clinicians act systematically on screening results. It also helps ensure that the healthcare system has appropriate resources for handling distress. Thorough clinical assessment and competent management should follow a positive screen [172]. Clinicians should be able to override screening protocols using their expert judgement if needed. Future studies will clarify the optimal methods that bring added value to clinical practice. They will also clarify the best mode of delivery (e.g. computerized, paper, verbal). Future studies should use representative samples, offer staff training and track uptake of subsequent interventions. New trials addressing some of these methodological issues are currently underway. Successful screening tools could be incorporated into screening programmes that also contain elements for measuring unmet needs, desire for help, clinical responses and longitudinal outcomes. Screening which is accurate, acceptable and has proven added value will have more likelihood of being seen as an integral part of essential clinical care.

Disclosures No author disclosures.

References

1. Mitchell AJ, Hardy S, Shiers D. Parity of esteem: addressing the inequalities between mental and physical healthcare. BJPsych Adv. 2017;23(3):196–205. https://doi.org/10.1192/apt.bp.114.014266.
2. Lesperance F, Frasure-Smith N, Talajic M. Major depression before and after myocardial infarction: its nature and consequences. Psychosom Med. 2000;58:99–110.
3. Penninx BW, Beekman AT, Honiq A, et al. Depression and cardiac mortality: results from a community-based longitudinal study. Arch Gen Psychiatry. 2001;58:221–7.
4. De Voogd JN, Wempe JB, Koeter GH, et al. Depressive symptoms as predictors of mortality in patients with COPD. Chest. 2009;135:619–25.
5. House A, Knapp P, Bamford J, et al. Mortality at 12 and 24 months after stroke may be associated with depressive symptoms at 1 month. Stroke. 2001;32:696–701.
6. Kimmel PL, Peterson RA, Weihs KL, et al. Multiple measurements of depression predict mortality in a longitudinal study of chronic hemodialysis outpatients. Kidney Int. 2000;57:2093–8.
7. Roest AM, Martens EJ, Denollet J, de Jonge P. Prognostic association of anxiety post myocardial infarction with mortality and new cardiac events: a meta-analysis. Psychosom Med. 2010;72(6):563–9. https://doi.org/10.1097/PSY.0b013e3181dbff97. Epub 2010 Apr 21.
8. Hayes JF, Miles J, Walters K, King M, Osborn DP. A systematic review and meta-analysis of premature mortality in bipolar affective disorder. Acta Psychiatr Scand. 2015;131(6):417–25. https://doi.org/10.1111/acps.12408. Epub 2015 Mar 3.
9. Kugathasan P, Jensen SE, Laursen TM, Aagaard J, Nielsen RE. Increased mortality following myocardial infarction in patients with schizophrenia: a national population based cohort study. Eur Heart J. 2017;38(Suppl 1):1408. ehx493.P6497.

10. Hjorthøj C, Stürup AE, McGrath JJ, Nordentoft M. Years of potential life lost and life expectancy in schizophrenia: a systematic review and meta-analysis. Lancet Psychiatry. 2017;4(4):295–301. https://doi.org/10.1016/S2215-0366(17)30078-0. Epub 2017 Feb 22.
11. Mujica-Mota RE, Roberts M, Abel G, Elliott M, Lyratzopoulos G, Roland M, Campbell J. Common patterns of morbidity and multi-morbidity and their impact on health-related quality of life: evidence from a national survey. Qual Life Res Int J Qual Life Asp Treat Care Rehabil. 2015;24(4):909–18.
12. Shim EJ, Mehnert A, Koyama A, et al. Health-related quality of life in breast cancer: cross-cultural survey of German, Japanese, and South Korean patients. Breast Cancer Res Treat. 2006;99:341–50.
13. Sareen J, Jacobi F, Cox BJ, Belik SL, Clara I, Stein MB. Disability and poor quality of life associated with comorbid anxiety disorders and physical conditions. Arch Intern Med. 2006;166(19):2109–16.
14. Royal College of Psychiatrists. Whole-person care: from rhetoric to reality achieving parity between mental and physical health. London: RCP; 2013. http://www.rcpsych.ac.uk/pdf/OP88.pdf
15. NHS England. Valuing mental health equally with physical health or "Parity of Esteem". London: NHS England. https://www.england.nhs.uk/mentalhealth/parity/
16. The Parliamentary Office of Science and Technology. Parity of esteem for mental health. London: Houses of Parliament; 2015.
17. Poulsen KM, Pachana NA, McDermott BM. Health professionals' detection of depression and anxiety in their patients with diabetes: the influence of patient, illness and psychological factors. J Health Psychol. 2016;21(8):1566–75. https://doi.org/10.1177/1359105314559618. Epub 2014 Dec 14.
18. Chew-Graham CA, Hogg T. Patients with chronic physical illness and co-existing and co-existing psychological morbidity: GPs' views on their role in detection and management. Prim Care Psychiatry. 2002;8(2):35–9.
19. Kessler D, Lloyd K, Lewis G, Gray DP. Cross sectional study of symptom attribution and recognition of depression and anxiety in primary care. Br Med J. 1999;318(7181):436–9.
20. Jones LE, Doebbeling CC. Suboptimal depression screening following cancer diagnosis. Gen Hosp Psychiatry. 2007;29:547–54.
21. Rodriguez KL, Bayliss N, Alexander SC, et al. How oncologists and their patients with advanced cancer communicate about health-related quality of life. Psychooncology. 2010;19(5):490–9.
22. Taylor S, Harley C, Campbell LJ, Bingham L, Podmore EJ, Newsham AC, Selby PJ, Brown JM, Velikova G. Discussion of emotional and social impact of cancer during outpatient oncology consultations. Psychooncology. 2011;20(3):242–51.
23. Mitchell AJ. Sensitivity × PPV is a recognized test called the clinical utility index (CUI+). Eur J Epidemiol. 2011;26(3):251–2. https://doi.org/10.1007/s10654-011-9561-x. Author reply 252. Epub 2011 Mar 26.
24. Mitchell AJ. How to design and analyse screening studies. In: Holland JC, Breitbart W, Jacobsen P, Lederberg MS, Loscalzo M, editors. Psycho-oncology. Oxford: Oxford University Press; 2010.
25. Bidstrup PE, Johansen C, Mitchell AJ. Screening for cancer-related distress: summary of evidence from tools to programmes. Acta Oncol. 2011;50(2):194–204.
26. Carlson LE, Groff SL, Maciejewski O, Bultz BD. Screening for distress in lung and breast cancer outpatients: a randomized controlled trial. J Clin Oncol. 2010;28(33):4884–91.
27. Mitchell AJ, Vaze A, Rao S. Clinical diagnosis of depression in primary care: a meta-analysis. Lancet. 2009;374(9690):609–19. https://doi.org/10.1016/S0140-6736(09)60879-5. Epub 2009 Jul 27.
28. Cepoiu M, McCusker J, Cole MG, Sewitch M, Belzile E, Ciampi A. Recognition of depression by non-psychiatric physicians—a systematic literature review and meta-analysis. J Gen Int Med. 2008;23:25–36.

29. Diagnostic and statistical manual of mental disorders. 4th ed. Washington, DC: American Psychiatric Publishing; 1994.
30. Read JR, Sharpe L, Modini M, Dear BF. Multimorbidity and depression: a systematic review and meta-analysis. J Affect Disord. 2017;221:36–46. https://doi.org/10.1016/j.jad.2017.06.009. Epub 2017 Jun 14.
31. Krishnan K, Delong M, Kraemer H, Carney R, Spiegel D, Gordon C, et al. Comorbidity of depression with other medical diseases in the elderly. Biol Psychiatry. 2002;52(6):559–88.
32. Mitchell AJ, Chan M, Bhatti H, Halton M, Grassi L, Johansen C, Meader N. Prevalence of depression, anxiety, and adjustment disorder in oncological, haematological, and palliative-care settings: a meta-analysis of 94 interview-based studies. Lancet Oncol. 2011;12(2):160–74. Epub 2011 Jan 19.
33. Knol M, Twisk J, Beekman A, et al. Depression as a risk factor for the onset of type 2 diabetes mellitus. A meta-analysis. Diabetologia. 2006;49:837–45.
34. Pederson JL, Warkentin LM, Majumdar SR, McAlister FA. Depressive symptoms are associated with higher rates of readmission or mortality after medical hospitalization: a systematic review and meta-analysis. J Hosp Med. 2016;11:373–80. https://doi.org/10.1002/jhm.2547.
35. Nicholson A, Kuper H, Hemingway H. Depression as an aetiologic and prognostic factor in coronary heart disease: a meta-analysis of 6362 events among 146 538 participants in 54 observational studies. Eur Heart J. 2006;27(23):2763–74.
36. Satin JR, Wolfgang Linden W, Phillips MJ. Depression as a predictor of disease progression and mortality in cancer patients. A meta-analysis. Cancer. 2009;115(22):5349–61.
37. Bui QUT, Ostir GV, Kuo YF, Freeman J, Goodwin JS. Relationship of depression to patient satisfaction: findings from the barriers to breast cancer study. Breast Cancer Res Treat. 2005;89(1):23–8.
38. Kennard BD, Smith SM, Olvera R, et al. Nonadherence in adolescent oncology patients: preliminary data on psychological risk factors and relationships to outcome. J Clin Psychol Med Settings. 2004;11:30–9.
39. Skarstein J, Aass N, Fossa SD, et al. Anxiety and depression in cancer patients: relation between the Hospital Anxiety and Depression Scale and the European Organization for Research and Treatment of Cancer Core Quality of Life Questionnaire. J Psychosom Res. 2000;49:27–34.
40. https://www.nice.org.uk/guidance/cg90
41. https://www.nice.org.uk/guidance/cg91
42. Siu AL, US Preventive Services Task Force (USPSTF), et al. Screening for depression in adults: US preventive services task force recommendation statement. JAMA. 2016;315(4):380–7. https://doi.org/10.1001/jama.2015.18392.
43. Thombs BD, Ziegelstein RC. Primary care doctors should not screen their patients for depression. Expert Rev Neurother. 2017;17(7):645–7. https://doi.org/10.1080/14737175.2017.1327356. Epub 2017 May 12.
44. https://canadiantaskforce.ca/the-canadian-task-force-on-preventive-health-care-releases-updated-guideline-on-screening-for-depression/
45. Vodermaier A, Linden W, Siu C. Screening for emotional distress in cancer patients: a systematic review of assessment instruments. J Nat Cancer Inst. 2009;101(21):1464–88.
46. Zealley AK, Aitken RCB. Measurement of mood. Proc R Soc Med. 1969;62:993–6.
47. Zigmond AS, Snaith RP. The hospital anxiety and depression scale. Acta Psychiatr Scand. 1983;67:361–70.
48. Luckett T, Butow PN, King MT, Oguchi M, Heading G, Hackl NA, Rankin N, Price MA. A review and recommendations for optimal outcome measures of anxiety, depression and general distress in studies evaluating psychosocial interventions for English-speaking adults with heterogeneous cancer diagnoses. Support Care Cancer. 2010;18(10):1241–62. Epub 2010 Jul 2.
49. Mitchell AJ, Meader N, Symonds P. Diagnostic validity of the hospital anxiety and depression scale (HADS) in cancer and palliative settings: a meta-analysis. J Affect Disord. 2010;126(3):335–48. Epub 2010 Mar 5.

50. Beck AT, Steer RA, Brown GK. Beck depression inventory. Manual. 2nd ed. San Antonio: The Psychological Corporation; 1996.
51. Cox J, Holden J, Sagovsky R. Detection of postnatal depression: development of 10 item Edinburgh postnatal depression scale. Br J Psychiatry. 1987;150:782–6.
52. Radloff LS. The CESD scale: a self report scale for research in the general population. Appl Psychol Measure. 1977;1:385–401.
53. Mitchell AJ, Meader N, Davies E, Clover K, Carter GL, Loscalzo MJ, Linden W, Grassi L, Johansen C, Carlson LE, Zabora J. Meta-analysis of screening and case finding tools for depression in cancer: evidence based recommendations for clinical practice on behalf of the depression in cancer care consensus group. J Affect Disord. 2012;140(2):149–60.
54. Mitchell AJ, Yadegarfar M, Gill J, Stubbs B. Case finding and screening clinical utility of the Patient Health Questionnaire (PHQ-9 and PHQ-2) for depression in primary care: a diagnostic meta-analysis of 40 studies. BJPsych Open. 2016;2(2):127–38.
55. Mitchell AJ, Coyne JC. Do ultra-short screening instruments accurately detect depression in primary care? A pooled analysis and meta-analysis of 22 studies. Br J Gen Pract. 2007;57(535):144–51.
56. Mitchell AJ. Are one or two simple questions sufficient to detect depression in cancer and palliative care? A Bayesian meta-analysis. Br J Cancer. 2008;98(12):1934–43.
57. Kariuki-Nyuthe C, Stein DJ. Anxiety and related disorders and physical illness in: Sartorius N, Holt RIG, Maj M (eds): Comorbidity of mental and physical disorders. Key issues Ment Health. Basel, Karger, 2015, 179, pp 81-87.
58. Whitehead D, Perkins-Porras L, Strike P, Steptoe A. Post-traumatic stress disorder in patients with cardiac disease: predicting vulnerability from emotional responses during admission for acute coronary syndromes. Heart. 2006;92(9):1225–9.
59. Stein MB, Roy-Byrne PP, Craske MG, et al. Quality of and patient satisfaction with primary health care for anxiety disorders. J Clin Psychiatry. 2011;72(7):970–6.
60. Weisberg RB1, Beard C, Moitra E, Dyck I, Keller MB. Adequacy of treatment received by primary care patients with anxiety disorders. Depress Anxiety. 2014;31(5):443–50. https://doi.org/10.1002/da.22209. Epub 2013 Nov 4.
61. Lane D, Carroll D, Ring C, Beevers D, Lip G. The prevalence and persistence of depression and anxiety following myocardial infarction. Br J Health Psychol. 2002;7(1):11–21.
62. Schoepf D, Heun R. Anxiety disorders and physical comorbidity: increased prevalence but reduced relevance of specific risk factors for hospital-based mortality during a 12.5-year observation period in general hospital admissions. Eur Arch Psychiatry Clin Neurosci. 2015;265(5):387–98. https://doi.org/10.1007/s00406-014-0566-9. Epub 2014 Dec 4.
63. El-Gabalawy R. Comorbidity and functional correlates of anxiety and physical conditions in Canadian Veterans. J Mil Vet Fam Health. 1(1). https://doi.org/10.3138/jmvfh.2014-03.
64. Mitchell AJ, Ferguson DW, Gill J, Paul J, Symonds P. Depression and anxiety in long-term cancer survivors compared with spouses and healthy controls: a systematic review and meta-analysis. Lancet Oncol. 2013;14(8):721–32. https://doi.org/10.1016/S1470-2045(13)70244-4. Epub 2013 Jun 5.
65. Brown LF, Kroenke K, Theobald DE, et al. The association of depression and anxiety with health-related quality of life in cancer patients with depression and/orpain. Psychooncology. 2010;19:734–41.
66. Frojd C, Lampic C, Larsson G, et al. Patient attitudes, behaviours, and other factors considered by doctors when estimating cancer patients' anxiety and desire for information. Scand J Caring Sci. 2007;21:523–9.
67. Mitchell AJ. Pooled results from 38 analyses of the accuracy of distress thermometer and other ultrashort methods of detecting cancer-related mood disorders. J Clin Oncol. 2007;25:4670–81.
68. Mitchell AJ, Baker-Glenn EA, Symonds P. Can the distress thermometer be improved by additional mood domains? Part I. Initial validation of the emotion thermometers tool. Psychooncology. 2010;19(2):125–33.
69. Andersen BL, DeRubeis RJ, Berman BS, Gruman J, Champion VL, Massie MJ, Holland JC, Partridge AH, Bak K, Somerfield MR, Rowland JH, American Society of Clinical

Oncology. Screening, assessment, and care of anxiety and depressive symptoms in adults with cancer: an American Society of Clinical Oncology guideline adaptation. J Clin Oncol. 2014;32(15):1605–19. https://doi.org/10.1200/JCO.2013.52.4611. Epub 2014 Apr 14.
70. https://www.nice.org.uk/guidance/cg123/chapter/1-Guidance
71. Slade T, Andrews G. DSM-IV and ICD-10 generalized anxiety disorder: discrepant diagnoses and associated disability. Soc Psychiatry Psychiatr Epidemiol. 2001;36(1):45–51.
72. NICE. Generalised anxiety disorder and panic disorder in adults: management. Clinical Guide [CG113]; 2011.
73. Carlson LE, Clifford SK, Groff SL, Maciejewski O, Bultz B. Screening for depression in cancer care. In: Mitchell AJ, Coyne JC, editors. Screening for depression in clinical practice. New York: Oxford University Press; 2010. p. 265–98.
74. Graves KD, Arnold SM, Love CL, Kirsh KL, Moore PG, Passik SD. Distress screening in a multidisciplinary lung cancer clinic: prevalence and predictors of clinically significant distress. Lung Cancer. 2007;55:215–24.
75. Shim EJ, Mehnert A, Koyama A, Cho SJ, Inui H, Paik NS, et al. Health-related quality of life in breast cancer: a cross-cultural survey of German, Japanese, and South Korean patients. Breast Cancer Res Treat. 2006;99:341–50.
76. von EL, Larsson G, Oberg K, Sjoden PO. 'Satisfaction with care': associations with health-related quality of life and psychosocial function among Swedish patients with endocrine gastrointestinal tumours. Eur J Cancer Care. 2002;11:91–9.
77. Faller H, Bulzebruck H, Drings P, Lang H. Coping, distress, and survival among patients with lung cancer. Arch Gen Psychiatry. 1999;56:756–62.
78. Chow E, Tsao MN, Harth T. Does psychosocial intervention improve survival in cancer? A meta-analysis. Palliat Med. 2004;18(1):25–31.
79. Smedslund G, Ringdal GI. Meta-analysis of the effects of psychosocial interventions on survival time in cancer patients. J Psychosom Res. 2004;57(2):123–31; discussion 133–5.
80. Roth AJ, Kornblith AB, Batel-Copel L, et al. Rapid screening for psychologic distress in men with prostate carcinoma: a pilot study. Cancer. 1998;82:1904–8.
81. NCCN clinical practice guidelines in oncology distress management V.1.2007. http://www.nccn.org/professionals/physician_gls/PDF/distress.pdf
82. Mitchell AJ. Short screening tools for cancer-related distress: a review and diagnostic validity meta-analysis. J Natl Compr Cancer Netw. 2010;8(4):487–94.
83. Morasso G, Costantini M, Baracco G, Borreani C, Capelli M. Assessing psychological distress in cancer patients: validation of a self-administered questionnaire. Oncology. 1996;53(4):295–302.
84. Lees N, Lloyd-Williams M. Assessing depression in palliative care patients using the visual analogue scale: a pilot study. Eur J Cancer Care. 1999;8(4):220–3.
85. Gil F, Grassi L, Travado L, et al. Southern European Psycho-Oncology Study Group. Use of distress and depression thermometers to measure psychosocial morbidity among Southern European cancer patients. Support Care Cancer. 2005;13:600–6.
86. Kupka RW, Altshuler LL, Nolen WA, Suppes T, Luckenbaugh DA, Leverich GS, Frye MA, Keck PE Jr, McElroy SL, Grunze H, Post RM. Three times more days depressed than manic or hypomanic in both bipolar I and bipolar II disorder. Bipolar Disord. 2007;9(5):531–5.
87. Picardi A. Rating scales in bipolar disorder. Curr Opin Psychiatry. 2009;22(1):42–9.
88. Hirschfeld R, Williams J, Spitzer R, Calabrese J, Flynn L, Keck P, et al. Development and validation of screening instrument for bipolar spectrum disorder: the mood disorder questionnaire. Am J Psychiatry. 2000;157:1873–5.
89. Wang HR, Woo YS, Ahn HS, Ahn IM, Kim HJ, Bahk WM. The validity of the mood disorder questionnaire for screening bipolar disorder: a meta-analysis. Depress Anxiety. 2015;32(7):527–38. https://doi.org/10.1002/da.22374. Epub 2015 May 22.
90. Tafalla M, Sanchez-Moreno J, Diez T, Vieta E. Screening for bipolar disorder in a Spanish sample of outpatients with current major depressive episode. J Affect Disord. 2009;114:299–304.
91. https://www.nice.org.uk/guidance/cg185/chapter/1-Recommendations#recognising-and-managing-bipolar-disorder-in-adults-in-primary-care-2

92. http://www.nhs.uk/dementia/Pages/Dementia.aspx
93. http://alzheimers.org.uk/site/scripts/documents.php?categoryID=200316
94. Lang L, Clifford A, Wei L, et al. Prevalence and determinants of undetected dementia in the community: a systematic literature review and a meta-analysis. BMJ Open. 2017;7:e011146. https://doi.org/10.1136/bmjopen-2016-011146.
95. Goldberg SE, Whittamore KH, Harwood RH, Bradshaw LE, Gladman JRF, Jones RG. The prevalence of mental health problems among older adults admitted as an emergency to a general hospital (advance access). Age Ageing. 2011;0:1–7.
96. Reynish EL, Hapca SM, De Souza N, Cvoro V, Donnan PT, Guthrie B. Epidemiology and outcomes of people with dementia, delirium, and unspecified cognitive impairment in the general hospital: prospective cohort study of 10,014 admissions. BMC Med. 2017;15:140.
97. Wilkinson D, Stave C, Keohane D, Vincenzino O. The role of general practitioners in the diagnosis and treatment of Alzheimer's disease: a multinational survey. J Int Med Res. 2004;32(2):149–59.
98. Riedel-Heller SG, Schork A, Matschinger H, Angermeyer MC. The role of referrals in diagnosing dementia at the primary care level. Int Psychogeriatr. 1999;11(3):251–62.
99. Bamford C, Lamont S, Eccles M, et al. Disclosing a diagnosis of dementia: a systematic review. Int J Geriatr Psychiatry. 2004;19(2):151–69.
100. Mitchell AJ. Reluctance to disclose difficult diagnoses: a narrative review comparing communication by psychiatrists and oncologists. J Support Care Cancer. 2007;15(7):819–28.
101. Laurila JV, Pitkala KH, Strandberg TE, Tilvis RS. Detection and documentation of dementia and delirium in acute geriatric wards. Gen Hosp Psychiatry. 2004;26(1):31–5.
102. Facing Dementia. 2004. http://www.alz.co.uk/media/dementiasurvey.html
103. Turner S, Iliffe S, Downs M, Wilcock J, Bryans M, Levin E, Keady J, O'Carroll R. General practitioners' knowledge, confidence and attitudes in the diagnosis and management of dementia. Age Ageing. 2004;33:461–7.
104. Bradford A, Kunik ME, Schulz P, et al. Missed and delayed diagnosis of dementia in primary care prevalence and contributing factors. Alzheimer Dis Assoc Disord. 1999;23(4):306–14.
105. Cordery R, Harvey R, Frost C, et al. National survey to assess current practices in the diagnosis and management of young people with dementia. Int J Geriatr Psychiatry. 2002;17(2):124–7.
106. Iracleous P, Nie JX, Tracy CS, et al. Primary care physicians' attitudes towards cognitive screening: findings from a national postal survey. Int J Geriatr Psychiatry. 2010;25(1):23–9.
107. Brodaty H, Howarth GC, Mant A, Kurrle SE. General practice and dementia. A national survey of Australian GPs. Medn J Aust. 1994;160:10–4.
108. National Audit Office. Improving dementia services in England—an interim report GP survey results. 2010.
109. Erkinjuntti T, Ostbye T, Steenhuis R, Hachinski V. The effect of different diagnostic criteria on the prevalence of dementia. N Engl J Med. 1997;337(23):1667–74.
110. Ngo J, Holroyd-Leduc JM. Systematic review of recent dementia practice guidelines. Age Ageing. 2015;44(1):25–33. https://doi.org/10.1093/ageing/afu143.
111. https://www.nice.org.uk/guidance/cg42/chapter/1-Guidance#risk-factors-prevention-and-early-identification
112. https://www.nice.org.uk/guidance/cg42/chapter/1-guidance
113. Inouye SK, Westendorp RG, Saczynski JS. Delirium in elderly people. Lancet. 2014;383:911–22. https://doi.org/10.1016/S0140-6736(13)60688-1.
114. Collins N, Blanchard MR, Tookman A, et al. Detection of delirium in the acute hospital. Age Ageing. 2010;39:131–5. https://doi.org/10.1093/ageing/afp201.
115. Teodorczuk A, Reynish E, Milisen K. Improving recognition of delirium in clinical practice: a call for action. BMC Geriatr. 2012;12:55. https://doi.org/10.1186/1471-2318-12-55.
116. Leonard M, McInerney S, McFarland J, et al. Comparison of cognitive and neuropsychiatric profiles in hospitalised elderly medical patients with delirium, dementia and comorbid delirium–dementia. BMJ Open. 2016;6:e009212. https://doi.org/10.1136/bmjopen-2015-009212.
117. Pendlebury ST, Lovett NG, Smith SC, et al. Observational, longitudinal study of delirium in consecutive unselected acute medical admissions: age-specific rates and associated

factors, mortality and re- admission. BMJ Open. 2015;5:e007808. https://doi.org/10.1136/bmjopen-2015-007808.
118. Davis DH, Muniz Terrera G, Keage H, et al. Delirium is a strong risk factor for dementia in the oldest-old: a population-based cohort study. Brain. 2012;135(Pt 9):2809–16. https://doi.org/10.1093/brain/aws190.
119. Breitbart W, Gibson C, Tremblay A. The delirium experience: delirium recall and delirium-related distress in hospitalized patients with cancer, their spouses/caregivers, and their nurses. Psychosomatics. 2002;43:183–94. https://doi.org/10.1176/appi.psy.43.3.183.
120. Inouye S. The dilemma of delirium: clinical and research controversies regarding diagnosis and evaluation of delirium in hospitalised medical patients. Am J Med. 1994;97:278–87.
121. Hshieh TT, Yue J, Esther OH, Puelle M, Dowal S, Travison T, Inouye SK. Effectiveness of multi-component non-pharmacologic delirium interventions: a meta-analysis. JAMA Intern Med. 2015;175(4):512–20.
122. Martinez F, Tobar C, Hill N. Preventing delirium: should non-pharmacological, multicomponent interventions be used? A systematic review and meta-analysis of the literature. Age Ageing. 2015;44(2):196–204. https://doi.org/10.1093/ageing/afu173. Epub 2014 Nov 25.
123. De J, Wand APF. Delirium screening: a systematic review of delirium screening tools in hospitalized patients. Gerontologist. 2015;55(6):1079–99. https://doi.org/10.1093/geront/gnv100. Epub 2015 Nov 5.
124. Guidelines for the prevention, diagnosis and management of delirium in older people in hospital. Revision January 2006. http://www.bgs.org.uk/Publications/Clinical%20Guidelines/clinical_1-2_delirium.htm. Accessed 30 Mar 2011.
125. Clinical practice guidelines for the management of delirium in older people. Revision October 2006. www.health.vic.gov.au/acute-agedcare/delirium-cpg.pdf. Accessed 30 Mar 2011.
126. Jacobi J, Fraser GL, Coursin DB, et al. Clinical practice guidelines for the sustained use of sedatives and analgesics in the critically ill adult. Crit Care Med. 2002;30:119–41.
127. https://www.nice.org.uk/guidance/cg103/chapter/1-Guidance
128. Delirium: diagnosis, prevention and management. Revision July 2010. www.nice.org.uk/CG103. Accessed 30 Mar 2011.
129. Wong CL, Holroyd-Leduc J, Simel DL, Straus SE. Does this patient have delirium?: value of bedside instruments. JAMA. 2010;304(7):779–86. https://doi.org/10.1001/jama.2010.1182.
130. Mitchell AJ, Shukla D, Ajumal HA, Stubbs B, Tahir TA. The mini-mental state examination as a diagnostic and screening test for delirium: systematic review and meta-analysis. Gen Hosp Psychiatry. 2014;36(6):627–33.
131. Mitchell AJ. The mini-mental state examination (MMSE): update on its diagnostic accuracy and clinical utility for cognitive disorders. In: Larner A, editor. Cognitive screening instruments. Cham: Springer; 2017. Print ISBN 978-3-319-44774-2.
132. Room R, Babor T, Rehm J. Alcohol and public health. Lancet. 2005;365:519–30.
133. Saitz R. Clinical practice. Unhealthy alcohol use. N Engl J Med. 2005;352:596–607.
134. Rehm J, Mathers C, Popova S, Thavorncharoensap M, Teerawattananon Y, Patra J. Global burden of disease and injury and economic cost attributable to alcohol use and alcohol-use disorders. Lancet. 2009;373:2223–33.
135. Compton WM, Conway KP, Stinson FS, Colliver JD, Grant BF. Prevalence, correlates, and comorbidity of DSM-IV antisocial personality syndromes and alcohol and specific drug use disorders in the United States: results from the national epidemiologic survey on alcohol and related conditions. J Clin Psychiatry. 2005;66:677–85.
136. National Institute on Alcohol Abuse and Alcoholism. Tenth special report to the U.S. Congress on alcohol and health, NIH publication No. 00-3769. Rockville, MD: Department of Health and Human Services; 2000.
137. Roche AM, Freeman T, Skinner N. From data to evidence, to action: findings from a systematic review of hospital screening studies for high risk alcohol consumption. Drug Alcohol Depend. 2006;83(1):1–14.
138. Coder B, Freyer-Adam J, Bischof G. Alcohol problem drinking among general hospital inpatients in northeastern Germany. Gen Hosp Psychiatry. 2008;30:147–54.

139. Berner MM, Zeidler C, Kriston L, et al. Diagnostic and treatment approaches to alcohol-related disorders. Results of a survey in general practices. Fortschritte Der Neurologie Psychiatrie. 2006;74(3):157–64.
140. Aalto M, Seppa K. Use of laboratory markers and the audit questionnaire by primary care physicians to detect alcohol abuse by patients. Alcohol Alcohol. 2005;40(6):520–3.
141. Wenrich MD, Paauw DS, Carline JD, Curtis JR, Ramsey PG. Do primary care physicians screen patients about alcohol intake using the CAGE questions? J Gen Intern Med. 1995;10:631–4.
142. Reid MC, Tinetti ME, Brown CJ, et al. Physician awareness of alcohol use disorders among older patients. J Gen Intern Med. 1998;13:729–34.
143. Spandorfer JM, Israel Y, Turner BJ. Primary care physicians' views on screening and management of alcohol abuse: inconsistencies with national guidelines. J Fam Pract. 1999;48(11):899–902.
144. Deitz D, Rohde F, Bertolucci D, Dufour M. Prevalence of screening for alcohol use by physicians during routine physical examinations. Alcohol Health Res World. 1994;18:162–8.
145. Taira DA, Safran DG, Seto TB, Rogers WH, Tarlov AR. The relationship between patient income and physician discussion of health risk behaviors. JAMA. 1997;278(17):1412–7.
146. Edlund MJ, Jürgen U, Wells KB. Clinician screening and treatment of alcohol, drug, and mental problems in primary care: results from healthcare for communities. Med Care. 2004;42(12):1158–66.
147. Hasin DS, Grant BF, Dufour MG, Endicott J. Alcohol problems increase while physician attention declines 1967 to 1984. Arch Intern Med. 1990;150(2):397–400.
148. McManus S, Hipkins J, Haddad P. Implementing an effective intervention for problem drinkers on medical wards. Gen Hosp Psychiatry. 2003;25(5):332–7.
149. Rush B, Ellis K, Crowe T, Powell L. How general practitioners view alcohol use: clearing up the confusion. Can Fam Physician. 1994;40:1570–8.
150. Cornuz J, Ghali WA, Di Carlantonio D, Pecoud A, Paccaud F. Physicians' attitudes towards prevention: importance of intervention-specific barriers and physicians' health habits. Fam Pract. 2000;17:535–40.
151. Wilson Graeme B, Lock Catherine A, Nick H, et al. Intervention against excessive alcohol consumption in primary health care: a survey of GPs' attitudes and practices in England 10 years on. Alcohol Alcohol. 2011;46(5):570–7.
152. Aira M, Kauhanen J, Laricaara P, Rautio P. Factors influencing inquiry about patients' alcohol consumption by primary health care physicians: qualitative semi-structured interview study. Fam Pract. 2003;20:270–5.
153. Bander KW, Goldman DS, Schwartz MA, Rabinowitz E, English JT. Survey of attitudes among three specialties in a teaching hospital toward alcoholics. J Med Educ. 1987;62: 17–24.
154. Ferguson L, Ries R, Russo J. Barriers to identification and treatment of hazardous drinkers as assessed by urban/rural primary care doctors. J Addict Dis. 2003;22:79–90.
155. Vinson DC, et al. Comfortably engaging: which approach to alcohol screening should we use? Ann Fam Med. 2004;2:398–404.
156. Institute of Medicine. Broadening the base of treatment for alcohol problems: report of a study by a committee of the institute of medicine, division of mental health and behavioral medicine. Washington, DC: National Academy Press; 1990.
157. National Institute on Alcohol Abuse and Alcoholism. The physician's guide to helping patients with alcohol problems. Washington, DC: National Institutes of Health; 1995. NIH publication 95-3769.
158. American Society of Addiction Medicine. Public policy statement on screening for addiction in primary care settings. ASAM News. 1997;17:17–8.
159. Scottish Intercollegiate Guidelines Network (SIGN). The management of harmful drinking and alcohol dependence in primary care. National clinical guidelines; 2003.
160. US Preventive Services Task Force. Guide to clinical preventive services. 2nd ed. Alexandria, VA: International Medical Publishing; 1998.

161. The physicians' guide to helping patients with alcohol problems. Washington, DC: US Dept of Health and Human Services, Public Health Service, National Institutes of Health, National Institute on Alcohol Abuse and Alcoholism; 1995.
162. Hui D, Bruera E. The Edmonton symptom assessment system 25 years later: past, present, and future developments. J Pain Symptom Manag. 2017;53(3):630–43. https://doi.org/10.1016/j.jpainsymman.2016.10.370. Epub 2016 Dec 29.
163. Beck KR, Tan SM, Lum SS, Lim LE, Krishna LK. Validation of the emotion thermometers and hospital anxiety and depression scales in Singapore: screening cancer patients for distress, anxiety and depression. Asia Pac J Clin Oncol. 2016;12(2):e241–9. https://doi.org/10.1111/ajco.12180.
164. Gaynes BN, DeVeaugh-Geiss J, Weir S, Gu H, MacPherson C, Schulberg HC, Culpepper L, Rubinow DR. Feasibility and diagnostic validity of the M-3 checklist: a brief, self-rated screen for depressive, bipolar, anxiety, and post-traumatic stress disorders in primary care. Ann Fam Med. 2010;8(2):160–9. https://doi.org/10.1370/afm.1092.
165. Houston JP, Kroenke K, Davidson JR, Adler LA, Faries DE, Ahl J, Swindle R, Trzepacz PT. PDI-4A: an augmented provisional screening instrument assessing 5 additional common anxiety-related diagnoses in adult primary care patients. Postgrad Med. 2011;123(5):89–95. https://doi.org/10.3810/pgm.2011.09.2463.
166. Wing JK, Curtis RH, Beevor AS. HoNOS: health of the nation outcome scales: report on research and development July 1993-December 1995. London: Royal College of Psychiatrists; 1996.
167. Pirkis JE, Burgess PM, Kirk PK, Dodson S, Coombs TJ, Williamson MK. A review of the psychometric properties of the health of the nation outcome scales (HoNOS) family of measures. Health Qual Life Outcomes. 2005;3:76.
168. Barkham M, Margison F, Leach C, Lucock M, Mellor-Clark J, Evans C, Benson L, Connell J, Audin K, McGrath G. Service profiling and outcomes benchmarking using the CORE-OM: toward practice-based evidence in the psychological therapies. J Consult Clin Psychol. 2001;69:184–96.
169. Thombs BD, Coyne JC, Cuijpers P, et al. Rethinking recommendations for screening for depression in primary care. Can Med Assoc J. 2011;184(4):413–8.
170. Valderas JM1, Kotzeva A, Espallargues M, Guyatt G, Ferrans CE, Halyard MY, Revicki DA, Symonds T, Parada A, Alonso J. The impact of measuring patient-reported outcomes in clinical practice: a systematic review of the literature. Qual Life Res. 2008;17(2):179–93. https://doi.org/10.1007/s11136-007-9295-0. Epub 2008 Jan 4.
171. Boyce MB1, Browne JP. Does providing feedback on patient-reported outcomes to healthcare professionals result in better outcomes for patients? A systematic review. Qual Life Res. 2013;22(9):2265–78. https://doi.org/10.1007/s11136-013-0390-0. Epub 2013 Mar 17.
172. Williams S, Dale J. The effectiveness of treatment for depression/depressive symptoms in adults with cancer: a systematic review. Br J Cancer. 2006;94:372–90.

Clinimetric Assessment in Psychosomatic Medicine

5

Fiammetta Cosci and Giovanni A. Fava

Abstract

"Clinimetrics" is the term introduced by Alvan R. Feinstein in the early 1980s to indicate a domain concerned with indexes, rating scales, and other expressions that are used to describe or measure symptoms, physical signs, and other clinical phenomena. Macroanalysis is a helpful clinimetric tool to identify the relationships between biological and psychosocial variables and the individual targets for medical intervention. The present chapter illustrates how clinimetrics may help expanding the narrow range of information that is currently used in psychosomatic medicine. It will focus on the clinimetric approach, on the limitations of the current traditional nosography (i.e., the DSM-5), and on the assessment of psychosocial syndromes via the Diagnostic Criteria for Psychosomatic Research (DCPR)—revised. They have been recently presented in an updated version based on insights derived from studies carried out so far and encompass allostatic overload, type A behavior, alexithymia, the spectrum of maladaptive illness behavior, demoralization, irritable mood, and somatic symptoms secondary to a psychiatric disorder. Clinimetrics represents a perspective of psychosomatic medicine providing an intellectual home for clinical judgment, whose implementation is likely to improve outcomes both in clinical research and practice.

F. Cosci
Department of Health Sciences, University of Florence, Florence, Italy

G. A. Fava (✉)
Department of Psychology, University of Bologna, Bologna, Italy

Department of Psychiatry, State University of New York at Buffalo, Buffalo, NY, USA
e-mail: giovanniandrea.fava@unibo.it

L. Grassi et al. (eds.), *Person Centered Approach to Recovery in Medicine*,
Integrating Psychiatry and Primary Care, https://doi.org/10.1007/978-3-319-74736-1_5

5.1 The Clinimetric Approach

In 1967, Alvan Feinstein dedicated a monograph to an analysis of clinical reasoning that underlies medical evaluations, such as the appraisal of symptoms, signs, and the timing of individual manifestations [1]. In 1982, he introduced the term "clinimetrics" to indicate a domain concerned with the measurement of clinical issues that do not find room in customary clinical taxonomy. Such issues include type, severity, and sequence of symptoms, rate of illness progression (i.e., staging), severity of comorbidity, problems of functional capacity, reasons for medical decisions (e.g., treatment choices), and many other aspects of daily life, such as well-being and distress [2]. Feinstein, in his book on clinimetrics [2], quotes Molière's bourgeois gentleman who was astonished to discover that he spoke in prose as an example of clinicians who may discover that they constantly communicate with clinimetric indices.

When Feinstein introduced the concept of comorbidity, he referred to any "additional co-existing ailment" separated from the primary disease, even in the case this secondary phenomenon does not qualify as a disease per se [3]. Indeed, in clinical medicine, the many methods that are available for measuring comorbidity are not limited to disease entities [4], and, as Cloninger remarked [5], mental disorders can be characterized as manifestations of complex adaptive systems that are multidimensional in their description, multifactorial in their origins, and involve nonlinear interactions in their development.

A new method, which follows the clinimetric principles, has been developed for organizing psychosocial data as variables in clinical reasoning. Emmelkamp et al. [6] introduced the concept of macroanalysis (i.e., a relationship between co-occurring syndromes and problems is established on the basis of where treatment should commence in the first place), and Fava and Sonino [7] applied macroanalysis to assess the relationship between medical and psychological variables.

Macroanalysis starts from the assumption that in most cases there are functional relationships with different more or less clearly defined problem areas [8] and that the targets of treatment may vary during the course of disturbances [7]. The hierarchical organization that is chosen may depend on a variety of contingent factors (e.g., urgency, availability of treatment) that include also the patient's preferences and priorities. Indeed, macroanalysis is not only a tool for the therapist but can be used to inform the patient about the relationship between different problem areas and motivate the patient to change [6]. Macroanalysis also requires reference to the staging method, whereby a disorder is characterized according to seriousness, extension, and longitudinal development [9]. Macroanalysis should be supplemented by microanalysis, a detailed analysis of specific symptoms (e.g., onset and course of the complaints, circumstances that worsen symptoms, and consequences) [6].

Feinstein [10] remarks that, when making a diagnosis, thoughtful clinicians seldom leap from a clinical manifestation to a diagnostic endpoint. The clinical reasoning goes through a series of "transfer stations," where potential connections between presenting symptoms and pathophysiological process are drawn. These stations are a pause for verification or change to another direction. Macroanalysis may allow to

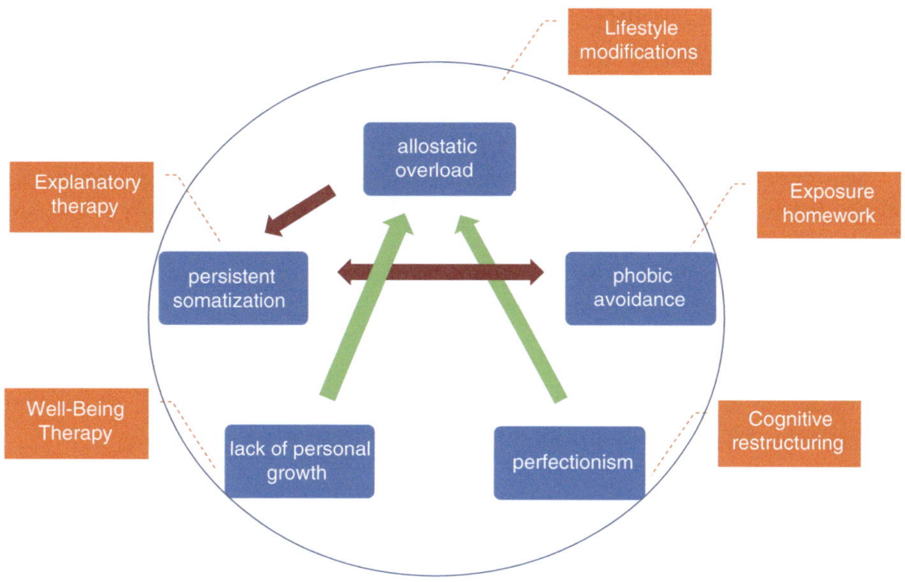

Fig. 5.1 Assessment by macroanalysis (blue boxes and arrows in the blues circle) and related therapeutic approaches (orange boxes)

identify modifiable factors and their interactions. The case which is illustrated in Box 5.1 and Fig. 5.1 exemplifies the use of macroanalysis in the setting of a functional bowel disorder. Symptoms of autonomic arousal are secondary to low sensation threshold and high suggestionability, thus indicating a syndrome of persistent somatization [11]. This category identifies patients in whom psychophysiological symptoms tend to cluster [11], as is frequently the case in patients with irritable bowel syndrome. As illustrated in Box 5.1 and in Fig. 5.1, the clinical psychologist approached the psychological problems according to a sequential approach [12], starting from lifestyle modification, proceeding to explanatory therapy and exposure, proposing cognitive restructuring, and well-being therapy [13]. The treatment team was multidisciplinary and involved the collaboration of a primary care physician who referred the patient to a psychiatrist, a gastroenterologist, and a clinical psychologist.

The issue is to take full advantage of clinimetric tools within the clinical process. It is not that certain disorders lack an organic explanation; it is that our assessment is inadequate in most clinical encounters, and this particularly strikes when information is not collected. In fields such as neurology and geriatrics, the main challenge is to classify disability rather than disease. Accordingly, clinimetric instruments have been developed for measuring pain, muscle functioning, gait and balance, dyskinesia, and delirium. On the contrary, psychiatric assessment [14] is focused on categorical diagnoses (DSM) [15] and does not take into account clinimetric concepts such as well-being and euthymia [16] or measure of resilience such as coping strategies [13, 17]. As Feinstein remarks, "even when the morphologic evidence shows the actual lesion that produces the symptoms of a functional disorder, a mere citation of the lesion does not explain the functional process by which the symptom is produced (...). Thus, the clinician may make an accurate diagnosis of gallstones, but if the diagnosed gallstones do not account for the abdominal pain, a cholecystectomy will not solve the patient's problem" [10; p. 270].

The emerging needs for a more complete and satisfactory assessment underscore the importance of patient-reported outcome scales [18, 19], such as the Psychosocial Index [20] or the Family Assessment Device [21]. In clinical medicine, there is the tendency to rely exclusively on "hard data," preferably expressed in the dimensional numbers of laboratory measurements, excluding "soft information" such as impairment, distress, and well-being [2]. This soft information, however, may now be reliably assessed by clinimetric methods. The new era of individualized patient care will require new ways of thinking; new types of data to describe clinical, social, and behavioral features of individuals; and new methods of analysis [22].

5.2 Traditional Nosography

Somatic symptoms disorder and other disorders with prominent somatic symptoms constitute the most specific classification of DSM-5 in the medically ill [15]. This category includes the diagnoses of somatic symptom disorder, illness anxiety disorder, conversion disorder, psychological factors affecting other medical conditions, factitious disorder, other specified somatic symptom and related disorder, and unspecified somatic symptom and related disorder [15]. According to the DSM-5, these disorders share as common feature the prominence of somatic symptoms associated with significant distress and impairment. However, DSM provides a very partial assessment of these disorders.

The main diagnosis, somatic symptom disorder, requires one or more distressing somatic symptoms (criterion A) and excessive thoughts, feelings, and behaviors related to these symptoms or associated health concerns (criterion B). It is assumed (criterion A) that these patients bear excessive health concerns about such symptoms. The DSM-5 justified this choice with the need to de-emphasize the role of medically unexplained symptoms. Criterion B was also justified by the need of including positive psychological features which are a requisite for diagnosing a mental disorder. However, psychological symptoms related to medically unexplained symptoms do not necessarily involve excessive anxiety and thoughts about the seriousness of symptoms. The persistence of distressing somatic symptoms may induce demoralization and irritability rather than anxiety about the meaning of the symptoms. In addition, the evaluation of the disproportion of thoughts on the seriousness of symptoms, as well as of time and energy spent for them (criterion B), entails a wide variability in the clinician's judgment [23].

The diagnosis of illness anxiety disorder is concerned with the preoccupation with having or acquiring a serious illness. It is characterized by absence or low intensity of somatic symptoms and health-seeking or avoidant behavior that is judged to be maladaptive [15]. The definition does not include hypervigilance to bodily symptoms but mentions that "the individual is easily alarmed about personal health status." Thus, no insight specifiers have been introduced [24]. A potential problem is the lack of clarity inherent in the overlapping criteria of somatic symptom disorder and illness anxiety disorder. A broader problem is that illness anxiety disorder does not depend on the presence of somatic symptoms and clearly shares clinical characteristics with disorders in other groupings [24]. In addition, according to F diagnostic criterion, illness-related preoccupation is not better explained by another mental disorder. A potential problem, in this case, is related to the differential diagnosis. Avoidance and repetitive safety-seeking behaviors are, for instance, common in patients with obsessive-compulsive disorder [25] and body dysmorphic disorder [26]. Similarly, the most common prodromal symptoms of panic are illness phobia, health anxiety, or fear of disease [9]. Thus, the application of criterion F might reduce significantly the possibility to formulate this diagnosis and might let clinician forget that illness anxiety is a dimensional rather than a categorical construct.

In conversion disorder, the essential feature is neurological symptoms that are incompatible with neurological pathophysiology [15]. The DSM-IV criterion B concerning the presence of psychological factors preceding the initiation or the exacerbation of symptoms was removed in DSM-5. This choice seems to be inconsistent with the proposal to de-emphasize the role of medically unexplained symptoms and to include positive psychological features in the diagnoses. According to the suggested criteria, each patient with medically unexplained symptoms or deficits of voluntary motor or sensory function may satisfy the diagnosis of conversion disorder. However, about 30% of outpatients who attend neurological facilities have symptoms not explained by medical findings [27]. In addition, the proposed diagnosis of conversion disorder might depend on the accuracy of the medical examinations.

The essential feature of psychological factors affecting other medical conditions is the presence of clinically significant psychological or behavioral factors that adversely affect a medical condition by increasing the risk for suffering, death, or disability [15]. These factors are poorly specified and add little to the diagnostic process.

The diagnosis of factitious disorder embodies persistent problems related to illness perception and identity [15]. Other specified somatic symptom and related disorders and unspecified somatic symptom and related disorder include conditions for which some, but not all, of the criteria for somatic symptom disorder or illness anxiety disorder are met [15].

The DSM-5 removed the diagnosis of hypochondriasis. The majority of patients with DSM-IV hypochondriasis would be subsumed under the rubric of somatic symptom disorder and the remaining part under the diagnosis of illness anxiety disorder [15]. Those with somatic symptom disorder are characterized by the presence of distressing somatic symptoms, while in patients with illness anxiety disorder, somatic symptoms are absent or, if present, are mild. The presence of somatic symptoms is the differential feature between the two diagnoses. Thus, the distinctive features of hypochondriasis, which include preoccupation, anxiety, bodily hypervigilance, and avoidance behaviors, were lost [23]. In addition, both in somatic symptom disorder and illness anxiety disorder, disease conviction is virtually neglected, and the diagnostic criteria are more representative of health anxiety than disease phobia.

In addition, there are two major ambiguities that may result in misleading clinical indications. One is concerned with the use of the term "somatic symptom." Even though the DSM-5 attempts to avoid the centrality of medically unexplained symptoms that occurred in the DSM-IV and acknowledges the potential occurrence of these clinical phenomena in established medical disorders, its use of the term "somatic symptoms" reflects an ill-defined concept of somatization, as the tendency to experience and communicate psychological distress in the form of physical symptoms and to seek medical help for them [28]. Anything that could not be explained by organic factors, with special reference to laboratory investigations, is thus likely to fall within the domains of somatization. For instance, conversion disorder is also named functional neurological symptom disorder; its B diagnostic criterion states "clinical findings provide evidence of incompatibility between the symptom and recognized neurological or medical conditions" [15], and its C criterion states "the symptom or deficit is not better explained by another medical or mental disorder" [15]. Thus, the DSM-5 maintains the misleading organic/functional dichotomy which is based on the assumption that if organic factors cannot be identified, there should be psychiatric reasons which may be able to fully explain the somatic symptomatology. In addition, it neglects that the presence of a non-functional medical disorder does not exclude, but indeed increases, the likelihood of psychological distress and abnormal illness behavior [29]. This old logic that, if it is not organic, it should be psychiatric is reinforced by the fact that these diagnostic categories are defined as psychiatric and exclusion criteria for other psychiatric disorders are endorsed. George Engel [30] was very critical on the disease concept of functional medical disorder or medically unexplained symptoms. For instance, he regarded the view that irritable bowel syndrome is caused by psychological influences as an oversimplification [30]. It clashes with the nature of psychosomatic medicine itself which is a comprehensive, interdisciplinary framework for the assessment of psychosocial factors affecting individual vulnerability, course, and outcome of any type of disease, the holistic consideration of patient care in clinical practice, and the specialist interventions to integrate psychological therapies in the prevention, treatment, and rehabilitation of medical disease [11].

A second major source of confusion in the DSM-5 classification system is given by the fact that it makes reference to abnormal illness behavior in all diagnostic rubrics, but it never provides a conceptual definition for it. Pilowsky [31] characterized abnormal illness behavior as the persistence of a maladaptive mode of experiencing, perceiving, evaluating, and responding to one's own health status, despite the fact that a doctor has provided a lucid and accurate appraisal of the situation and management to be followed (if any), with opportunity for discussion, negotiation, and clarification, based on adequate assessment of all relevant biological, psychological, social, and cultural factors. Its formulation takes into account the role of the patient-doctor interaction in determining illness behavior. We recently proposed a conceptualization of illness behavior as a unifying viewpoint of psychosomatic medicine [32]. The simple fact that, in the presence of certain physical symptoms, some persons immediately seek medical help while others wait a long time before consulting a physician determines the likelihood of early recognition of a life-threatening disease and its prompt treatment and prognosis [33]. In addition, once the symptoms of a medical disease are experienced by a person, or she has been told by a doctor that he/she is ill even if symptoms are absent, this disease-related information gives rise to psychological responses which are likely to influence the course, therapeutic response, and outcome of a given illness episode. Illness behavior is one of the factors that demarcate major prognostic and therapeutic differences among patients who otherwise seem to be deceptively similar since they share the same diagnosis [33]. Thus, illness behavior is a core characterization in psychosomatic medicine and provides an explanatory model for clinical phenomena that do not find room in customary taxonomy [32].

The clinical inadequacy of DSM-5 is not limited to somatic symptom and related disorders; critiques have been raised also for anxiety and depressive disorders chapters. The main limitation is that DSM-5 maintains the categorical diagnoses, since, ultimately, the diagnosis is largely dependent on a "yes" or "no" decision. Thus, comorbidity is still common, and there is some question as to whether comorbid conditions such as depression and anxiety are distinct or different expressions of some shared underlying dysfunction [34]. Second, although clinicians had used the "not otherwise specified" disorders 30–50% of the time, the category "unspecified disorder" was maintained indicating that a sizable proportion of phenomena will still have a varied presentation that existing categories do not capture [35]. This is problematic because "unspecified" is not informative in terms of describing the condition or making decisions about treatments, even in case of use of specifiers. Finally, a categorical system assumes that each disorder is homogenous and that disorder occurs at the particular cut point. There is no recognition of prodromes, of residual symptoms, and of different stages of the same illness [9]. This view is at odds with clinimetrics as well as with a bulk of the literature showing that symptoms vary considerably in terms of severity and accompanying features. In this vein, categorical assignment loses potentially useful clinical information about the condition and about what treatment strategies might be indicated. There has been considerable debate on various diagnostic aspects of mood and anxiety disorders [36–41].

5.3 Assessment of Psychosocial Syndromes

Current emphasis in psychiatry is still about assessment of symptoms resulting in syndromes identified by diagnostic criteria (DSM). However, growing awareness has shown that also symptoms which do not reach the threshold of a psychiatric disorder may affect quality of life and entail pathophysiological and therapeutic implications. This awareness led to the development of the Diagnostic Criteria for Psychosomatic Research (DCPR) [42] together with a specific diagnostic interview [43]. The DCPR have helped to translate psychosocial variables that derived from

Table 5.1 Diagnostic Criteria for Psychosomatic Research revised version (DCPR-R) [11]

Allostatic overload	Stress
Type A behavior	Personality
Alexithymia	
Hypochondriasis	Illness behavior
Disease phobia	
Thanatophobia	
Health anxiety	
Persistent somatization	
Conversion symptoms	
Anniversary reaction	
Illness denial	
Demoralization	Psychological
Irritable mood	
Secondary somatic symptoms	

psychosomatic research into operational tools. They were introduced in 1995 and tested in various clinical settings in different countries [42–49]. Their value in the psychosomatic assessment, regardless of "organic" or "functional" nature of the illness, has been largely documented [43, 50]. The DCPR have been recently revised [11] based on insights derived from their use in two decades and different settings [43, 50]. The DCPR-revised (DCPR-R) syndromes will be here briefly described in relation to the clinical domains they pertain to (Table 5.1).

5.3.1 Stress

The role of life change and stress has evolved from a simplistic linear model to a more complex multivariant conception embodied in the "allostatic" construct [51, 52], allostasis being the ability of the organism to achieve stability through change. *DCPR-R allostatic overload* refers to the wear and tear that results from either too much stress or from insufficient coping, such as not turning off the stress response when it is no longer needed. Biological parameters of allostatic load have been linked to cognitive and physical functioning and mortality [53]; and the human reward system has been conceptualized as the main antagonist of the stress system, thus allowing to understand health and stress-related disease from a wellness perspective [19]. Frequently post-stress symptoms occur during leisure periods such as weekends and vacation [54].

5.3.2 Personality

DCPR-R type A behavior is derived from the "specific emotional complex" observed in patients with heart conditions in the late 1950s [55] and has been recognized in 36.1% of subjects at risk of coronary heart disease and in 10.8% of patients with non-cardiac diseases [56]. *DCPR-R alexithymia* appears to be linked to increased risk and worsened outcome of medical conditions such as cardiovascular diseases, gastrointestinal disorders, cancer, and altered immune response to stress [57, 58].

5.3.3 Illness Behavior

DCPR-R include the DSM diagnosis of *hypochondriasis*, which was omitted in the DSM-5 classification [15], and its prevalent variant, *disease phobia*. Disease phobia and *thanatophobia* may be components of a hypochondriacal syndrome, yet they may also occur independently. Disease phobia differs from hypochondriasis for three characteristics: (a) fears concern a specific disease and are unlikely to be shifted to another disease or organ system [32], (b) fears tend to manifest themselves in attacks rather than in constant worries as in hypochondriasis [59], and (c) disease phobia often results in the avoidance of internal and external illness-related stimuli, while hypochondriasis usually involves reassurance-seeking or checking behaviors [60]. *Health anxiety* is characterized by worries and attitudes concerning illness and pain that are less specific than in hypochondriasis and disease phobia and respond to medical reassurance. Both the DSM somatization disorder and undifferentiated somatoform disorder are replaced by the DCPR-R *persistent somatization*, conceptualized as a clustering of somatic symptoms involving different organ systems [61]. *DCPR-R conversion symptoms* may be redefined according to Engel's stringent criteria [62], involving features such as ambivalence, histrionic personality, and precipitation of symptoms by psychological stress of which the patient is unaware. In a sample of 1498 patients from various medical settings [63], DCPR conversion symptoms were found in 4.5% of subjects. In the same study [63], *anniversary reaction*, which is a special form of somatization or conversion specifically linked to an anniversary, had a prevalence of 3.6%. DCPR-R *illness denial* corresponds to the persistent denial of having a medical disorder and needing treatment which frequently occurs in the medical setting [64].

5.3.4 Psychological

The original DCPR definition of demoralization integrated Frank's demoralization syndrome [65] and Schmale and Engel's giving up-given up complex [66]. Demoralization and major depression can be differentiated on clinical grounds; they may occur together or independently; and major depression does not necessarily involve demoralization [67]. The revised DCPR criteria for *demoralization* include two different expressions: helplessness (i.e., the individual maintains the capacity to react but lacks adequate support) and hopelessness (i.e., the individual feels he/she alone is responsible for the situation, and there is nothing he/she or anyone else can do to overcome the problem) [68]. Hopelessness/giving-up would be more likely linked to depressive illness and may provide a severity connotation to the diagnosis of major depressive disorder.

The DCPR-R *irritable mood* refers to the concept of irritability which may be part of psychiatric syndromes; it is always unpleasant for the individual, and its overt manifestation lacks a cathartic effect [69]. Several studies found a significant impact of irritable mood on the course of medical disorders as well as on the adoption of unhealthy lifestyles [70, 71].

Psychiatric illness appears to be strongly associated with physical diseases: mental disorders increase the risk for communicable and noncommunicable diseases, many health conditions increase the risk for mental disturbances, and comorbidity complicates recognition and treatment of medical disorders [72]. The potential relationship between medical disorders and psychiatric symptoms ranges from a purely coincidental occurrence to a direct causal role of organic factors. The latter may be subsumed under the rubric of symptomatic affective disorder whose key feature is the resolution of psychiatric disturbances upon specific treatment of the organic condition [73]. The relationship between depression and medical illness [74–76] as well as between anxiety disorders and medical illness has been found to entail important clinical implications [77, 78]. The revised DCPR diagnosis of *secondary somatic symptoms* acknowledges their hierarchical relationship to psychiatric disorders, particularly mood and anxiety disturbances. With the DCPR-R syndrome of somatic symptoms secondary to a psychiatric disorder, the physician formulates the hypothesis that the bulk of somatic symptomatology may remit upon remission of the psychiatric disorder [78].

The advantage of this classification is that it departs from the organic/functional dichotomy and from the misleading and dangerous assumption that if organic factors cannot be identified, there should be psychiatric reasons which may be able to fully explain the somatic symptomatology. In 2004, Tinetti and Fried [79] suggested that time has come to abandon disease as the primary focus of medical care. When disease became the focus of medicine in the past two centuries, the average life expectation was 47 years, and most clinical encounters were for acute illness. Today the life expectancy in Western countries is much higher, and most of clinical activities are concentrated on chronic disease or non-disease-specific complains. Disease-specific guidelines provide very limited indicators for patients with multiple conditions [80]. Tinetti and Fried [79] suggested that the goal of treatment should be the attainment of individual goals and the identification and treatment of all modifiable biological and non-biological factors, according to Engel's biopsychosocial model [81].

5.4 Clinical Implications

A satisfactory psychosomatic assessment may entail several implications for management of medical disorders:

(a) *Presence of psychological disturbances* (e.g., demoralization, irritable mood) or *abnormal illness behavior* (from hypochondriasis to illness denial passing through cyberchondria [82]) which interferes with treatment or leads to frequent health-care utilization.
(b) *Subtyping according to psychological variables* since psychological variables such as depressed mood in the medically ill are associated with a worse prognosis and deserve specific consideration [83].
(c) *Impaired quality of life and functioning* not entirely justified by the medical condition. An increasing body of evidence links the progression of severe medical disorders to specific lifestyle behaviors [e.g., 84]. The benefits of modifying lifestyle have been particularly demonstrated in coronary heart disease [85] and

type 2 diabetes [86]. A basic psychosomatic assumption is the consideration of patients as partners in managing disease. The partnership paradigm includes collaborative care (i.e., a patient-physician relationship in which physicians and patients make health decisions together) and self-management (i.e., a plan that provides patients with problem-solving skills to enhance their self-efficacy).

(d) *Treatment of psychiatric comorbidity*. Psychiatric disorders, and particularly major depression, are frequently unrecognized and untreated in medical settings, with widespread harmful consequences for the individual and the society. Treatment of psychiatric comorbidity such as depression, with either pharmacological or psychotherapeutic interventions, may improve symptoms, health-related functioning, and the patient's quality of life, even though an effect on medical outcome has not been demonstrated [11].

(e) *Psychosocial interventions*. The use of psychotherapeutic strategies (i.e., cognitive-behavioral therapy, stress management procedures, brief dynamic therapy) in controlled investigations has yielded a substantial improvement in a number of medical disorders [87, 88]. Examples are interventions that increase social support, improve mood and enhance health-related behavior in patients with cancer [89], foster self-control and self-management in chronic pain [90] and asthma [91], and improve emotional disclosure [92].

(f) *Treatment of abnormal illness behavior*. For many years abnormal illness behavior has been viewed mainly as an expression of personality predisposition and considered to be refractory to treatment by psychotherapeutic methods. There is now evidence to challenge such pessimistic stance. For instance, several controlled studies indicated that hypochondriasis is a treatable condition by the use of cognitive strategies [93].

Conclusions

The need to include consideration of functioning in daily life, productivity, performance of social roles, intellectual capacity, emotional stability, and well-being has emerged as a crucial part of clinical investigation and patient care. Feinstein urged clinicians to develop a "basic science" of their own "to study clinical phenomena directly, to specify the importance of different types of clinical data, to improve the scientific quality of the data, to identify (or create) appropriate systems of taxonomy for classifying the information, and to develop intellectual models and pragmatic methods that would articulate the clinical process, recapitulate it, and use the results for quantified analyses" [94; p.800]. Yet, such "basic" scientific challenges have been generally overlooked in the past decades, where emphasis has been placed on models derived from basic sciences [2].

Psychosocial aspects have become particularly important in chronic diseases, where cure cannot take place and also extend over family caregivers of chronically ill patients and health providers. Both in primary care and specialty fields, the traditional morphologic constraints (e.g., cardiology, gastroenterology) appear to be more and more inadequate in dealing with symptoms and problems that cut across organ system subdivisions. These inadequacies appear to be particularly pronounced in the large proportion of patients who lack an organic explanation for their disturbances [95]. Patients have become increasingly aware of these issues.

The commercial success of books on complementary and mind-body medicine exemplifies the receptivity of the general public to messages of well-being pursuit by alternative medical practices. Psychosomatic interventions may respond to these emerging needs within the established medical system and may play an important role in supporting the healing process. Further, there is increasing need of expanding the concept of recovery merely based on laboratory and/or imaging parameters to consideration of the level of functioning in daily life. Patients, for instance, may display a normalization of hormone parameters and yet feel impairment and distress [7, 96]. These issues are well known in rehabilitation medicine [97].

In health care, the product is clearly health, and the patients are one of the producers, not just a customer [98]. As a result, "optimally efficient health production depends on a general shift of patients from their traditional roles as passive or adversarial consumers, to become producers of health jointly with their health professionals" [98]. The partnership paradigm includes both collaborative care and self-management. As Kroenke argued [99], neither chronic medical nor psychiatric disorders can be managed adequately in the current environment of general practice, where the typical patient must be seen in 10–15 min or less. It is idealistic to pursue shared decision and self-management, when time for interaction is so minimal.

Box 5.1: A 34-Year-Old Woman with Irritable Bowel Syndrome[1]

Ms. X is a 34-year-old woman who was diagnosed with **irritable bowel syndrome** (abdominal pain, diarrhea) on the basis of her symptomatology, after extensive negative medical work-up. She was in a situation of chronic stress because in the previous 12 months, she made several attempts to get pregnant, without success. She was then referred for psychiatric consultation. Interviewing did not identify a specific psychiatric disorder but disclosed the presence of an **allostatic overload** (she felt overwhelmed by the several medical examinations she was running to clarify the reasons of her difficulties in getting pregnant), a tendency to **perfectionism, phobic avoidance** (she did not use public buses because she felt unsafe there), and **lack of personal growth** (i.e., seeing her future without a child or overcoming the difficulties of getting pregnant). No psychotropic drugs were prescribed. She was referred to a clinical psychologist who found **persistent somatization** and first introduced some lifestyle modifications as to her allostatic overload. The psychologist then addressed abnormal illness behavior with explanatory therapy for correcting hypochondriacal fears and beliefs, phobic avoidance with exposure, perfectionism with cognitive restructuring, and lack of personal growth with well-being therapy. After 6 months, there was a remarkable general improvement, which was maintained at a 1-year follow-up.

[1] The various elements of macroanalysis are highlighted (bold letters) and shown in Fig. 5.1.

References

1. Feinstein AR. Clinical judgment. Baltimore: Williams & Wilkins; 1967.
2. Feinstein AR. Clinimetrics. New Haven: Yale University Press; 1987.
3. Feinstein AR. The pre-therapeutic classification of comorbidity in chronic disease. J Chronic Dis. 1970;23:455–68.
4. deGroot V, Beckerman H, Lankhorst GJ, Bouter LM. How to measure comorbidity: a critical review of available methods. J Clin Epidemiol. 2003;56:221–9.
5. Cloninger CR. Implications of comorbidity for the classification of mental disorders: the need for a psychobiology of coherence. In: Maj M, Gaebel W, Lopez-Ibor JJ, Sartorius N, editors. Psychiatric diagnosis and classification. Chichester: Wiley; 2002. p. 79–105.
6. Emmelkamp PMG. The additional value of clinimetrics needs to be established rather than assumed. Psychother Psychosom. 2004;73:142–4. https://doi.org/10.1159/000076450.
7. Fava GA, Sonino N. Psychosomatic assessment. Psychother Psychosom. 2009;78:333–41. https://doi.org/10.1159/000235736.
8. Emmelkamp PMG, Bouman TK, Scholing A. Anxiety disorders. Chichester: Wiley; 1993.
9. Cosci F, Fava GA. Staging of mental disorders: systematic review. Psychother Psychosom. 2013;82:20–34. https://doi.org/10.1159/000342243.
10. Feinstein AR. An analysis of diagnostic reasoning. I. The domains and disorders of clinical macrobiology. Yale J Biol Med. 1973;46:212–32.
11. Fava GA, Cosci F, Sonino N. Current psychosomatic practice. Psychother Psychosom. 2017;86:13–30. https://doi.org/10.1159/000448856.
12. Fava GA, Tomba E, Grandi S. The road to recovery from depression. Psychother Psychosom. 2007;76:260–5. https://doi.org/10.1159/000104701.
13. Fava GA. Well-being therapy: current indications and emerging perspectives. Psychother Psychosom. 2016;85:136–45. https://doi.org/10.1159/000444114.
14. Fava GA, Rafanelli C, Tomba E. The clinical process in psychiatry: a clinimetric approach. J Clin Psychiatry. 2012;73:177–84. https://doi.org/10.4088/JCP.10r06444.
15. American Psychiatric Association. Diagnostic and statistical manual of mental disorders. 5th ed. Washington: American Psychiatric Association; 2013.
16. Fava GA, Bech P. The concept of euthymia. Psychother Psychosom. 2016;85:1–5. https://doi.org/10.1159/000441244.
17. Hasler G. Well-being: an important concept for psychotherapy and psychiatric neuroscience. Psychother Psychosom. 2016;85:255–61. https://doi.org/10.1159/000447268.
18. Bech P. Clinimetric dilemmas in outcome scales for mental disorders. Psychother Psychosom. 2016;85:323–6. https://doi.org/10.1159/000448810.
19. Basch E. Patient-reported outcomes- harnessing patients' voices to improve clinical care. N Engl J Med. 2017;376:105–8. https://doi.org/10.1056/NEJMp1611252.
20. Piolanti A, Offidani E, Guidi J, Gostoli S, Fava GA, Sonino N. Use of the psychosocial index: a sensitive tool in research and practice. Psychother Psychosom. 2016;85:337–45. https://doi.org/10.1159/000447760.
21. Cosci F, Svicher A, Bech P. The family assessment device: a clinimetric analysis. Psychother Psychosom. 2016;85:241–3. https://doi.org/10.1159/000445438.
22. Horwitz RI, Hayes-Conroy A, Singer BH. Biology, social environment, and personalized medicine. Psychother Psychosom. 2017;86:5–10. https://doi.org/10.1159/000452134.
23. Sirri L, Fava GA. Diagnostic criteria for psychosomatic research and somatic symptom disorders. Int Rev Psychiatry. 2013;25:19–30. https://doi.org/10.3109/09540261.2012.726923.
24. van den Heuvel OA, Veale D, Stein DJ. Hypochondriasis: considerations for ICD-11. Rev Bras Psiquiatr. 2014;36:21–7.
25. Calkins AW, Berman NC, Wilhelm S. Recent advances in research on cognition and emotion in OCD: a review. Curr Psychiatry Rep. 2013;15:357. https://doi.org/10.1007/s11920-013-0357-4.

26. Veale D, Gournay K, Dryden W, Boocock A, Shah F, Willson R, et al. Body dysmorphic disorder: a cognitive behavioural model and a pilot randomised controlled trial. Behav Res Ther. 1996;34:717–29.
27. Stone J, Carson A, Duncan R, Coleman R, Roberts R, Warlow C, et al. Symptoms "unexplained by organic disease" in 1144 new neurology out-patients: how often does the diagnosis change at follow-up? Brain. 2009;132:2878–88. https://doi.org/10.1093/brain/awp220.
28. Lipowski ZJ. Somatization: the experience and communication of psychological distress as somatic symptoms. Psychother Psychosom. 1987;47:160–7.
29. Härter M, Baumeister H, Reuter K, Jacobi F, Höfler M, Bengel J, et al. Increased 12-month prevalence rates of mental disorders in patients with chronic somatic diseases. Psychother Psychosom. 2007;76:354–60. https://doi.org/10.1159/000107563.
30. Engel GL. Psychological aspects of gastrointestinal disorders. In: Reiser MF, editor. American handbook of psychiatry. New York: Basic Books; 1975. p. 653–92.
31. Pilowsky I. Abnormal illness behaviour. Chichester: Wiley; 1997.
32. Cosci F, Fava GA. The clinical inadequacy of the DSM-5 classification of somatic symptom and related disorders: an alternative trans-diagnostic model. CNS Spectr. 2016;21:310–7. https://doi.org/10.1017/S1092852915000760.
33. Sirri L, Fava GA, Sonino N. The unifying concept of illness behavior. Psychother Psychosom. 2013;82:74–81. https://doi.org/10.1159/000343508.
34. Lilienfeld SO, Smith SF, Watts AL. Issues in diagnosis: conceptual issues and controversies. In: Craighead WE, Miklowitz DJ, Craighead LW, editors. Psychopathology: history, diagnosis, and empirical foundations. 2nd ed. Hoboken: Wiley; 2013. p. 1–35.
35. Widiger TA. Classification and diagnosis: historical development and contemporary issues. In: Maddux JE, Winstead BA, editors. Psychopathology: foundations for contemporary understanding. Mahwah: Lawrence Erbaum Associates; 2005. p. 69–91.
36. Shear MK, Simon N, Wall M, Zisook S, Neimeyer R, Duan N, et al. Complicated grief and related bereavement issues for DSM-5. Depress Anxiety. 2011;28:103–17. https://doi.org/10.1002/da.20780.
37. Pies RW. The bereavement exclusion and DSM-5: an update and commentary. Innov Clin Neurosci. 2014;11:19–22.
38. Fava GA. Rational use of antidepressant drugs. Psychother Psychosom. 2014;83:197–204. https://doi.org/10.1159/000362803.
39. Millon T. On the nature of taxonomy in psychopathology. In: Last CG, Hersen M, editors. Issues in diagnostic research. New York: Plenum Press; 1987. p. 3–85.
40. Tyrer P, Seivewright N, Ferguson B, Tyrer J. The general neurotic syndrome: a coaxial diagnosis of anxiety, depression and personality disorder. Acta Psych Scand. 1992;58:201–6.
41. Tyrer P, Tyrer H, Guo B. The general neurotic syndrome: a re-evaluation. Psychother Psychosom. 2016;85:193–7. https://doi.org/10.1159/000444196.
42. Fava GA, Freyberger HJ, Bech P, Christodoulou G, Sensky T, Theorell T, et al. Diagnostic criteria for use in psychosomatic research. Psychother Psychosom. 1995;63(1):1–8. https://doi.org/10.1159/000288931.
43. Porcelli P, Sonino N. Psychological factors affecting medical conditions. A new classification for DSM-V. Basel: Karger; 2007.
44. Porcelli P, Bellomo A, Quartesan R, Altamura M, Inso S, Ciannameo I, et al. Psychosocial functioning in consultation-liaison psychiatry patients. Psychother Psychosom. 2009;78:352–8. https://doi.org/10.1159/000235739.
45. Wise TN. Diagnostic criteria for psychosomatic research are necessary for DSM-V. Psychother Psychosom. 2009;78:330–2. https://doi.org/10.1159/000235735.
46. Basińska MA, Woźniewicz A. Occurrence of diagnostic criteria for psychosomatic research syndromes in polish patients with chronic illness. Psychother Psychosom. 2016;8:386–7. https://doi.org/10.1159/000447243.
47. De Caro MF, Laera D, De Robertis F, Taurino A. Diagnostic criteria for psychosomatic research and psychosocial functioning in multiple sclerosis. Psychother Psychosom. 2016;85:384–5. https://doi.org/10.1159/000446706.

48. Desai G, Chaturvedi SK. Do diagnostic criteria for psychosomatic research explain diagnosis of medically unexplained somatic symptoms. Psychother Psychosom. 2016;85:121–2. https://doi.org/10.1159/000441063.
49. Huang WL, Liao SC. Psychometric properties of the chinese version of the diagnostic criteria for psychosomatic research. Psychother Psychosom. 2017;86:119–20. https://doi.org/10.1159/000450714.
50. Porcelli P, Guidi J. The clinical utility of the diagnostic criteria for psychosomatic research: a review of studies. Psychother Psychosom. 2015;84:265–72. https://doi.org/10.1159/000430788.
51. McEwen BS, Stellar E. Stress and the individual. Mechanisms leading to disease. Arch Intern Med. 1993;153:2093–101.
52. McEwen BS. Epigenetic interactions and the brain-body communication. Psychother Psychosom. 2017;86:1–4.
53. McEwen BS. Physiology and neurobiology of stress and adaptation: central role of the brain. Physiol Rev. 2007;87:873–904. https://doi.org/10.1152/physrev.00041.2006.
54. Waeldin S, Vogt D, Linden M, Hellhammer DH. Frequency of perceived poststress symptoms in inpatients, outpatients and healthy controls: the role of perceived exhaustion and stress. Psychother Psychosom. 2016;85:36–44. https://doi.org/10.1159/000438866.
55. Friedman M, Rosenman RH. Type a behavior and your heart. New York: Knopf; 1974.
56. Sirri L, Fava GA, Guidi J, Porcelli P, Rafanelli C, Bellomo A, et al. Type a behavior: a reappraisal of its characteristics in cardiovascular disease. Int J Clin Pract. 2012;66:854–61. https://doi.org/10.1111/j.1742-1241.2012.02993.x.
57. De Vries AM, Forni V, Voellinger R, Stiefel F. Alexithymia in cancer patients: review of the literature. Psychother Psychosom. 2012;81:79–86. https://doi.org/10.1159/000330888.
58. Porcelli P, Bagby RM, Taylor GJ, De Carne M, Leandro G, Todarello O. Alexithymia as predictor of treatment outcome in patients with functional gastrointestinal disorders. Psychosom Med. 2003;65:911–8.
59. Fava GA, Grandi S. Differential diagnosis of hypochondriacal fears and beliefs. Psychother Psychosom. 1991;55:114–9.
60. Noyes R, Carney CP, Langbehn DR. Specific phobia of illness: search for a new subtype. J Anxiety Disord. 2004;18:531–45. https://doi.org/10.1016/S0887-6185(03)00041-0.
61. Kellner R. Psychosomatic syndromes, somatization and somatoform disorders. Psychother Psychosom. 1994;61:4–24.
62. Engel GL. Conversion symptoms. In: Mac Bryde CM, Blacklow RS, editors. Signs and symptoms. Philadelphia: Lippincott; 1970. p. 650–99.
63. Porcelli P, Fava GA, Rafanelli C, Bellomo A, Grandi S, Grassi L, et al. Anniversary reactions in medical patients. J Nerv Ment Dis. 2012;200:603–6. https://doi.org/10.1097/NMD.0b013e31825bfb2e.
64. Goldbeck R. Denial in physical illness. J Psychosom Res. 1997;43:575–93.
65. Frank JD. Persuasion and healing. Baltimore: Johns Hopkins University Press; 1961.
66. Schmale AH, Engel GL. The giving up-given up complex illustrated on film. Arch Gen Psychiatry. 1967;17:133–45.
67. Tecuta L, Tomba E, Grandi S, Fava GA. Demoralization: a systematic review on its clinical characterization. Psychol Med. 2015;45:673–91. https://doi.org/10.1017/S0033291714001597.
68. Sweeney DR, Tinling DC, Schmale AH. Differentiation of the "giving-up" affects- helplessness and hopelessness. Arch Gen Psychiatry. 1970;23:378–82.
69. Snaith RP, Taylor CM. Irritability. Br J Psychiatry. 1985;147:127–36.
70. Fava GA. Irritable mood and physical illness. Stress Med. 1987;3:293–9. https://doi.org/10.1080/00223890701629649.
71. Chida Y, Steptoe A. The association of anger and hostility with future coronary heart disease: a meta-analytic review of prospective evidence. J Am Coll Cardiol. 2009;53:936–46.
72. Sartorius N, Holt RIG, Maj M. Comorbidity of mental and physical disorders. Basel: Karger; 2015.
73. Fava GA, Sonino N. Depression associated with medical illness. CNS Drugs. 1996;5:175–89.
74. Rafanelli C, Sirri L, Grandi S, Fava GA. Is depression the wrong treatment target for improving outcome in coronary artery disease? Psychother Psychosom. 2013;82:285–91. https://doi.org/10.1159/000351586.

75. Katon WJ. Clinical and health services relationships between major depression, depressive symptoms and general medical illness. Biol Psychiatry. 2003;54:216–26.
76. Cosci F, Fava GA, Sonino N. Mood and anxiety disorders as early manifestations of medical illness: a systematic review. Psychother Psychosom. 2015;84:22–9. https://doi.org/10.1159/000367913.
77. Fava GA, Porcelli P, Rafanelli C, Mangelli L, Grandi S. The spectrum of anxiety disorders in the medically ill. J Clin Psychiatry. 2010;71:910–4. https://doi.org/10.4088/JCP.10m06000blu.
78. Niles AN, Dour HJ, Stanton AL, Roy-Byrne PP, Stein MB, Sullivan G, et al. Anxiety and depressive symptoms and medical illness among adults with anxiety disorders. J Psychosom Res. 2015;78:109–15. https://doi.org/10.1016/j.jpsychores.2014.11.018.
79. Tinetti ME, Fried T. The end of the disease era. Am J Med. 2004;116:179–85.
80. Tinetti ME, Bogardus ST, Agostini JV. Potential pitfalls of disease—specific guidelines for patients with multiple conditions. N Engl J Med. 2004;351:2870–4. https://doi.org/10.1056/NEJMsb042458.
81. Engel GL. The need for a new medical model: a challenge for biomedicine. Science. 1977;196:129–36.
82. Starcevic V. Cyberchondria: challenges of problematic online searches for health-related information. Psychother Psychosom. 2017;86:129–33. https://doi.org/10.1159/000465525.
83. Rapp MA, Rieckmann N, Lessman DA, Tang CY, Paulino R, Burg MM, et al. Persistent depressive symptoms after acute coronary syndrome are associated with compromised white matter integrity in the anterior cingulate: a pilot study. Psychother Psychosom. 2010;79:149–55. https://doi.org/10.1159/000286959.
84. Forman JP, Stampfer MJ, Curhan GC. Diet and lifestyle risk factors associated with incident hypertension in women. JAMA. 2009;302:401–11. https://doi.org/10.1001/jama.2009.1060.
85. Rozanski A, Blumenthal JA, Kaplan J. Impact of psychological factors on the pathogenesis of cardiovascular disease and implications for therapy. Circulation. 1999;99:2192–217.
86. Narayan KMV, Kanaya AM, Gregg EW. Lifestyle intervention for the prevention of type 2 diabetes mellitus. Treat Endocrinol. 2003;2:315–20.
87. Abbass A, Kisely S, Kroenke K. Short-term psychodynamic psychotherapy for somatic disorders. Psychother Psychosom. 2009;78:265–74. https://doi.org/10.1159/000228247.
88. Balon R. Cognitive-behavioral therapy, psychotherapy and psychosocial interventions in the medically ill. Psychother Psychosom. 2009;78:261–4. https://doi.org/10.1159/000228246.
89. Andersen BL, Yang HC, Farrar WB, Golden-Krentz DM, Emery CF, Thornton LM, et al. Psychologic intervention improves survival for breast cancer patients. Cancer. 2008;113:3450–8. https://doi.org/10.1002/cncr.23969.
90. Turk DC, Swanson KS, Tunks ER. Psychological approaches in the treatment of chronic pain patients. Can J Psychiatr. 2008;53:213–23. https://doi.org/10.1177/070674370805300402.
91. Lahmann C, Nickel M, Schuster T, Sauer N, Ronel J, Noll-Hussong M, et al. Functional relaxation and guided imagery as complementary therapy in asthma: a randomized controlled clinical trial. Psychother Psychosom. 2009;78:233–9. https://doi.org/10.1159/000214445.
92. van Middendorp H, Geenen R, Sorbi MJ, van Doornen LJ, Bijlsma JW. Health and physiological effects of an emotional disclosure intervention adapted for application at home: a randomized clinical trial in rheumatoid arthritis. Psychother Psychosom. 2009;78:145–51. https://doi.org/10.1159/000206868.
93. Fava GA, Grandi S, Rafanelli C, Fabbri S, Cazzaro M. Expanatory therapy of hypochondriasis. J Clin Psychiatry. 2000;61:317–22.
94. Feinstein AR. Clinical judgment revisited: the distraction of quantitative models. Ann Intern Med. 1994;120:799–805.
95. Fava GA, Tomba E, Sonino N. Clinimetrics: the science of clinical measurements. Int J Clin Pract. 2012;66(1):11–5. https://doi.org/10.1111/j.1742-1241.2011.02825.x.
96. Sonino N, Peruzzi P. A psychoneuroendocrinology service. Psychother Psychosom. 2009;78:346–51. https://doi.org/10.1159/000235738.
97. Wade DT, Smeets RJEM, Werbunt JA. Research in rehabilitation medicine. Methodological challenges. J Clin Epidemiol. 2010;63:69–74. https://doi.org/10.1016/j.jclinepi.2009.07.010.
98. Hart JT. Clinical and economic consequences of patients as producers. J Public Health Med. 1995;17:383–6.
99. Kroenke K. Psychological medicine. BMJ. 2002;324:1536–7.

Part II

The Clinical Contexts of Psychosomatic Medicine

Dignity-Conserving Care in Medicine

6

Luigi Grassi, Harvey Chochinov, Giuseppe Moretto, and Maria Giulia Nanni

> *"The patient enters the hospital as if he were entering a business concern, to be served in the best possible way by an impersonal apparatus. And the physician of modernity acts as if he were a collectivity, which cares for the patient without a physician's entering into the treatment in any personal way. […]"*
>
> *(Jaspers, 1959, The physician in the technological age, p. 254)*

L. Grassi (✉)
Institute of Psychiatry, Department of Biomedical and Specialty Surgical Sciences, University of Ferrara, Ferrara, Italy
e-mail: luigi.grassi@unife.it

H. Chochinov
Department of Psychiatry, University of Manitoba, Winnipeg, MB, Canada

Manitoba Palliative Care Research Unit, CancerCare Manitoba, Winnipeg, MB, Canada

Research Institute of Oncology and Hematology, CancerCare Manitoba, Winnipeg, MB, Canada

G. Moretto
Division of Neurology, Palliative Care Programme, Integrated University Hospital, Verona, Italy

M. G. Nanni
Department of Biomedical and Specialty Surgical Sciences, Institute of Psychiatry, University of Ferrara, Ferrara, Italy

University Hospital Psychiatry Unit, Program on Psycho-Oncology and Psychiatry in Palliative Care, Integrated Department of Mental Health, S. Anna Hospital and Local Health Authorities, Ferrara, Italy
e-mail: luigi.grassi@unife.it

L. Grassi et al. (eds.), *Person Centered Approach to Recovery in Medicine*, Integrating Psychiatry and Primary Care, https://doi.org/10.1007/978-3-319-74736-1_6

Abstract

Dignity-conserving care is a multifactorial construct, consisting of three primary domains, i.e. illness-related concerns, such as symptom distress; dignity-conserving perspectives and practices, such as continuity of the self, maintenance of pride and hopefulness; and social dimensions of dignity, such as privacy concerns, burden to others and aftermath concerns. Dignity-conserving care has recently been the focus of research in both somatic and mental care settings. In patients suffering from somatic disorders, particularly chronic and progressive disorders, loss of dignity is often manifested by loss of identity, shattering of their self-image or having psychological, interpersonal, spiritual and existential needs that are not being adequately addressed. Similar issues apply to psychiatric patient healthcare, where stereotypes, prejudice and discrimination continue to exist. Fractured dignity has been associated with increasing levels of physical and psychological symptoms, including spiritual pain. The delivery of dignity-conserving care is essential in achieving a holistic and healing approach, improving the satisfaction of patients, families and healthcare professionals alike.

6.1 Introduction

Dignity, as a core tenant of human life and human rights, has been studied in many different areas from philosophy to bioethics, from law to sociology as well as medicine and the healthcare system in general [1, 2]. The term "dignity" derives from the Latin nouns *decus* (ornament, distinction, honour, glory, but also worthiness of honour and esteem) and *dignitas*, which is "an individual or group's sense of self-respect and self-worth, physical and psychological integrity and empowerment" [3, 4].

Human dignity has been the object of essays and reflection starting from Pico della Mirandola *Oration on the Dignity of Man* (*De hominis dignitate*) [5] that, as the Manifesto of the Renaissance, remapped the human landscape to centre all attention on human capacity and human perspective. He said that "human vocation is a mystical vocation that has to be realized in three stages, which comprehends necessarily moral transformation, intellectual research and final perfection in the identity with the absolute reality. This paradigm is universal, because it can be retraced in every tradition". The Kantian perspective of dignity is more aligned with the moral imperative stipulating that we should treat human beings not as instruments but as ends in and of themselves, having ultimate moral worth [6]. Marcel, from a different perspective, situated dignity in inter-human relationships and in the fragile vulnerable finitude of the human individual, which contrasts with his effort to recognize his unique human values.

Although the concept of dignity in medicine is complex, in general, we can consider that dignity relates to the dimension of intrinsic worth, that is, the inherent and inalienable value that belongs to every human being simply by virtue of being human [7]. The other notion of dignity invokes the dimension of worthiness of respect or attributable dignity that demands affirmation and calls for action, approval and support [8]. Sulmasy [9] also identifies similar concepts when speaking of *intrinsic dignity*, which refers to worth, stature or value that human beings have simply because they are human, and *attributed dignity*, thus a created dignity, which refers to worth, stature or value that human beings confer upon others by acts of affirmation. These two aspects of dignity are sometimes referred to as *dignity-of-self* (the dignity we attach to ourselves as integrated and autonomous persons) and *dignity-in-relation* (the dignity that the individual perceives or does not perceive in the eyes of others within interpersonal relationships) [8].

In modern medicine, the importance of dignity has not been taken much into consideration within the relationship between patients and their healthcare professionals. As Jaspers pointed out over 60 years ago, advances in the natural sciences and in technology have had a transformative influence on the art of clinical medicine and its ancient Hippocratic ideal, which has seen medicine become largely rooted in science and technology and less so in the humanity of the physician. He indicates that this leads to the patient being perceived as an "object" without any specific individuality and uniqueness (also referred as personhood),[1] while, at the samte time, the physician's identity is threatened since he becomes victim of his technological instruments. This results in a doctor-patient relationship that is deprived of considerations such as dignity [10]. More recently, Pellegrino [11] echoes these risks by underlining the need to preserve dignity and prevent indignity in medicine, namely, patients easily losing their identity, not being able to recover their self-image challenged by the illness, losing all sense of personal worth and feeling ashamed and vulnerable. He states:

> Physicians cannot ignore those many assaults on human dignity, intrinsic as well as attributed, that are taken for granted in the bureaucratic, commercialized, and impersonal places that hospitals have, all too often, become. [...] A more collective sense of shared responsibility for the 'dehumanization,' the 'depersonalization,' or the 'alienation' that the sick feel in today's health and medical care institutions must fall on the physician. [...] The need to sensitize physicians and other health professionals is an urgent one in today's mechanized experience of illness. (p. 2 532)

In spite of the fact that guidelines for several clinical specialties and other healthcare professionals include ethical codes that underscore the importance of maintaining and respecting patient dignity, there are a myriad of ways in which dignity can be compromised. These include rudeness, indifference, condescension, dismissal, disregard, intrusion, objectification, restriction, labelling, contempt, discrimination, revulsion, deprivation and assault [12]. These can emerge in the context of asymmetrical relationships between patients and healthcare professionals [10]. Also, the structure of the healthcare system, as underscored in many different reports, can result in bureaucratic organizations in which workers experience increasing demands and caseloads, inadequate resources and uncertainty about the best way to approach their work. These are all obstacles to a dignified, compassionate and humanized approach. Task-based culture prioritizes meeting targets over the provision of patient-centred care, spending time filling out forms rather than attending to the psychological and spiritual dimensions of patient suffering and priveliging

[1] Personhood here is intended as the status of being a person, a human person as the natural inherent capacity to give rise to human functions, whether or not those functions are ever attained.

models of care which value "doing" things rather than "reflecting" on the holistic nature of the patient experience [13–15].

The challenge of modern medicine is how to embrace the human side of the profession, while not abandoning the empirical scientific approach, hence allowing healthcare professionals to more fully address the multitude of individual patient needs.

6.2 Dignity and the Dimensions of Care in Medicine

An attempt to redefine the mission of medicine was proposed by Tournier, who emphasized the need for personalized medicine [16] as a holistic clinical approach. The latter denotes an integration of the scientific method along with psychological insights that are infused with transcendental/existential awareness and the search for meaning and purpose [17]. In Tournier's conceptualization of medicine, all the dimensions of the person as a whole, namely, the biological, psychological, social and spiritual aspects of individuals in health and illness, should be part of medicine, by referring to the uniqueness and dignity of man, also in his suffering, with his resources and not just deficits, with all his desires to be accepted, experiencing sincere validation and finding purpose in life [18].

The medical literature, particularly the palliative care literature, has begun to examine these holistic dimensions of healthcare. Patients affected by chronic conditions (including psychiatric and medical disorders) and life-threatening diseases usually present and report a series of interpersonal, psychological and spiritual unmet needs. Spiritual pain, a notion that aligns with an undermining of dignity, has been defined by Murata [19] as the pain caused by extinction of the being and the meaning of the self and characterized by a threat to three dimensions of being human: namely, a being founded on temporality, a being in relationship and a being with autonomy. For these reasons, spiritual pain and undermining of dignity in patients with chronic and disabling conditions (medical, psychiatric as well as at the end of life) are characterized by a sense of meaninglessness of life, loss of identity and worthlessness of living derived from loss of the future, loss of others and loss of autonomy.

6.2.1 Dignity in Somatic Disorders

In different medical settings, such as cardiology, neurology, infectious disease (e.g. HIV infection), nephrology, respirology and oncology, studies have shown that patients' needs are not being addressed by multidisciplinary healthcare teams, causing an increase of suffering [20–23]. About 50% of patients with advanced stages of cancer indicated that overcoming their fears, finding hope, finding meaning in life, finding spiritual resources and having someone to talk to about finding peace of mind were significant needs to be responded to [24]. According to Chochinov et al. [25], a very high percentage of patients in an advanced stage of cancer would consider spiritual and interpersonal problems as needing attention from healthcare professionals, such as feeling a burden to others (87.1%), feeling of not making a meaningful and/or lasting contribution in one's own life (83.7%) and not feeling worthwhile or valued (81.4%). More recently, Chochinov et al. [26] examined patients with amyotrophic lateral sclerosis (ALS), chronic obstructive pulmonary disease (COPD) and end stage renal disease (ESRD) and found that some aspects of dignity, such as feeling of being a burden to others, anxiety and depression, uncertainty and feeling of not having control over one's own life, differed across these conditions. Physicians tend to have a limited vision of dignity, wherein they consider the physical aspects of suffering most influential in preserving dignity, while patients' caregivers have a broader perspective that includes the significant role of psychosocial aspects in preserving dignity at the end of life [27].

In patients with chronic medical disorders, Van Gennip et al. [28] found three different trajectories of dignity over time: a dynamic equilibrium in which the individual's sense of dignity was temporarily diminished followed by a return to previous levels, a downward trend in which the sense of dignity was diminished with progression of the disease without a return to previous levels, and stability in which the sense of dignity remained unaltered despite changes in circumstances. In their longitudinal study, dignity remained unaffected by the disease experience in a small percentage of cases, while most patients experienced more frequent problems in maintaining or regaining their sense of dignity in the face of progressive loss.

Loss of dignity has been associated with both physical (e.g. lack of energy, pain, shortness of breath) and psychological symptoms (e.g. anxiety, sadness, irritability) [29]. In contrast, treating patients with dignity is an independent factor related to higher satisfaction, adherence and receptivity to preventive care [30].

Spirituality and its components related to dignity have also been investigated in many different chronic diseases, including cancer [31, 32], cardiovascular disorders [33], HIV infection [34, 35], critical care medicine [36] and palliative medicine [37]. A number of studies have indicated that spiritual well-being, particularly the dimensions of meaning and peace, is related to better quality of life, adaptation to illness and physical, emotional and interpersonal well-being [38]. Williams [39] has underlined the fundamental importance of spirituality at the end of life and highlighted the need for a shift to spiritually oriented care considering that the existing end-of-life frameworks tend to neglect spiritual work and research that focus on spirituality.

6.2.2 Dignity in Psychiatric Disorders

Issues related to dignity have not been specifically examined in psychiatry, although the theme has been indirectly addressed under the rubric of stigma [40] and violations of human rights [41]. There is much work to be done in order to achieve health and equality among patients with severe mental illness (SMI), given their experience is still characterized by multiple overlapping layers of inequality and discrimination within society and the health system itself [42].

Stereotype, prejudice and discrimination continue to exist within the healthcare setting and can enter into relational encounters in daily life and among healthcare providers [43]. Institutional stigma (i.e. organizational policies or a culture of negative attitudes and beliefs about mental illness), public stigma (i.e. a set of negative attitudes and beliefs that motivate individuals to fear, reject, avoid and discriminate against people with mental illness), self-stigma (i.e. the internalization of public stigma and prejudices influencing an individual's self-conception with secondary feelings of shame, anger, hopelessness or despair) and label avoidance (i.e. the choice not to pursue mental health services because patients do not want to suffer the prejudice and discrimination that the label entails) are part of stigma [44–46]. Such layers of inequality and discrimination within society and the healthy system itself have led to the recovery movement within psychiatry.

It has been reported that severe internalized stigma is related to lower self-esteem, self-efficacy and likelihood of recovery. Severe psychiatric symptom has a negative impact on sense of coherence, sense of hope and quality of life among people affected by SMI, irrespective of the diagnosis [47–49]. A lack of compassion in healthcare setting can worsen this situation [50].

The literature regarding the relationship between dignity and stigma among mentally ill patients includes the notion suffering related to feeling inferior and suffering in pursuit of maintaining one's own dignity as weel as the need to be treated as an equal huamn being [51]. In this respect, patients with SMI perceive stigma and discrimination as omnipresent potential problems to which they remain eternally vigilant, taking various preventive behavioural and psychological measures, such as conscious and strenuous efforts to look, act and behave "normal" [52].

Research shows that patients with mental illness tend to perceive spirituality as a source of giving and receiving love and care and as an inherent part of a person's well-being, rehabilitation and life in general [53]. Spirituality is considered essential in providing meaning in life in about 25% of patients with SMI and is associated with better functioning, self-esteem, psychological and social quality of life, fewer negative symptoms and higher endorsement of values such as universalism, tradition, devoutness and benevolence, as well as a more meaningful perspective in life [54]. It has also reported that patients with schizophrenia or schizoaffective disorder often use spirituality and religion to their benefit to cope with their illness [55]. In patients with depressive disorders, higher spirituality has been found to independently contribute to favourable treatment responses [56], as well as to lower levels of hopelessness and severity of depression [57].

6.3 The Need for a Dignity Care Approach in Medicine

Dignity can inform the approach to patients affected by medical or psychiatric disorders, given that healthcare providers have a profound influence on how patients experience illness [58] and that *caring*, besides curing, plays a major role in preserving the dignity of the patients. As reported by some scholars [59], the patient-healthcare professional relationship is an opportunity for a careful and active defence of patient's dignity.

A specific perspective has been taken by Chochinov et al. [60, 61] in their examination of dignity in the setting of palliative care. This model indicates that it is possible to structure a dignity-centred approach that promotes a state of physical, mental, social and spiritual well-being. According to this model, dignity has three primary domains:

- Illness-related concerns (i.e. concerns related to symptoms of physical and psychological distress, functional capacity, cognitive acuity) that threaten or impinge on the individual sense of dignity
- The dignity-conserving perspectives and practices (dignity-conserving repertoire) (i.e. continuity of the self, role preservation, maintenance of pride, hopefulness, autonomy/control, acceptance, resilience, living in the moment, seeking spiritual help, maintaining normality)
- The social aspects of dignity (i.e. privacy boundaries, social support, care tenor, burden to others, aftermath concerns)

Chochinov [62] has proposed an easily remembered core framework of dignity-conserving care, to be applied more broadly in medicine (i.e. A B C D, with A for attitude, B for behaviour, C for compassion, D for dialogue), which can guide physicians and all healthcare professionals in better relating and communicating with their patients. This framework represents a roadmap for maintaining dignity and improving patient experience.

A = Attitude: It is critical that healthcare professionals examine their own attitudes and assumptions towards patients, including asking questions about themselves (e.g. how would I be feeling in this patient's situation? Could my attitude towards the patient be based on something to do with my own experiences, anxieties or fears?)

B = Behaviour: It is necessary to acknowledge that certain communication behaviours (e.g. contact, respect, sitting at a comfortable distance for conversation, at the patient's eye level when possible, small acts of kindness, like getting the patient a glass of water) have a significant impact in the relationship with the patients and enhance the trust and connection between patients and their healthcare providers.

C = Compassion: Compassion refers to a deep awareness of the suffering of another coupled with the wish to relieve it. It can be conveyed in various ways—spoken or unspoken—that shows some recognition of the person and not simply their illness ().

D = Dialogue: Dialogue includes the acknowledgement of personhood beyond the illness and recognizes the emotional impact that accompanies illness (see Table 6.1).

Table 6.1 The ABCD sequence for a dignity-conserving care in medicine (from Chochinov [60])

Attitudes (questions to be asked)
• How would I be feeling in this patient's situation? • What is leading me to draw those conclusions? • Have I checked whether my assumptions are accurate? • Am I aware how my attitude towards the patient may be affecting him or her? • Could my attitude towards the patient be based on something to do with my own experiences, anxieties or fears? • Does my attitude towards being a healthcare provider enable or disenable me to establish open and empathic professional relationships with my patients? • Actions to be taken • Make a conscious effort to make these questions a part of your reflection on the care of each and every patient • Discuss the issue of healthcare providers' attitudes and assumptions and how they influence caring for patients, as a regular part of case reviews and clinical teaching • Include ongoing professional development activities that have you challenge and question your attitudes and assumptions as they might affect patient care • Create a culture among your colleagues and within your healthcare setting in which acknowledgement and discussion of these issues become a standard part of providing care
Behaviours (disposition)
• Treat contact with patients as you would any potent and important clinical intervention • Professional behaviours towards patients must always include respect and kindness • Lack of curative options should never rationalize or justify a lack of ongoing patient contact • Clinical examination • Always ask the patient's permission to perform a physical examination • Always ask the patient's permission to include students or trainees in the clinical examination • Although an examination may be part of routine care, it is rarely routine for the patient, so always, as far as possible, take time to set the patient at ease and show that you have some appreciation for what they are about to go through (e.g. "I know this might feel a bit uncomfortable"; "I'm sorry that we have to do this to you"; "I know this is an inconvenience"; "This should only hurt for a moment"; "Let me know if you feel we need to stop for any reason"; "This part of the examination is necessary because…") • Limit conversations with patients during an examination (aside from providing them with instruction or encouragement) until they have dressed or been covered appropriately • Facilitating communication • Act in a manner that shows the patient that he or she has your full and complete attention • Always invite the patient to have someone from his or her support network present, particularly when you plan to discuss or disclose complex or "difficult" information • Personal issues should be raised in a setting that attempts to respect the patient's need for privacy • When speaking with the patient, try to be seated at a comfortable distance for conversation, at the patient's eye level when possible • Given that illness and changing health status can be overwhelming, offer patients and families repeated explanations as requested • Present information to the patient using language that he or she will understand; never speak about the patient's condition within their hearing distance in terms that they will not be able to understand • Always ask if the patient has any further questions and assure them that there will be other opportunities to pose questions as they arise

Table 6.1 (continued)

Compassion (getting in touch with one's own feelings requires the consideration of human life and experience)
• Reading stories and novels and observing films, theatre and art that portray the pathos of the human condition
• Discussions of narratives, paintings and influential, effective role models
• Considering the personal stories that accompany illness
• Experiencing some degree of identification with those who are ill or suffering
• Ways to show compassion
• An understanding look
• A gentle touch on the shoulder, arm or hand
• Some form of communication, spoken or unspoken, that acknowledges the person beyond their illness
Dialogue (acknowledging personhood)
• "This must be frightening for you"
• "I can only imagine what you must be going through"
• "It's natural to feel pretty overwhelmed at times like these"
• Knowing the patient
• "What should I know about you as a person to help me take the best care of you that I can?"
• "What are the things at this time in your life that are most important to you or that concern you most?"
• "Who else (or what else) will be affected by what's happening with your health?"
• "Who should be here to help support you?" (friends, family, spiritual or religious support network, etc.)
• "Who else should we get involved at this point, to help support you through this difficult time?" (psychosocial services, group support, chaplaincy, complementary care specialists, etc.)

Although other proposals and models exist, all of them have a common framework that is intended to increase awareness that the relationship with the patient is a special human encounter, in which empathy and compassion represent part of a patient-centred approach [63].

Compassion has been explored, particularly in the nursing literature [64], affirming the overlap between these concepts and various elements of dignity, as reported in a report by the Prime Minister's Commission on the Future of Nursing and Midwifery in England [65]. This report affirms that "truly compassionate care is skilled, competent, value-based care that respects individual dignity" (p. 3). For some authors [66] compassion pertains to a sequence of layers (not necessarily a step-by-step process), including routine care (i.e. a minimal engagement in a respectful dialogue with patients), "detached" empathy (i.e. learning how to effectively communicate care and concern for the patient and family in a "detached way", thus only at a cognitive level, but not at an emotional level), affective or emotional empathy (i.e. the professional's ability to both cognitively understand what the patient is going through and experience a non-verbal resonance with the patient emotionally) and compassionate care (i.e. a deep response at an affective level and appropriate action to relieve it). For others, such as Sinclair et al. [67, 68], who have specifically examined what patients perceive in terms of compassionate care, "compassion seems to reside between objective and affective understanding oriented to an other (empathy) and subjective responses oriented to the self, rooted in pity toward an other (sympathy). It requires emotion and action on the part of respondents, finds its basis in love, vulnerability, and reciprocity, and is actualized in the disadvantaging of oneself for the benefit of another" [69]. In this way, a model of compassion has been developed consisting of a series of components related to genuine communication (e.g. authenticity, honesty, openness, kindness) in a relational space in which a series of intentions (e.g. seeking to understand the person and his/her needs) and actions (e.g. in terms of demeanour, affect, behaviour, engagement) can be expressed [67].

This is in line with other research indicating that compassion is not only a feeling or a state of mind or a moral virtue but a practice that imbues the approach to suffering within a profound connection and understanding between two or more human beings [70, 71]. Similar dimensions or themes identified within the compassion framework are reported to be communication, patients involvement, connection and connectedness with patients, empathy and being empathetic and caring, competence and professionalism, recognizing suffering and acting to alleviate this suffering [72]. Sinclair et al. [68] and others [73, 74] have indicated the differences between empathy (i.e. the ability to understand and accurately acknowledge the feelings of another, leading to an attuned response from the observer), sympathy (i.e. the emotional reaction of pity towards the misfortune of another, especially those who are perceived as suffering unfairly) and compassion as core elements of person-centred care.

When speaking about the relationship between the patients, their families and healthcare professionals, six components have been delineated by the Institute of Medicine [75] as essential to respectful, personalized care in medicine. These are summarized by Cox [76] as:

1. Compassion, empathy, responsiveness to needs, values and expressed preferences
2. Co-ordination and integration
3. Information, communication and education
4. Physical comfort
5. Emotional support, relieving fear and anxiety
6. Involvement of family and friends

A similar framework by Rushton et al. [77, 78] posits that within the clinical context, responses to the suffering of the patient, healthcare professionals are thought to enter in the relationship with empathy (*emotional attunement*), perspective taking (*cognitive attunement*), moral sensitivity (*ethical attunement*) and memory (*personal experience*). For these authors, if these four dimensions are closely aligned, the intensity and valence of emotional arousal will influence ethical appraisal and discernment by engaging a robust view of the ethical issues, conflicts and possible solutions, thus cultivating compassionate action and resilience. On the other hand, if these dimensions are not aligned, ethical appraisal and discernment will be deficient, with the risk of creating emotional dysregulation and potentially leading to personal and moral distress, self-centred attitudes and behaviours, moral outrage, burnout and secondary stress.

6.3.1 Training in Dignity Orientation

A dignity in care approach is critical if healthcare systems are to be transformed from their techno-bureaucratical orientation to a more humanized, healing perspective, improving the satisfaction of clients [79], HCPs and healthcare outcomes [80]. It is recognized that education in medicine should focus on many approaches (e.g. mindfulness, self-reflection and emotional skills) that are essential components to recognize, regulate and behaviourally demonstrate empathy and compassion within clinical and professional encounters [81], including general medicine [82], nursing [83] and mental healthcare [84].

According to Chochinov [85], dignity in care can be taught, and healthcare systems can be changed. Chochinov et al. [86] have also examined facets of communication that are needed to achieve optimal therapeutic effectiveness, consistent with a dignity-conserving, person-centred approach. Three primary elements of optimal therapeutic communication include:

- Therapeutic approaches (i.e. skills and techniques used by clinicians to help them communicate and support patients experiencing distress)
- Creation of a safe space (i.e. an environment or setting in which patients feel safe and secure)
- Personal growth and self-care (i.e. characteristics of the clinicians, which contributes to the therapeutic process). This includes the professional's capacity to maintain emotional health, including self-reflection, openness to personal growth and acknowledgement of one's own feelings of vulnerability.

Other elements of this model include therapeutic humility (e.g. the capacity to not avoid emotion, tolerate clinical ambiguity, explore difficult topics, avoid the urge to have to fix), therapeutic pacing (e.g. utilizing approaches that set the clinical tempo and modulate—based on the client's need—between emotionally containing and evocative strategies) and therapeutic presence (e.g. characteristics of the clinician that foster the creation of a safe therapeutic space, being compassionate and empathetic, being respectful and nonjudgemental, being genuine and authentic, valuing intrinsic worth of client) [84].

Eliciting information regarding patient personhood can be achieved by way of the Patient Dignity Question (PDQ), which entails asking patients "What do I need to know about you as a person to give you the best care possible?" Ninety three percent of palliative care patients and families felt that their response was important information for healthcare professionals to know, and 99% would recommend the PDQ for others [87]. Among healthcare professionals, 90% indicated that they learned something new from the PDQ, 64% that they were emotionally affected by it, 59% that it influenced their sense of empathy and 44% that it influenced their care

Table 6.2 The TIME (This Is ME) interview (from Pan et al. [86])

• Are there particular relationships or personal connections you would like us to be aware of?
• Are there specific accomplishments or roles you would like us to be aware of?
• Are there important values you would like us to know about?
• Are there particular qualities or characteristics that you would like us to know about?
• Are there specific beliefs, religious or spiritual practices that we should know about?
• Are there particular worries or concerns you would like us to be aware of?
• Are there particular responsibilities or obligations you would like us to be aware of?
• Are there things we should know about you, which might influence how to provide your care (e.g. vision or hearing challenges, problems with thinking, mental health issues and others)?
• Is there anything else about you as a person that you would like us to know, in order to give you the best care possible?

[85]. In nursing homes, the application of a short tool to address personhood, the TIME (This Is ME) questionnaire (Table 6.2), favourably influenced healthcare professionals by way of their attitude, care, respect and empathy towards the residents, as well as enhanced a sense of connectedness they feel towards residents and their satisfaction in providing care [88]. This is in keeping with patient needs, with compassion being identified as a quality that can be nurtured through experiential learning and reflective practices. These can be taught through compassion training (e.g. patient-centred communication, self-reflection exercises and compassionate role modelling) [89]. This is also important from a neuroscientific perspective. It has been shown that empathy and compassion can be modulated through education and training and are associated with positive emotions, a sense of affiliation, reward and prosocial behaviours. Neural networks may generate shared representations of directly experienced and observed feelings, sensations and actions. This can generate a heightening of empathic concern or compassion and altruistic motivation to help, accompanied by activation of areas in the brain associated with affiliation and reward. Activation of these neural networks is sensitive to multiple inter- and intrapersonal influences (e.g. ability to focus one's attention, to receive and accurately interpret input about distress, to recognize and regulate one's own emotions, to attend to one's own well-being through self-care and self-compassion and effective communication) [90].

6.3.2 The Assessment of Dignity in Routine Care

Since dignity is a multifactorial and complex construct, research has been conducted to explore and evaluate the dimensions of dignity. The Patient Dignity Inventory (PDI) has been developed based on Chocinov's model of dignity. As said, this model is comprised of three primary elements, specifically illness-related concerns (e.g. concerns related to symptoms of physical and psychological distress, functional capacity) that threaten or impinge on the individual sense of dignity, the dignity-conserving perspectives and practices (e.g. continuity of the self, role preservation, maintenance of pride, hopefulness) and the social aspects of dignity (e.g. social support, privacy concerns, burden to others, aftermath concerns and care tenor) [91]. Factor analysis of the original PDI resulted in a five-factor solution, including symptom distress, existential distress, dependency, peace of mind and social support. The PDI has been translated and validated in several countries to test its role from a cross-cultural perspective. Studies, carried out in Germany [95], Greece [96], Iran [92], Italy [93, 94], Spain [97] and The Netherlands [98], have shown the PDI to have good psychometric properties.

From the clinical point of view, the PDI can assist clinicians to routinely detect dignity-related distress and guide clinical intervention. By using the PDI, one or more previously unreported concerns were found in 76% of patients in varying stages of cancer; and in 81% of instances, clinicians reported that the PDI facilitated their work [99]. Similarities in the dignity-related problems reported by cancer patients and care home residents were shown by Hall et al. [100], suggesting a common existential pathway leading towards death for malignant and non-malignant diseases. Among cancer patients, loss of dignity was associated with physical problems and demoralization, indicating that early recognition of dignity-related existential concerns and interventions to enhance the sense of dignity could be useful in the prevention of demoralization in oncology settings [101]. Loss of dignity has been also associated with both physical (e.g. lack of energy, pain, shortness of breath) and psychological symptoms (e.g. anxiety, sadness, irritability), with psychological distress correlating with all dimensions of dignity [29]. The PDI has shown that physicians tend to have a limited vision of dignity, wherein they consider the physical aspects of suffering most influential in preserving dignity, whereas caregivers tend to focus on the significant role of psychosocial aspects in preserving dignity at the end of life [27]. Also, the application of the PDI has been shown to have an intrinsic therapeutic value and provides a way of examining issues related to dignity and the meaning of life within the context of advanced-stage illness [102]. In a study regarding the application of the PDI involving the couples (patients with advanced stages of illness and their partners), the PDI provided important and valuable insight favouring the communication and connection between couples facing end-of-life issues [103].

In geriatric care, where interventions to improve the dignity of older people in hospitals are lacking [104], Chochinov et al. [105] showed that patients with advanced chronic medical diseases and institutionalized frail elderly residents face unique challenges as they move towards the end of life. The PDI can help in understanding the intricacies of distress and how they differ across different groups of patients. Among patients with cardiovascular disease in an Iranian general hospital, patients' indignity was associated with psychological distress, suggesting the need for policy makers and health services administrators to establish and implement plans to maintain and enhance patients' dignity in hospitals [106, 107].

The PDI has been used to help staff elicit dignity perceptions in a psychiatric inpatient unit for acute psychiatric disorders, helping professionals to improve quality of care and patients to accept treatments [108]. Also, dimensions of dignity were associated with spirituality and psychological well-being among patients with SMI, indicating the need to examine these variables and accordingly implement treatment to achieve recovery-based outcomes [109].

Conclusion

Evidence-based medicine is slowly making way for value-based paradigms, as a way counterbalancing modern biotechnological reductionism. Person-centred medicine has many aspects in common with a dignity-centred medicine, affirming personhood of the patients and their family members [110, 111]. As underscored elsewhere [112], the artificial separation between curing and caring reflects the problem of a Cartesian and post-Cartesian dualistic model, which can only be overcome by a personalized approach that eliminates the paradoxical impossibility of "non-curative caring" and "non-carative curing" [113]. Thus, *curing* should not be confined in a "physicalizing tendency" towards an un-affective (unhuman) (cold science, objective, quantitative, high-tech) style of relation dealing only with the quantifiable, material body. Likewise, *caring* should not be confined in a "dematerializing tendency" towards a "disembodied" (subjective, qualitative, high-touch) attitude[2] [114, 115]. Cure and care are complementary parts of the medical profession and without both, the integrity of the profession collapses [116]. Along with communication skills and compassion, understanding the multiple dimensions of dignity offers healthcare providers a means by which to more fully engage their patients and better attend to their physical, psychological and existential needs.

References

1. Barclay L. In sickness and in dignity: a philosophical account of the meaning of dignity in health care. Int J Nurs Stud. 2016;61:136–41.
2. Jacobson N. Dignity and health: a review. Soc Sci Med. 2007;64:292–302.
3. Rosen M. Dignity. His history and meaning. Cambridge, MA: Harvard University Press; 2012.
4. Lebech M. On the problem of human dignity. A Hermenutical and Phenomenolgical Investigation: Königshausen und Neumann, Würzburg; 2009.
5. Pico della Mirandola G. Discorso sulla dignità dell'uomo (Oratio de hominis dignitate) 1496 (Italian re-edition: Dignità dell'uomo (De hominis dignitate), by Bruno Cicognani, Le Monnier, Firenze, 1942; English Translation Oration on the dignity of man by Robert A. Caponigri, Henry Regnery Company, Chicago, ILL, 1956).
6. Sensen O. Kant on human dignity. Berlin: Walter De Gruyter Inc.; 2011.
7. Spiegelberg H. Human dignity: a challenge to contemporary philosophy. J New Paradigm Res. 1971;9:39–64.

[2] What I feel regarding my body, that is, the intentional, living aspects of my body, is often described in terms of *Leib* to be differentiated by *Körper*, where *Leib* is the intentional lived body, to be a body, and *Körper* is the material body, to have a body. These concepts, which are important in a psychosomatic approach in medicine, were introduced by Husserl and re-proposed by Merleau-Ponty and are still crucial in the mind-body problem.

8. Malvestiti B. Human dignity as a status vs. human dignity as a value. A double nature. Spring School and International Conference; 2011 June 7–9; Milan: University Vita-Salute San Raffaele.
9. Sulmasy DP. The varieties of human dignity: a logical and conceptual analysis. Med Health Care Philos. 2013;16(4):937–44.
10. Jaspers K. Der Arzt im technischen Zeitalter. Universitas: Zeitschrift für Wissenschaft, Kunst und Literatur. 1959;14(4):337–54. (English translation by Arthur A. Grugan, The physician in the technological age. Theoretical Medicine and Bioethics, 1989;10(3):251–267).
11. Pellegrino E. The lived experience of human dignity. In: Human dignity and bioethics. Essays commissioned by the President's Council of Bioethics, Washington DC; 2008. p. 513–40.
12. Jacobson N. Dignity violation in health care. Qual Health Res. 2009;19(11):1536–47.
13. Stenhouse R, Ion R, Roxburgh M, Devitt PF, Smith SDM. Exploring the compassion deficit debate. Nurse Educ Today. 2016;39:12–5.
14. Deery R, Fisher P. Professionalism and person-centredness: developing a practice based approach to leadership within NHS maternity services in the UK. Health Sociol Rev. 2017;26:143–59.
15. Barron K, Deery R, Sloan G. Community mental health nurses' and compassion: an interpretative approach. J Psychiatr Ment Health Nurs. 2017;24:211–20.
16. Tournier P. Médicine de la personne. (English Tr. The Healing of Persons. Harper Collins Pub, 1965).
17. Pfeifer H-R. Paul Tournier and 'Médecine de la Personne'—the man and his vision. Int J Integr Care. 2010;10:60–2.
18. Cox JL. Towards an evidence-based 'Medicine of the Person': the contribution of psychiatry to health care provision. J Eval Clin Pract. 2008;14:694–8.
19. Murata H. Spiritual pain and its care in patients with terminal cancer: construction of a conceptual framework by philosophical approach. Palliat Support Care. 2003;1(1):15–21.
20. Luddington L, Cox S, Higginson I, Livesley B. The need for palliative care for patients with non-cancer diseases: a review of the evidence. Int J Palliat Nurs. 2001;7(5):221–6.
21. Solano JP, Gomes B, Higginson IJ. A comparison of symptom prevalence in far advanced cancer, AIDS, heart disease, chronic obstructive pulmonary disease and renal disease. J Pain Symptom Manag. 2006;31(1):58–69.
22. Oliver DJ, Borasio GD, Caraceni A, de Visser M, Grisold W, Lorenzl S, Veronese S, Voltz R. A consensus review on the development of palliative care for patients with chronic and progressive neurological disease. Eur J Neurol. 2016;23:30–8.
23. Lloyd-Williams M, Mogan C, Dening KH. Identifying palliative care needs in people with dementia. Curr Opin Support Palliat Care. 2017. [Epub ahead of print].
24. Moadel A, Morgan C, Fatone A, Grennan J, Carter J, Laruffa G, Skummy A, Dutcher J. Seeking meaning and hope: self-reported spiritual and existential needs among an ethnically-diverse cancer patient population. Psychooncology. 1999;8(5):378–85.
25. Chochinov HM, Krisjanson LJ, Hack TF, Hassard T, McClement S, Harlos M. Dignity in the terminally ill: revisited. J Palliat Med. 2006;9(3):666–72.
26. Chochinov HM, Johnston W, McClement SE, Hack TF, Dufault B, Enns M, Thompson G, Harlos M, Damant RW, Ramsey CD, Davison S, Zacharias J, Milke D, Strang D, Campbell-Enns HJ, Kredentser MS. Dignity and distress towards the end of life across four non-cancer populations. PLoS One. 2016;11(1):e0147607. https://doi.org/10.1371/journal.pone.0147607.
27. Albers G, de Vet HC, Pasman HR, Deliens L, Onwuteaka-Philipsen BD. Personal dignity in the terminally ill from the perspective of caregivers: a survey among trained volunteers and physicians. J Palliat Med. 2013;16(9):1108–14.
28. van Gennip IE, Pasman HR, Oosterveld-Vlug MG, Willems DL, Onwuteaka-Philipsen BD. Dynamics in the sense of dignity over the course of illness: a longitudinal study into the perspectives of seriously ill patients. Int J Nurs Stud. 2015;52(11):1694–704.
29. Oechsle K, Wais MC, Vehling S, Bokemeyer C, Mehnert A. Relationship between symptom burden, distress, and sense of dignity in terminally ill cancer patients. J Pain Symptom Manag. 2014;48(3):313–21.

30. Beach MC, Sugarman J, Johnson RL, Arbelaez JJ, Duggan PS, Cooper LA. Do patients treated with dignity report higher satisfaction, adherence, and receipt of preventive care? Ann Fam Med. 2005;3:331–8.
31. Visser A, Garssen B, Vingerhoets A. Spirituality and well-being in cancer patients: a review. Psychooncology. 2010;19(6):565–72.
32. Salsman JM, Pustejovsky JE, Jim HS, Munoz AR, Merluzzi TV, George L, Park CL, Danhauer SC, Sherman AC, Snyder MA, Fitchett G. A meta-analytic approach to examining the correlation between religion/spirituality and mental health in cancer. Cancer. 2015;121(21):3769–78.
33. Naghi JJ, Philip KJ, Phan A, Cleenewerck L, Schwarz ER. The effects of spirituality and religion on outcomes in patients with chronic heart failure. J Relig Health. 2012;51(4):1124–36.
34. Dalmida SG. Spirituality, mental health, physical health, and health-related quality of life among women with HIV/AIDS: integrating spirituality into mental health care. Issues Ment Health Nurs. 2006;27(2):185–98.
35. Szaflarski M. Spirituality and religion among HIV-infected individuals. Curr HIV/AIDS Rep. 2013;10(4):324–32.
36. Puchalski C. Spirituality in health: the role of spirituality in critical care. Crit Care Clin. 2004;20(3):487–504.
37. Delgado-Guay MO. Spirituality and religiosity in supportive and palliative care. Curr Opin Support Palliat Care. 2014;8(3):308–13.
38. Park CL, Masters KS, Salsman JM, Wachholtz A, Clements AD, Salmoirago-Blotcher E, Trevino K, Wischenka DM. Advancing our understanding of religion and spirituality in the context of behavioral medicine. J Behav Med. 2017;40(1):39–51.
39. Williams AL. Perspectives on spirituality at the end of life: a meta-summary. Palliat Support Care. 2006;4(4):407–17.
40. Livingston JD, Boyd JE. Correlates and consequences of internalized stigma for people living with mental illness: a systematic review and meta-analysis. Soc Sci Med. 2010;71(12):2150–61.
41. Bhugra D, Ventriglio A, Pathare S. Freedom and equality in dignity and rights for persons with mental illness. Lancet Psychiatry. 2016;3(3):196–7.
42. Burns JK. Mental health and inequity: a human rights approach to inequality, discrimination, and mental disability. Health Hum Rights. 2009;11(2):19–31.
43. Mestdagh A, Hansen B. Stigma in patients with schizophrenia receiving community mental health care: a review of qualitative studies. Soc Psychiatry Psychiatr Epidemiol. 2014;49(1):79–87.
44. Corrigan PW, Watson AC. Understanding the impact of stigma on people with mental illness. World Psychiatry. 2002;1(1):16–20.
45. Corrigan PW, Watson AC. The paradox of self-stigma and mental illness. Clin Psychol Sci Pract. 2002;9:35–53.
46. Corrigan PW, Wassel A. Understanding and influencing the stigma of mental illness. J Psychosoc Nurs Ment Health Serv. 2008;46(1):42–8.
47. Mashiach-Eizenberg M, Hasson-Ohayon I, Yanos PT, Lysaker PH, Roe D. Internalized stigma and quality of life among persons with severe mental illness: the mediating roles of self-esteem and hope. Psychiatry Res. 2013;208(1):15–20.
48. Świtaj P, Grygiel P, Chrostek A, Nowak I, Wciórka J, Anczewska M. The relationship between internalized stigma and quality of life among people with mental illness: are self-esteem and sense of coherence sequential mediators? Qual Life Res. 2017;26(9):2471–8. https://doi.org/10.1007/s11136-017-1596-3.
49. Oliveira SE, Carvalho H, Esteves F. Internalized stigma and quality of life domains among people with mental illness: the mediating role of self-esteem. J Ment Health. 2016;25(1):55–61.
50. Crawford P, Gilbert P, Gilbert J, Gale C, Harvey K. The language of compassion in acute mental health care. Qual Health Res. 2013;23(6):719–27.
51. Skorpen F, Thorsen AA, Forsberg C, Rehnsfeldt AW. Suffering related to dignity among patients at a psychiatric hospital. Nurs Ethics. 2014;21(2):148–62.

52. Whitley R, Campbell RD. Stigma, agency and recovery amongst people with severe mental illness. Soc Sci Med. 2014;107:1–8.
53. Ho RT, Chan CK, Lo PH, Wong PH, Chan CL, Leung PP, Chen EY. Understandings of spirituality and its role in illness recovery in persons with schizophrenia and mental-health professionals: a qualitative study. BMC Psychiatry. 2016;16:86.
54. Huguelet P, Mohr SM, Olié E, Vidal S, Hasler R, Prada P, Bancila M, Courtet P, Guillaume S, Perroud N. Spiritual meaning in life and values in patients with severe mental disorders. J Nerv Ment Dis. 2016;204(6):409–14.
55. Mohr S, Borras L, Nolan J, Gillieron C, Brandt PY, Eytan A, Leclerc C, Perroud N, Whetten K, Pieper C, Koenig HG, Huguelet P. Spirituality and religion in outpatients with schizophrenia: a multi-site comparative study of Switzerland, Canada, and the United States. Int J Psychiatry Med. 2012;44(1):29–52.
56. Kim NY, Huh HJ, Chae JH. Effects of religiosity and spirituality on the treatment response in patients with depressive disorders. Compr Psychiatry. 2015;60:26–34.
57. Peselow E, Pi S, Lopez E, Besada A, Ishak WW. The impact of spirituality before and after treatment of major depressive disorder. Innov Clin Neurosci. 2014;11(3–4):17–23.
58. Chochinov HM. Dignity-conserving care—a new model for palliative care: helping the patient feel valued. JAMA. 2002;287(17):2253–60.
59. Andorno R. The dual role of human dignity in bioethics. Med Health Care Philos. 2013;16(4):967–73.
60. Chochinov HM, Hack T, McClement S, Kristjanson L, Harlos M. Dignity in the terminally ill: a developing empirical model. Soc Sci Med. 2002a;54(3):433–43.
61. Hack TF, Chochinov HM, Hassard T, Kristjanson LJ, McClement S, Harlos M. Defining dignity in terminally ill cancer patients: a factor-analytic approach. Psychooncology. 2004;13:700–8.
62. Chochinov HM. Dignity and the essence of medicine: the A, B, C, and D of dignity conserving care. BMJ. 2007;335(7612):184–7.
63. Lown BA, McIntosh S, Gaines ME, McGuinn K, Hatem DS. Integrating compassionate, collaborative care (the "Triple C") into health professional education to advance the triple aim of health care. Acad Med. 2016;91(3):310–6.
64. McCaffrey G, McConnell S. Compassion: a critical review of peer-reviewed nursing literature. J Clin Nurs. 2015;24:3006–15.
65. Prime Minister's Commission on the Future of Nursing and Midwifery in England Front Line Care. The Future of Nursing and Midwifery in England. Report of the Prime Minister's Commission on the Future of Nursing and Midwifery in England. http://webarchive.nationalarchives.gov.uk/20100331110400/http:/cnm.independent.gov.uk/wp-content/uploads/2010/03/front_line_care.pdf.
66. Post SG, Ng LE, Fischel JE, Bennett M, Bily L, Chandran L, Joyce J, Locicero B, McGovern K, McKeefrey RL, Rodriguez JV, Roess MW. Routine, empathic and compassionate patient care: definitions, development, obstacles, education and beneficiaries. J Eval Clin Pract. 2014;20:872–80.
67. Sinclair S, Torres MB, Raffin-Bouchal S, Hack TF, McClement S, Hagen NA, Chochinov HM. Sympathy, empathy, and compassion: a grounded theory study of palliative care patients' understandings, experiences, and preferences. Palliat Med. 2017;31(5):437–47.
68. Sinclair S, McClement S, Raffin-Bouchal S, Hack TF, Hagen NA, McConnell S, Chochinov HM. Compassion in health care: an empirical model. J Pain Symptom Manag. 2016;51(2):193–203.
69. Sinclair S, Norris JM, McConnell SJ, Chochinov HM, Hack TF, Hagen NA, McClement S, Bouchal SR. Compassion: a scoping review of the healthcare literature. BMC Palliat Care. 2016;15:6.
70. van der Cingel M. Compassion: the missing link in quality of care. Nurse Educ Today. 2014;34:1253–7.
71. van der Cingel M. Compassion and professional care: exploring the domain. Nurs Philos. 2009;10:124–36.

72. Papadopoulos I, Ali S. Measuring compassion in nurses and other healthcare professionals: an integrative review. Nurse Educ Pract. 2016;16:133–9.
73. Svenaeus F. The relationship between empathy and sympathy in good healthcare. Med Health Care Philos. 2015;18:267–77.
74. Jeffrey D. Empathy, sympathy and compassion in healthcare: is there a problem? Is there a difference? Does it matter? J R Soc Med. 2016;109(12):446–52.
75. Institute of Medicine. Crossing the quality chasm: a new health system for the 21st century. Washington, DC: National Academy Press; 2001.
76. Cox J. Medicine of the person and personalized care: a stitch in time saves nine? J Eval Clin Pract. 2010;16:315–7.
77. Rushton CH, Kaszniak AW, Halifax JS. A framework for understanding moral distress among palliative care clinicians. J Palliat Med. 2013a;16(9):1074–9.
78. Rushton CH, Kaszniak AW, Halifax JS. Addressing moral distress: application of a framework to palliative care practice. J Palliat Med. 2013b;16(9):1080–8.
79. Hojat M, Louis DZ, Maxwell K, Markham F, Wender R, Gonnella JS. Patient perceptions of physician empathy, satisfaction with physician, interpersonal trust, and compliance. Int J Med Educ. 2010;1:83–7.
80. Street RL, Makoul G, Arora NK, Epstein RM. How does communication heal? Pathways linking clinician–patient communication to health outcomes. Patient Educ Couns. 2009;74:295–301.
81. Raab K. Mindfulness, self-compassion, and empathy among health care professionals: a review of the literature. J Health Care Chaplain. 2014;20(3):95–108.
82. Burks DJ, Kobus AM. The legacy of altruism in health care: the promotion of empathy, prosociality and humanism. Med Educ. 2012;46(3):317–25.
83. Crawford P, Brown B, Kvangarsnes M, Gilbert P. The design of compassionate care. Clin Nurs. 2014;23(23–24):3589–99.
84. Spandler H, Stickley T. No hope without compassion: the importance of compassion in recovery-focused mental health services. J Ment Health. 2011;20(6):555–66.
85. Chochinov HM. Dignity in care: time to take action. J Pain Symptom Manag. 2013;46(5):756–9.
86. Chochinov HM, McClement SE, Hack TF, McKeen NA, Rach AM, Gagnon P, Sinclair S, Taylor-Brown J. Health care provider communication: an empirical model of therapeutic effectiveness. Cancer. 2013;119(9):1706–13.
87. Chochinov HM, McClement S, Hack T, Thompson G, Dufault B, Harlos M. Eliciting personhood within clinical practice: effects on patients, families, and health care providers. J Pain Symptom Manag. 2015;49(6):974–80.
88. Pan JL, Chochinov H, Thompson G, McClement S. The TIME questionnaire: a tool for eliciting personhood and enhancing dignity in nursing homes. Geriatr Nurs. 2016;37(4):273–7.
89. Sinclair S, Torres MB, Raffin-Bouchal S, Hack TF, McClement S, Hagen NA, Chochinov HM. Compassion training in healthcare: what are patients' perspectives on training healthcare providers? BMC Med Educ. 2016;16:169.
90. Lown BA. A social neuroscience-informed model for teaching and practising compassion in health care. Med Educ. 2016;50(3):332–42.
91. Chochinov HM, Hassard T, McClement S, et al. The patient dignity inventory: a novel way of measuring dignity-related distress in palliative care. J Pain Symptom Manag. 2008;36:559–71.
92. Abbaszadeh A, Borhani F, Rabori R. Patient dignity in coronary care: psychometrics of the Persian version of the patient dignity inventory. Br J Med Med Res. 2015;8(5):463–9.
93. Ripamonti CI, Buonaccorso L, Maruelli A, et al. Patient dignity inventory (PDI) questionnaire: the validation study in Italian patients with solid and hematological cancers on active oncological treatments. Tumori. 2012;98:491–500.
94. Grassi L, Costantini A, Caruso R, Brunetti S, Marchetti P, Sabato S, Nanni MG. Dignity and psychosocial-related variables in advanced and nonadvanced cancer patients by using the patient dignity inventory-Italian version. J Pain Symptom Manag. 2017;53(2):279–87.
95. Sautier L, Vehling S, Mehnert A. Assessment of patient dignity in cancer care: preliminary psychometrics of the German version of the patient dignity inventory (PDI-G). J Pain Symptom Manag. 2014;47:181–8.

96. Parpa E, Kostopoulou S, Tsilika E, Galanos A, Katsaragakis S, Mystakidou K. Psychometric properties of the Greek version of the patient dignity inventory in advanced cancer patients. J Pain Symptom Manag. 2017;54(3):376–82.
97. Rullán M, Carvajal A, Núñez-Córdoba JM, Martínez M, Carrasco JM, et al. Spanish version of the patient dignity inventory: translation and validation in patients with advanced cancer. J Pain Symptom Manag. 2015;50:874–81.
98. Albers G, Pasman HR, Rurup ML, de Vet HC, Onwuteaka-Philipsen BD. Analysis of the construct of dignity and content validity of the patient dignity inventory. Health Qual Life Outcomes. 2011;9:45.
99. Chochinov HM, McClement SE, Hack TF, et al. The patient dignity inventory: applications in the oncology setting. J Palliat Med. 2012;15:998–1005.
100. Hall S, Davies JM, Gao W, Higginson IJ. Patterns of dignity-related distress at the end of life: a cross-sectional study of patients with advanced cancer and care home residents. Palliat Med. 2014;28:1118–27.
101. Vehling S, Mehnert A. Symptom burden, loss of dignity, and demoralization in patients with cancer: a mediation model. Psychooncology. 2014;23(3):283–90.
102. Rullán M, Arantzamendi M, Carvajal A, Martínez M, Saenz de Ormijana A, Centeno C. The patient dignity inventory: just another evaluation tool? Experiences with advanced cancer patients. Palliat Support Care. 2018;16(1):73–9. https://doi.org/10.1017/S1478951517000517.
103. Mowll J, Lobb EA, Lane L, Lacey J, Chochinov HM, Kelly B, Agar M, Links M, Kearsley JH. A preliminary study to develop an intervention to facilitate communication between couples in advanced cancer. Palliat Support Care. 2015;13(5):1381–90.
104. Zahran Z, Tauber M, Watson HH, Coghlan P, White S, Procter S, Addis G, Norton C. Systematic review: what interventions improve dignity for older patients in hospital? J Clin Nurs. 2016;25(3–4):311–21.
105. Chochinov HM, Johnston W, McClement SE, et al. Dignity and distress towards the end of life across four noncancer populations. PLoS One. 2016;11:e0147607.
106. Borhani F, Abbaszadeh A, Moosavi S. Status of human dignity of adult patients admitted to hospitals of Tehran. J Med Ethics Hist Med. 2014;7:20. Epub 2014 Dec 1.
107. Mehdipour-Rabori R, Abbaszadeh A, Borhani F. Human dignity of patients with cardiovascular disease admitted to hospitals of Kerman, Iran, in 2015. J Med Ethics Hist Med. 2016;9:8. eCollection 2016.
108. Di Lorenzo R, Cabri G, Carretti E, Galli G, Giambalvo N, Rioli G, Saraceni S, Spiga G, Del Giovane C, Ferri P. A preliminary study of Patient Dignity Inventory validation among patients hospitalized in an acute psychiatric ward. Neuropsychiatr Dis Treat. 2017;13:177–90.
109. Grassi L, Nanni MG, Pavanati M, Caruso R. Dignity and spiritual issues among patients with severe mental illness. Submitted.
110. Laine C, Davidoff F. Patient-centered medicine. A professional evolution. JAMA. 1996;275:152–6.
111. Charon R. The patient-physician relationship. Narrative medicine: a model for empathy, reflection, profession, and trust. JAMA. 2001;286:1897–902.
112. Grassi L. Quam bene vivas referre: curing and caring in psycho-oncology. Psychooncology. 2013;22(8):1679–87.
113. Webb C. Caring, curing, coping: towards an integrated model. J Adv Nurs. 1996;23:960–8.
114. Aho JA, Aho K. Body matters: a phenomenology of sickness, disease, and illness. Lanham, MD: Lexington Books; 2008.
115. Bullington J. The expression of the psychosomatic body from a phenomenological perspective, SpringerBriefs in philosophy. New York: Springer. p. 19–37.
116. de Valck C, Bensing J, Bruynooghe R, Batenburg V. Cure-oriented versus care-oriented attitudes in medicine. Pat Edu Counsel. 2001;45:119–26.

Cross-Cultural Issues

7

Ilaria Tarricone, Iris T. Graef-Calliess, Nasim Chaudhry, Marianne Kastrup, Domenico Berardi*, Dinesh Bhugra*, Mauro Braca*, Ronald Burian*, Albert Diefenbacher*, Silvia Ferrari*, Nusrat Husain*, Adil Qureshi*, Meryam Schouler-Ocak*, and Sarah Tosato*

*Cross-cultural CLP Group

I. Tarricone (✉)
Bologna Transcultural Psychosomatic Team (BoTPT), Department of Medical and Surgical Sciences (DIMEC), Alma Mater Studiorum Bologna University, Bologna, Italy
e-mail: ilaria.tarricone@unibo.it

I. T. Graef-Calliess
Department of Psychiatry, Hannover Medical School, Social Psychiatry and Psychotherapy, Hannover, Germany
e-mail: iristatjana.graef-calliess@krh.eu

N. Chaudhry
Dow University of Health Sciences, Pakistan Institute of Living and Learning, Karachi, Pakistan

M. Kastrup
Copenhagen, Denmark
e-mail: marianne.kastrup@dadlnet.dk

D. Berardi
Dipartimento di Scienze Biomediche e Neuromotorie (DIBINEM), Alma Mater Studiourum Bologna University, Bologna, Italy
e-mail: domenico.berardi@unibo.it

D. Bhugra
Emeritus Professor of Mental Health and Cultural Diversity at the Institute of Psychiatry, Psychology and Neuroscience at King's College London, London, UK
e-mail: dinesh.bhugra@kcl.ac.uk

M. Braca
Department of Mental Health, AUSL Bologna, Bologna, Italy
e-mail: m.braca@ausl.bologna.it

R. Burian · A. Diefenbacher
Department of Psychiatry, Psychotherapy and Psychosomatics, Evangelisches Krankenhaus Königin Elisabeth Herzberge, Berlin, Germany
e-mail: r.burian@keh-berlin.de; a.diefenbacher@keh-berlin.de

L. Grassi et al. (eds.), *Person Centered Approach to Recovery in Medicine*, Integrating Psychiatry and Primary Care, https://doi.org/10.1007/978-3-319-74736-1_7

S. Ferrari
Department of Diagnostics, Clinical and Public Health Medicine,
University of Modena and Reggio Emilia, Modena, Italy
e-mail: silvia.ferrari@unimore.it

N. Husain
University of Manchester, Lancashire Care Early Intervention Service, Manchester, UK
e-mail: nusrathusain@btopenworld.com

A. Qureshi
Hospital Universitari Vall d'Hebron, Servei de Psiquiatria, Barcelona, Spain

M. Schouler-Ocak
Psychiatric University Clinic of Charité at St. Hedwig's Hospital, Berlin, Germany
e-mail: meryam.schouler-ocak@charite.de

S. Tosato
Section of Psychiatry, Department of Neurosciences, Biomedicine and Movement Sciences,
University of Verona, Verona, Italy
e-mail: sarah.tosato@univr.it

Abstract

Migrants and ethnic minorities are at higher risk to develop mental disorders compared to native population. Culture has an important impact on the symptom presentation, diagnostic process and treatment strategies in all populations. Cultural competence represents good clinical practice and can be defined as a two-way learning encounter where clinician acknowledges the patient's culture as well as his own cultural values and prejudices. Cultural competent response to the mental health care requires knowledge, skills and attitudes. Both individual and organizational cultural competences are needed to improve the effectiveness of psychiatric treatment. In this chapter, we revised the WPA Guidance on Mental Health and Mental Health Care for Migrants and the EPA Guidance on Mental Health Care for Migrants and list a series of recommendations for policy-makers, service providers and clinicians. Cultural competent experiences in the treatment of somatization and other psychiatric disorders across several countries in Europe are also presented.

7.1 Introduction

Health-care professionals regularly have contact with patients from different cultural backgrounds, whose mental health is seriously affected by the social conditions in the receiving countries in which they live [1, 2]. Moreover, if they are immigrants, their mental health could be affected by the conditions under which they travel or by the reasons of migration. The social determinants of their health, including mental health, are often different from those of the settled community and may require a different, cultural adapted approach from health-care professionals [3–6]. Cultural factors play an important role in the symptoms' presentation of distress and illness, on the diagnostic process and on treatment strategies in all populations [2, 7–11].

One of the leading reasons for under-recognition and under-treatment of mental disorders among people of different ethnic or cultural backgrounds both at the primary and secondary level of care is somatization [12]. Several studies conducted in primary care show that common mental disorders (CMDs) are less recognized and treated in ethnic minorities than in native-born populations, even in cases where rates of consultation are higher [6, 13–16]. The reasons of poor levels of detection and treatment of CMDs among migrants in primary care have been related to difficulty in recognizing somatically presented CMDs [17, 18]. Patients with CMDs are less referred to mental health services (MHS) [16, 17] by general practitioners (GPs); moreover, members of certain ethnic minority groups show lower rates of initiation of appropriate drug therapy [18–21], especially when mental disorders are presented somatically. This primarily somatic presentation of mental disorders in turn appears to be related to underutilization of MHS by immigrants and to higher use of emergency services [2, 22, 23]. Thus, there are important reasons to try to develop culturally competent skills and interventions aimed at overcoming barriers to effective mental health treatment for migrants and ethnic minorities.

In this chapter, we propose to outline some of the key issues related to cultural competence and how to deal with these issues [24]. Cultural competency refers to good clinical practice so that all patients, including those from minority groups and/or with migration history, feel acknowledged and supported even when their cultural backgrounds differ from that of the health professionals [24]. Cultural competence is a way of capturing the capacity to provide appropriate care for diverse patients, overcoming sociocultural differences and other systemic challenges to reduce disparities [5, 24–29]. Cultural competency is not about learning the language of the patient or necessarily knowing details about the specific cultural values of a migrant, but about respecting differences and making sure that these are bridgeable [26, 29–34]. For the purposes of this chapter, cultural competence is best understood as a process and a therapeutic interaction or even a sort of meta-theory rather than a specific attainable skill set. We adopted the recommendations from the EPA and WPA guidance [3, 24, 35] and added new recommendations from the literature.

7.2 Cultural Competence: Framework

Cultural competence is defined as the ability to understand and be aware of cultural factors in the therapeutic interaction between the clinician and the patient [8, 25, 35–39]. Often it is erroneously assumed that only patients belong to ethnic minorities "have cultures" [24], while a cultural competent clinician acknowledges the patient's culture as well as his own cultural values and prejudices [24]. Clinicians are experts in biomedicine as well as patients in their own experience of distress. Thus, clinical encounters ought to be viewed as two-way learning encounters.

Clinically competent mental health professionals are both interested in the patient's cultural biases and their world view which is strongly coloured by cultural values. They should be also aware of their own personal cultural strengths/weaknesses and prejudices which may affect their responses to specific patients [27, 29, 38–43]. Moreover, cultural competence should be considered at both the individual/clinical level and at the institutional level [1, 9, 27, 29, 44–46].

Cultural competence is not a static phenomenon but a developmental process moving along a continuum [47, 48]. This spectrum includes stages of cultural destructiveness, cultural incapacity, cultural blindness, cultural pre-competence, cultural competence and eventually cultural proficiency [24]. It must be remembered that cultural competency should be tempered with what has been termed "cultural humility" [49, 50]: attaining a level of cultural proficiency indicates a level of cultural competence, but this is not absolute and will need ongoing development [24].

Indeed institutional cultural competence requires not only a recognition of barriers to quality care at a systemic, organizational and institutional level but also a project aimed at overcoming these barriers [1, 24, 25]. Some of these barriers are relatively straightforward, such as not having enough professionals who speak the same language of the patient, lack of physical access to services by public transportation, restricted opening hours of the mental health centre and so forth [24]. Thus organizational cultural competence will need to make appropriate changes accordingly [1, 9, 27, 45, 51, 52]. In fact it is extremely important to undertake the effort to make the mental health centre more accessible and comfortable for patients of minority groups through not only linguistically and culturally diverse staff but also the physical environment.

In order to increase cultural competence, (mental) health-care systems need to value diversity, to assess an individual's own cultural values, to be aware of cultural interactions, to incorporate cultural knowledge and to adjust service delivery accordingly [24]. Health-care systems should mark themselves on the cultural competency continuum [47, 48, 52]. Cultural competence also includes access to suitable well-trained interpreters and clinician's ability to work with them [24]. Bilingual professionals can add that extra bit, even if this may not always be possible due to limited resources. Moreover, in some countries, cultural mediators can be utilized: they can offer linguistic interpretation but also mediate between health professionals and service users [53]. In fact, having to communicate distress with language barriers can be a significant reason for nonengagement and increased levels of dissatisfaction.

In conclusion, cultural competence represents a comprehensive response to the mental health needs of care of immigrant patients and requires knowledge, skills and attitudes which can improve the effectiveness of psychiatric treatment [24, 25, 27, 40, 52, 54, 55].

We describe in the paragraphs below basic components of cultural competence at the level of clinician, service provider and policy-maker.

7.3 Cultural Competence Basic Components at the Clinician Level

7.3.1 Cultural Knowledge

Cognitive cultural competence, otherwise known as "knowledge", involves awareness of the various ways in which culture, immigration status and geographical origin impact on psychosocial development, psychopathology and therapeutic interactions. It is not always possible to be fully cognizant of all the cultures, but nowadays it will be possible to get the correct information from multiple sources. However, risks of stereotyping and as such losing sight of the patient as an individual [27, 41, 55–58] must be remembered.

7.3.2 Cultural Skills

Technical competence or skills are essential in applying the knowledge in the clinical context [24]. These key skills include a proficiency in intercultural communication, the capacity to develop a therapeutic relationship with a culturally different patient and the ability to adapt diagnosis and treatment in response to cultural differences between the psychiatrist and the patient [3, 27, 35, 48, 55]. These skills require the awareness of cultural differences and their role in the expression and explanation of mental distress but also of similarities among cultures. The nature of human cognition and perception helps us to recognize the impact of cultural filters on both sides, on oneself and on others [24]. This, subsequently, forms the basis for a flexible response that is adaptable to the cultural context of the patient [2, 27, 59].

7.3.3 Cultural Attitudes

Attitudes and beliefs, including personal prejudices, will be affected by knowledge and will also affect behaviours [2, 4, 27]. Intercultural work requires the clinicians to challenge their own perceptions of "reality"; to explore their own cultural identity, prejudices and biases; and to be willing to adapt to distinct cultural practices [24].

7.4 Cultural Competence Basic Components at the Service Provider Level

7.4.1 Providing Therapies for Minority Groups

It was reported that outcomes of therapies in various settings are poor for minority groups [24]. It was found that the proportion of immigrants in admission psychiatric wards of hospitals were roughly similar to that of immigrants in the general population in Germany [60] and in Italy [61]. However, few immigrant patients were found in psychotherapeutic settings [61]. Two recent meta-analyses [4, 62] enlightened evidences for the effectiveness of the implementation of cultural adaptations in mental health interventions. In details, four common methods of cultural adaptation [62] were showed. First, the cultural values of the immigrant patient should be incorporated into therapy; second, immigrant patients can be matched with therapists of the same cultural or ethnic group; third, mental health interventions should be easily accessible and targeted to immigrant patients' circumstances; and fourth, support resources available within immigrant patients' community, extended family members and tradition should be incorporated into therapy interventions. The results of the meta-analytic review [62] indicate a moderate to strong benefit of culturally adapted interventions. It was found that interventions targeted to a specific cultural group were four times more effective than interventions provided to groups consisting of patients from a variety of cultural backgrounds. Interventions conducted in patients' native or primary language were twice as effective as interventions conducted in English. Further, the results of additional analysis indicated that the format of intervention (individual therapy, group interventions) did not moderate the overall results [62].

7.4.2 Using Interpreters

Communication between professionals and patients from different cultural origins and without knowledge of each other's language is not possible without the help of interpreters. Psychotherapy in native languages cannot be realized everywhere because the number of qualified psychotherapists who speak a native language is limited. Moreover, each culture has different idioms of distress which are employed to communicate with clinicians. For example, many languages do not have equivalent words to describe depression, but the words "sadness" or "unhappiness" can be easily used and verified. Finally, there is a profound danger in applying diagnostic tools developed in a specific country blindly without taking conceptual equivalence into account. Not only does this affect diagnostic patterns but also does it introduce concepts of what Kleinman calls category fallacy [41, 63].

Non-professional translators (family members, members of hospital staff, etc.) can have a negative impact upon medical treatment via false translation, most commonly by the failure to add "creative elements" from their own interpretation to what has been said. Sometimes the "creative elements" have the aim to protect the patient by avoiding to translate what has been said. Minors are at special psychological risk when asked to help interpreting while a migrant parent with a mental disorder is seeking for mental health care. This issue is of crucial importance in traumatized refugee families. As a consequence, it is generally preferred using professional interpreters. It has been shown that professional translation improves the quality of treatment and patients' satisfaction with treatment [64].

Therefore, the work with psychologically trained interpreters is of great importance. Culture brokers or cultural mediators may provide an insight into different cultures and enable clinicians to provide better and more acceptable services [24]. In a European expert Delphi study, it was shown that the adequate use of interpreters constitutes the most important factor of influence for the provision of high-quality mental health care [65].

Psychiatrists and other mental health professionals should develop conceptual models, skills and experience for conducting cross-language interviews by the use of interpreters [66]. Tribe [67] describes four modes of interpreting as psychotherapeutic or constructionist, linguistic, advocate or adversarial/community and cultural broker/bicultural. It is helpful to know which model is being used and that sometimes interpreters may hold back information if they feel that sharing something may bring disrepute to the culture [24].

Three challenging issues were pointed out with regard to intercultural clinical settings with interpreters: (1) the vital role of interpreters for the diagnostic process, (2) difficulties to establish confidence and (3) a higher risk for marginalization [68].

7.5 Cultural Competence Basic Components at the Policy-Maker Level

7.5.1 Working on Intercultural Barriers

A key barrier for immigrants could often be inadequate legal entitlements [69]. Sometimes these barriers are mistakenly attributed to cultural differences and misunderstandings, and the term culture may be used as a putative politically correct expression reifying social differences and neglecting discrimination [70]. It is also helpful to recall that institutions have their own cultures which can produce barriers of various kinds, and minority groups may well face strongest barriers to health-care access [38, 39, 61]. Inequitable variation in the use and accessibility of health-care services for immigrants, indigenous populations and other minorities in EU countries remains a matter of concern for both health-care providers and policy-makers as variations in health-care usage between majority and minority populations have been noted [65]. Responsiveness to diversity is being recommended in European countries to improve access and quality of care for minority populations [71–75]. A study conducted in Italy showed that migrants' pathways to psychiatric services vary across cities. Particularly, social services were important sources of migrants' referrals for services providing cultural competent consultation-liaison activities [13]. With regard to massive disparities in the provision of adequate mental health care to refugees and asylum seekers with emotional distress or mental disorders in Europe, the European Psychiatric Association (EPA) established a task force working on this issue. Health-care providers have an obligation and responsibility to ensure that all service users irrespective of their background get highest quality services according to their needs [24].

Focusing on cultural competency, we believe that the recommendations listed in Table 7.1 will help.

Table 7.1 Recommendations for cultural competence implementation

Service providers
• The service providers must initiate a culture change within the institutions to make services culturally accessible and sensitive • Training all staff in cultural competency, cultural empathy and cultural sensitivity is an absolute must • Regular additional training must be part of continuous professional development for all staff members • Providers may consider the likelihood of employing culture brokers or cultural mediators which will benefit both the clinical team and the local communities • Regular cross-cultural supervision must be made available directly or using tele-psychiatry • Culturally sensitive services such as food and physical spaces be made available if relevant • Health education as well as prevention and mental health promotion must be a part of the overall services targeting minority groups • Information for immigrants by means of pamphlets in their preferred languages must be easily accessible and available • The institutions should consider having a nominated lead clinician responsible for cultural competency training and delivery • Qualified interpreters should be available for patients not mastering the language of the host country
Clinicians
• Training and ongoing education for all mental health professionals in understanding diagnosis, illness behaviours and culturally sensitive interventions must be mandatory when needed • Ensuring quality standards for expert court opinions for minority groups in the context of criminal, civil and social law is available and employed in relevant settings • Depending upon the needs of the local community, appropriate knowledge about culture-based medicine, culture-specific, illness-specific and migration-specific aspects should be offered to mental health professionals • Information for minority groups in their preferred languages about their rights, psychiatric disorders and treatment options must be made available • Cultural psychiatry should be an integral part of all curricula from undergraduate levels to continuing professional development • Specific research dealing with the needs of minority groups must be encouraged and appropriately funded
Policy-makers
• Policy-makers must take a lead on ensuring that clear messages on equality and diversity are enshrined in law with non-discriminatory health policies • Mandatory policies should cover all minority groups • More quantitative and qualitative research on aetiological factors, interventions and outcomes must be part of setting up services • Integrated services should be the preferred norm with culturally specific resources allocated according to patients' needs

Adapted from EPA guidance on cultural competence training [24]

7.6 Several Experiences on Somatizations Among Immigrants in Europe

Since 2007, a group of clinicians and researchers within the scientific network of the European Association of Psychosomatic Medicine (EAPM, former EACLPP) started sharing their common interest and curiosity about the mental health of migrants [24]. Common ideas and experiences as well as specificities and differences deriving from different sociocultural contexts and organizations of health-care provision were discussed, also by means of scientific symposia offered during the EAPM meetings. The group progressively acquired a more stable and formal structure culminating in the formal institution of the Cultural CLP Special Interest Group (SIG), in 2010, that aims at promoting multinational exchange of experience and inspiring clinical and research projects at the interface of cultural and CL psychiatry and psychosomatics. The members of the SIG are involved in research projects addressing different sub-items and presentations of mental health of migrants [76–84]. These previous experiences were relevant as they suggested what the best further objectives for the SIG should be. The SIG has proved to be a useful forum where to discuss transcultural issues, exchange experiences in establishing mental health services for migrant patients in different European countries, be able to advice others on training, share and disseminate research findings and promote high standard of practice. We briefly present here some example of researches and clinical experiences in Europe.

7.6.1 Somatization Among Migrants at the Bologna Transcultural Psychiatry Team, Bologna, Italy

The Bologna Transcultural Psychosomatic Team (BoTPT) [85] of the Bologna University works together with the local community mental health service [85]. The BoTPT is a multidisciplinary study and research centre of the Department of Medical and Surgical Sciences—Bologna University. The team provides consultations in partnership with the Department of Mental Health of Bologna designed to identify the mental and psychosocial needs of migrants and to direct them to appropriate services. The consultation includes psychiatrists, researchers, psychologists, medical doctors, students, psychiatry registrars and medical anthropologists, and if needed, a cultural mediator joins the team [85]. In addition, the BoTPT delivers training and support activities to informal carers, general practitioners, psychiatrists and mental health operators, social workers, medical students and psychiatric trainees. Training is specially directed to social and voluntary workers working with asylum seekers and traumatized immigrants [86].

A clinical survey and a 6-month follow-up were carried out on immigrants who consecutively attended the Bologna West Community Mental Health Centre between 1 July 1999 and 31 December 2007. An ad hoc schedule collecting socio-demographic, clinical and health service utilization data was specifically designed and adopted. Moreover, at the end of the first visit, the psychiatrists filled out sections 4 and 5 of the *Manual for the Assessment and Documentation of Psychopathology* (AMDP-SYSTEM) [87, 88]. Psychiatric diagnosis was provided according to ICD-10 criteria and confirmed by the Schedule for Clinical Assessment of Neuropsychiatry (SCAN) [89]. According to their birth area, patients were grouped under Maghreb, Sub-Saharan Africa, Asia, Eastern Europe and Central or South America. Following the AMDP structure, psychopathological items were grouped under three psychopathological syndromes: depressive, paranoid-hallucinatory and apathy syndromes [90, 91]; somatic items (nausea, breathing difficulties, dizziness, palpitations, cardiac pain, increased sweating, headache, hot flashes) were grouped together into the psychopathological definition of non-delusional hypochondria and autonomic syndrome [91]. The AMDP already showed good reliability and validity in samples of migrants [92].

Of the 180 migrant patients referred to BoTPT, 159 needed psychiatric care. Most of those patients came from North Africa (29%) and Sub-Saharan Africa (26%). At baseline, higher somatic scores were shown by Asian migrants (1.9 ± 3.6 vs. 1 ± 1.8, $p = 0.1$), workers (1.6 ± 2.9 vs. 1 ± 1.9, $p = 0.005$) and patients referred by GPs (2.1 ± 2.8 vs. 1.1 ± 2.3, $p = 0.06$). Somatization appeared to cut across the discrete categories of ICD-10: 40% of patients with anxiety or adjustment and 30% of patients with mood or psychotic disorders showed at least one somatic complain. At 6-month follow-up, a significant improvement of somatization without differences among ethnic or socio-demographic groups was found. Differences in levels of somatization severity persisted among ethnic groups (higher score for Asian migrants).

Functional somatic symptoms showed high prevalence in all diagnostic groups. Somatization severity at the baseline appeared to be related to pathways to care and socio-demographic features, as well as cultural/ethnic background. The BoTPT multidisciplinary approach showed transcultural effectiveness on reducing somatization severity.

7.6.2 Somatization and Self-Harm Behaviours in Migrants: The Experience in Modena, Italy

As the wave of immigration progressively increased in the last 20 years across Italy, health-care services had to adapt and react accordingly. Among the various expressions of this adaptation, there was, in the province of Modena, the institution of a transdisciplinary clinical group, within the local Department of Mental Health, dedicated to mental health of the immigrants as well as many research activities on this topic promoted by the psychiatry section of the University of Modena and Reggio Emilia.

One of these researches explored the differences between natives and foreigners, in a general population sample, regarding the prevalence and the clinical features of somatic symptoms, and analysed possible explanatory factors. After recruiting subjects in both public places and by a mail survey sent by GPs, somatic symptoms were assessed by means of the Bradford Somatic Inventory, short version (BSI-21), a self-administered questionnaire, created and validated to be used cross-culturally [93, 94]. BSI-21 mean scores and positive cases (subjects above the cut-off of probable mental disorder) were compared, and confounding and explanatory variables tested with logistic regression model. A sample of 229 Italians and 193 immigrants was recruited. Immigrants had a higher BSI-21 mean score (8.02 vs. 5.64, $p = 0.004$) and more positive cases (19.4% vs. 6.6%, $p < 0.001$). Differences were explained by adjustment for satisfaction about oneself and about relationship with Italians, presence of spouse and for reporting as cause of symptoms, poverty, the condition of foreigner, separation from friends and relatives or job (aOR = 1.11, 95% CI 0.48–2.57). This preliminary project suggested that immigrants from low-income countries, independently by origin, experienced more non-organic somatic symptoms than natives, and this seemed to be primarily due to their precarious social conditions and adaptation problems.

Self-harm behaviours among migrants were also felt as a major topic of investigation. At this regard, a retrospective analysis of migrants committing not lethal self-harm behaviours referred to psychiatric consultation at the local A&E department vs. completed (lethal) suicides recorded in the database of the Modena Forensic Medicine Service was conducted. Migrants with self-harm behaviours were 34% (102/297), whereas completed suicides of migrants were 5% (7/122). More recently, one research project was developed to study self-harm behaviours among migrants in jail and impulsivity and trauma as possible associated factors. A prospective cohort study was designed, which assessed 54 migrants (M = 96.3%, mean age 32.5 ± 8.68 years) recently admitted to the local jail for different crimes. At admission, subjects underwent a diagnostic assessment and were asked to fill in three psychometric instruments: the Jail Screening Assessment Tool [95], the LiMEs (List of Migration Experiences) [96] and the Barratt Impulsiveness Scale (BIT-11) [97]. After a 3-month follow-up, incidence of self-harm behaviours was calculated and analysed according to baseline data. According to the LiMEs, the prevalence of exposure to trauma related to war or conflict, in the premigration phase, was of 32.1%. The prevalence of trauma suffered by relatives and worries about the safety of relatives, in the post-migration phase, was 77.4%. The 72.2% of the initial sample was available for follow-up after 3 months, and nine subjects (16% of the initial sample) had presented self-harm behaviours in the meanwhile. A statistically significant association was found between self-harm behaviours and exposure to trauma related to war/conflict before migration or exposure to worries about trauma for family members.

7.6.3 From Epidemiology to Intervention in Somatization: A Brief Report from Manchester, UK

People of Pakistani origin form the largest ethnic minority group in Manchester. Evidence from earlier research shows high rates of distress in Pakistani Muslims [80, 81]. Higher rates of depression and anxiety in British Indians and Pakistanis as compared to the larger white population and higher rates of presentations with physical complaints have been reported in various works of research, although there has been contrasting evidence from other works of research [82] underlining the need for further analysis. A study was therefore conducted in Manchester, looking at rates of depression and access to primary care among people of Pakistani origin vs. white Europeans [83].

Cross-sectional population-based survey, followed by a prospective cohort study of depressed subjects, was conducted in order to determine whether the consultations were for somatic or psychological presentations and a description of GPs' interventions. In the first phase, patients were assessed with the Self-Reporting Questionnaire (SRQ) [98]. The SRQ has been successfully used in the Pakistani Muslim population and has shown good sensitivity and specificity for this group. In the second phase, all high scorers (score of 7 or more on SRQ) and a 1 in 4 sample of low scorers were contacted for an interview using the Schedule for Clinical Assessment in Neuropsychiatry (SCAN) to assess whether subjects met the criteria for either ICD-10 or DSM-IV depressive disorders [99]. A pain picture where the respondents were asked to mark any site where they would have experienced pain that lasted for more than a day in the previous 30 days was also used. Using the general practitioners' case notes, all consultations in primary care for 1 year prior to the 6-month follow-up were identified. All instruments were translated into Urdu, and these were reviewed by a bilingual focus group of mental health specialists and lay people according to a standard procedure [99].

Rates of depression were higher in women of Pakistani origin compared to white European women. There was no difference in somatic scores on the SRQ between the two ethnic groups whether depressed or nondepressed. Nor was there any difference in the psychological scores on the SRQ or on the pain scores or levels of distress. The correlation between total SRQ scores and pain was also exactly the same in the two groups. However, people of Pakistani origin had more frequent visits with their GPs for bodily symptoms. Although the prevalence of depression was significantly higher in the Pakistani population and there was no difference in symptoms of anxiety and depression presentations to the GPs in the two groups, people of Pakistani origin were less likely to be prescribed antidepressants and were less likely to be offered psychotherapy compared to the white European group.

The workgroup in Manchester is also currently working on the development of a culturally appropriate guidance on the delivery of cognitive behavioural therapy (CBT) for use with British South Asian women with medically unexplained symptoms. The guidance will include a manual, training programme and referral mechanism. It will be evidence-based and developed in partnership with service users. This is preliminary to an exploratory controlled trial of a ten-session, CBT-based, culturally adapted psychological intervention, which will focus on understanding the participant's model of illness, discussing physical manifestations of an existing mental state, modification of illness behaviour, cognitive restructuring to address dysfunctional cognitions and improving interpersonal relationships.

7.6.4 Social and Cultural Factors Affecting Physical and Psychosocial Wellbeing in Hospitalized Migrants in Barcelona, Spain ADIL

In Barcelona, in a sample of Latin American immigrants admitted in a general hospital, a study exploring the relationship between acculturation, social integration and social context with psychosocial and physical wellbeing was performed. Specifically, the focus is to explore the degree to which one or another acculturation strategy was more or less related to psychosocial and physical wellbeing and to see if that relationship was mitigated by acculturative stress.

The sample consisted of 290 Latin American immigrants who sought medical attention in a tertiary care hospital in Barcelona. Somatization was registered using the somatic symptoms subscale of the Patient Health Questionnaire (PHQ). Information about the patients' clinical outcomes, socio-demographic details, acculturative stress, social adaptation and legal status, anxiety and depression levels, acculturation and perceived stress was gathered.

The study revealed that acculturative stress and social integration (i.e. language, basic needs covered and legal status) play an important role in the psychosocial and physical wellbeing of the patient. Furthermore, none of the acculturative strategies appeared to be related to an improvement in psychosocial or physical wellbeing. Immigrants with higher levels of social support presented fewer symptoms of depression. After controlling for perceived stress, clinical outcomes and anxiety, legal status was the most predictive social integration variable for physical wellbeing (measured as somatization).

In conclusion, although culture may play an important role in somatic expression of distress, barriers to achieving immigration goals, or what could be considered strong stressors, seem to be what increase somatization.

7.6.5 Somatic and Depressive Symptom Variation in First-Generation Vietnamese and Native German Patients in a CL-Psychiatric Outpatient Clinic in Berlin, Germany

Vietnamese migrants are the largest group of immigrants from East Asia in Germany, and in Berlin they constitute the seventh largest immigrant group. In comparison to larger migrant groups, mental health-care utilization by first-generation (FG) Vietnamese migrants in Germany has been very low, and studies on symptom presentation and somatization in depression in Vietnamese immigrants were completely lacking. On the one hand, the Berlin working group aims to improve psychiatric and psychosomatic treatment facilities for Vietnamese migrants in Berlin [84]; on the other hand, these clinical activities are accompanied by research projects to study the complexity of migration processes and mental health [100].

A study that aims at exploring whether first-access FG Vietnamese CLP outpatients had a tendency to present more somatic symptoms and less psychological symptoms in depression and whether only a subset of symptoms was responsible for differences in the somatic or depressive symptom scores was reported [101].

All patients were simultaneously assessed with a semi-structured clinical interview according to DSM-IV by a team of native Vietnamese psychiatrists and a German psychiatrist. Psychological or affective symptoms of depression were assessed by the depression scale of the Patient Health Questionnaire (PHQ-9), and somatic symptoms were assessed by the somatic symptom scale of the PHQ-15. Both PHQ scales were presented in either German language or as a translated Vietnamese version, as appropriate. PHQ assessments of Vietnamese patients were further validated for understanding with a native Vietnamese psychiatrist. To minimize possible confounders, only patients who met DSM-IV criteria for major depressive episode (MDE) were included in the study. First-access German outpatients at the same outpatient clinic were matched for age, gender and clinical diagnosis of MDE.

A sample of 110 first-generation migrant Vietnamese patients and 109 native German outpatients was included. While no significant differences on the total score of the PHQ-9 between both groups were found, FG Vietnamese outpatients had an overall significant and markedly higher score on the somatic symptom scale PHQ-15. When analysing single somatic items, FG Vietnamese outpatients were significantly more likely to report somatic symptoms of headache, chest pain, dizziness and fainting than the native-born group. There was a trend towards higher scores on the item from the depression scale (PHQ-9): "moving or speaking so slowly that other people could have noticed" in Vietnamese outpatients, which might reflect a tendency to external orientation, as reported in other East Asian samples.

Depressed Vietnamese outpatients reported psychological symptoms at similar levels of severity or at a single item level as matched native German outpatients. That was in contrast to the first hypothesis that stated that native German depressed outpatients were more likely to report psychological symptoms. Confirming the second hypothesis, depressed Vietnamese outpatients had a higher total score for somatic symptoms using the PHQ-15. Emphasis on certain somatic symptoms does not reflect a minimization of depressive symptoms in FG Vietnamese immigrant outpatients. Limited language proficiency was shown to be linked to higher somatic symptom reporting. Cultural differences in somatization should be interpreted in the context of culturally shaped and migration-related experiences of help-seeking behaviour, also related to pathways to care.

7.7 Conclusions and Implication for Psychosomatic Medicine

With increasing globalization, there is an urgent need of adequate diagnoses and treatment strategies for patients with a migration background. Migrants and ethnic minorities show a higher prevalence of mental disorders when compared to natives or fellow countrymen without migratory experiences. Thus, it is very important for clinicians and mental health-care specialists to be aware of the wider determinants of the mental health of immigrants and to be trained in cultural competence. If a health-care system wants to increase its cultural competence, it needs to value diversity, be able to assess itself culturally, be aware of how cultures interact, incorporate and institutionalize cultural knowledge and adjust service delivery in order to understand and be aware of diversity between and within cultures.

A multidisciplinary and bio-psycho-social-cultural approach to illness is pivotal in the understanding of complexity and may promote cross-cultural effectiveness in detecting and adequately managing symptoms of somatization among migrants.

References

1. Fung K, Lo HT, Srivastava R, Andermann L. Organizational cultural competenceconsultation to a mental health institution. Transcult Psychiatry. 2012;49(2):165–84.
2. Mahoney JS, Carlson E, Engebretson JC. A framework for cultural competence in advanced practice psychiatric and mental health education. Perspect Psychiatr Care. 2006;42(4):227–37.
3. Bhugra D, Gupta S, Bhui K, Craig T, Dogra N, Ingleby JD, et al. WPA guidance on mental health and mental health care in migrants. World Psychiatry. 2011;10(1):2–10.
4. Bhui K, Warfa N, Edonya P, McKenzie K, Bhugra D. Cultural competence in mental health care: a review of model evaluations. BMC Health Serv Res. 2007;7:15.
5. Brach C, Fraser I. Can cultural competency reduce racial and ethnic health disparities? A review and conceptual model. Med Care Res Rev. 2000;57:181–217.
6. Johnsen BH, Meeùs P, Meling J, Rogde T, Eid J, Esepevik R, et al. Cultural differences in emotional intelligence among top officers on board merchant ships. Int Marit Health. 2012;63(2):90–5.
7. Andresen J. Cultural competence and health care: Japanese, Korean, and Indian patients in the United States. J Cult Divers. 2001;8(4):109–21.
8. Flores G. Culture and the patient-physician relationship: achieving cultural competency in health care. J Pediatr. 2000;136(1):14–23.
9. Siegel CE, Wanderling J, Haugland G, Laska EM, Case BG. Access to and use of non-inpatient services in New York State among racial-ethnic groups. Psychiatr Serv. 2013;64(2):156–64.
10. Tarricone I, Mimmi S, Paparelli A, Rossi E, Mori E, Panigada S, et al. First episode psychosis at the West Bologna Community Mental Health Centre: results of an 8-year prospective study. Psychol Med. 2012;42(11):2255–64.
11. Warren BJ. How culture is assessed in the DSM-5. J Psychosoc Nurs Ment Health Serv. 2013;51(4):40–5.
12. Ferrari S, Burian R, Hahn E, Chaudhry N, Chaudhry IB, Husain N, Ta TM, Diefenbacher A, Qureshi A, Berardi D, Braca M, Tarricone I. Somatization among ethnic minorities and immigrants: why does it matter to Consultation Liaison Psychiatry? J Psychosom Res. 2015;79(1):85–6.
13. Tarricone I, Stivanello E, Poggi F, Castorini V, Marseglia MV, Fantini MP, et al. Ethnic variation in the prevalence of depression and anxiety in primary care: a systematic review and meta-analysis. Psychiatry Res. 2012;195:91–106.
14. Commander MJ, Dharan SP, Odell SM, Surtees PG. Access tomental health care in an inner-city health district. II: association with demographic factors. Br J Psychiatry. 1997;170:317–20.
15. Borowsky SJ, Rubenstein LV, Meredith LS, Camp P, Jackson-Triche M, Wells KB. Who is at risk of nondetection of mental health problems in primary care? J Gen Intern Med. 2000;15:381–8.
16. Husain N, Waheed W, Tomenson B, Creed F. The validation of personal health questionnaire amongst people of Pakistani family origin living in the United Kingdom. J Affect Disord. 2007;97:261–4.

17. Gillam SJ, Jarman B, White P, Law R. Ethnic differences in consultation rates in urban general practice. BMJ. 1989;299:953–7.
18. Bhui K, Bhugra D, Goldberg D, Sauer J, Tylee A. Assessing the prevalence of depression in Punjabi and English primary care attenders: the role of culture, physical illness and somatic symptoms. Transcult Psychiatry. 2004;41:307–22.
19. Cornwell J, Hull S. Do GPs prescribe antidepressants differently for South Asian patients? Fam Pract. 1998;15:S16–8.
20. Melfi CA, Croghan TW, Hanna MP, Robinson RL. Racial variation in antidepressant treatment in a Medicaid population. J Clin Psychiatry. 2000;61:16–21.
21. Hull SA, Cornwell J, Harvey C, Eldridge S, Bare PO. Prescribing rates for psychotropic medication amongst east London general practices: low rates where Asian populations are greatest. Fam Pract. 2001;18:167–73.
22. Padgett DK, Patrick C, Burns BJ, Schlesinger HJ. Ethnicity and the use of outpatient mental health services in a national insured population. Am J Public Health. 1994;84:222–6.
23. Zhang M, Booth BM, Smith GR. Services utilization before and after the prospective payment system by patients with somatization disorder. J Behav Health Serv Res. 1998;25:76–82.
24. Schouler-Ocak M, Graef-Calliess IT, Tarricone I, Qureshi A, Kastrup MC, Bhugra D. EPA guidance on cultural competence training. Eur Psychiatry. 2015;30(3):431–40. https://doi.org/10.1016/j.eurpsy.2015.01.012.
25. Betancourt JR, Green AR, Carrillo JE, et al. Cultural competence and health care disparities: key perspectives and trends. Health Aff. 2005;24:499–505.
26. Mendez JL, Westerberg D. Implementation of a culturally adapted treatment to reduce barriers for Latino parents. Cultur Divers Ethnic Minor Psychol. 2012;18(4):363–72.
27. Qureshi A, Collazos F, Ramos M, Casas M. Cultural competency training in psychiatry. Eur Psychiatry. 2008;23(1):49–58.
28. Vega WA. Higher stakes ahead for cultural competence. Gen Hosp Psychiatry. 2005;27(6):446–50.
29. Yamada AM, Brekke JS. Addressing mental health disparities through clinical competence not just cultural competence: the need for assessment of sociocultural issues in the delivery of evidence-based psychosocial rehabilitation services. Clin Psychol Rev. 2008;28(8):1386–99.
30. Hornberger JC, Gibson CD Jr, Wood W, Dequeldre C, Corso I, Palla B, et al. Eliminating language barriers for non-English-speaking patients. Med Care. 1996;34(8):845–56.
31. Samu KS, Suaalii-Sauni T. Exploring the 'cultural' in cultural competencies in Pacific mental health. Pac Health Dialog. 2009;15(1):120–30.
32. Schouler-Ocak M, Reiske S-L, Rapp M, Heinz A. Cultural Factors in the diagnosis and treatment of traumatised migrant patients from Turkey. Transcult Psychiatry. 2008;45(4):652–70.
33. Vardar A, Kluge U, Penka S. How to express mental health problems—Turkish immigrants in Berlin compared to native Germans in Berlin and Turks in Istanbul. Eur Psychiatry. 2012;27(2):S50–6.
34. Williams MT, Domanico J, Marques L, Leblanc NJ, Turkheimer E. Barriers to treatment among African Americans with obsessive-compulsive disorder. J Anxiety Disord. 2012;26(4):555–63.
35. Bhugra D, Gupta S, Schouler-Ocak M, Graeff-Calliess I, Deakin NA, Qureshi A, et al. EPA guidance mental health care of migrants. Eur Psychiatry. 2014;29(2):107–15.
36. Bhui K, Abdi A, Abdi M, Pereira S, Dualeh M, Robertson D, et al. Traumatic events, migration characteristics and psychiatric symptoms among Somali refugees-preliminary communication. Soc Psychiatry Psychiatr Epidemiol. 2003;38(1):35–43.
37. Lederbogen F, et al. City living and urban upbringing affect neural social stress processing in humans. Nature. 2011;474:498–501.
38. Kim SP. Culture and child and adolescent psychiatry. In: Tseng WS, Streltzer J, editors. Cultural competence in clinical psychiatry. Arlington: American Psychiatric Publishing, Inc.; 2004.
39. Tseng WS, Streltzer J. Cultural competence in health care. A guide for professionals. New York: Springer Science + Business Media, LLC; 2008.

40. Kirmayer LJ. Rethinking cultural competence. Transcult Psychiatry. 2012;49(2):149–64.
41. Kleinman A, Benson P. Anthropology in the clinic: the problem of cultural competency and how to fix it. PLoS Med. 2006;3(10):e294.
42. Neelam K, Duddu V, Chaudhry IB, Antonysamy AS, Husain N. A survey of British senior psychiatry trainees' ethnocultural personal values. Acad Psychiatry. 2009;33(5):423–6.
43. Shaw SJ, Armin J. The ethical self-fashioning of physicians and health care systems in culturally appropriate health care. Cult Med Psychiatry. 2011;35(2):236–61.
44. Brannigan MC. Connecting the dots in cultural competency: institutional strategies and conceptual caveats. Camb Q Health Ethics. 2008;17(2):173–84.
45. Gregory H Jr, Van Orden O, Jordan L, Portnoy GA, Welsh E, Betkowski J, et al. New directions in capacity building: incorporating cultural competence into the interactive systems framework. Am J Community Psychol. 2012;50(3–4):321–33.
46. Penka S, Kluge U, Vardar A, Borde T, Ingleby D. The concept of "intercultural opening": the development of an assessment tool for the appraisal of its current implementation in the mental health care system. Eur Psychiatry. 2012;27(2):S63–9.
47. Cross T, Bazon B, Isaacs M. Towards a culturally competent system of care, volume I. Washington, DC: Georgetown University Child Development Center, CASSP Technical Assitance Center; 1989.
48. Kastrup M. Staff competence in dealing with traditional approaches. Eur Psychiatry. 2008;23(1):59–68.
49. Hoke MM, Robbins LK. Continuing the cultural competency journey through exploration of knowledge, attitudes, and skills with advanced practice psychiatric nursing students: an exemplar. Nurs Clin North Am. 2011;46(2):201–5.
50. Tervalon M, Murray-García J. Cultural humility versus cultural competence: a critical distinction in defining physician training outcomes in multicultural education. J Health Care Poor Underserved. 1998;9(2):117–25.
51. Dastjerdi M. The case of Iranian immigrants in the greater Toronto area: a qualitative study. Int J Equity Health. 2012;11:9.
52. Harris TL, McQuery J, Raab B, Elmore S. Multicultural psychiatric education: using the DSM-IV-TR Outline for Cultural Formulation to improve resident cultural competence. Acad Psychiatry. 2008;32(4):306–12.
53. Rechel B, Mladovsky P, Ingleby D, Mackenbach JP, McKee M. Migration and health in an increasingly diverse Europe. Lancet. 2013;381(9873):1235–45.
54. Kirmayer LJ. Cultural competence and evidence-based practice in mental health: epistemic communities and the politics of pluralism. Soc Sci Med. 2012;75:249–56.
55. Kirmayer LJ, Fung K, Rousseau C, Lo HT, Menzies P, Guzder J, et al. Guidelines for training in cultural psychiatry—position paper. Can J Psychiatr. 2012;57(3):1–17.
56. Cattacin S, Chimienti M et al. Difference sensitivity in the field of migration and health. National policies compared. Geneva: Working Paper No. 1 of the Department of sociology of the University of Geneva; 2007.
57. Chiarenza A. Developments in the concept of cultural competence. In: Ingleby D, Chiarenza A, Devillé W, Kotsioni I, editors. Inequalities in health care for migrants and ethnic minorities. Antwerp: Garant; 2012. p. 66–81.
58. Morawska A, Fletcher R, Pope S, Heathwood E, Anderson E, McAuliffe C. Evaluation of mental health first aid training in a diverse community setting. Int J Ment Health Nurs. 2013;22(1):85–92.
59. Sue S, Zane N. The role of culture and cultural techniques in psychotherapy. A critique and reformulation. Am Psychol. 1987;42(1):37–45.
60. Schouler-Ocak M, Bretz HJ, Penka S, Koch E, Hartkamp N, Siefen RG, et al. Patients of immigrant origin in inpatient psychiatric facilities. Eur Psychiatry. 2008;23(Suppl 1):S21–7.
61. Rucci P, Piazza A, Perrone E, Tarricone I, Maisto R, Donegani I, et al. Disparities in mental health care provision to immigrants with severe mental illness in Italy. Epidemiol Psychiatr Sci. 2014;30:1–11.

62. Griner D, Smith TB. Culturally adapted mental health intervention: a meta-analytic review. Psychotherapy (Chic). 2006;43(4):531–48.
63. Kleinman A. Major conceptual and research issues for cultural (anthropological) psychiatry. Cult Med Psychiatry. 1980;4(1):3–23.
64. Bauer AM, Alegría M. Impact of patient language proficiency and interpreter service use on the quality of psychiatric care: a systematic review. Psychiatr Serv. 2010;61(8):765–73.
65. Devillé W, Greacen T, Bogic M, Dauvrin M, Dias S, Gaddini A, Koitzsch Jensen N, Karamanidou C, Kluge U, Mertaniemi R, Puigpinos I, Riera R, Sárváry A, Soares JJF, Stankunas M, Strassmayr C, Welbel M, Priebe S. Health care for immigrants in Europe: is there still consensus among country experts about principles of good practice? A Delphi study. BMC Public Health. 2011;11:699.
66. Westermeyer J. Working with an interpreter in psychiatric assessment and treatment. J Nerv Ment Dis. 1990;178(12):745–9.
67. Tribe R. Bridging the gap or damming the flow? Some observations on using interpreters/bicultural workers when working with refugee clients, many of whom have been tortured. Br J Med Psychol. 1999;72(Pt4):567–76.
68. Sandhu S, Bjerre NV, Dauvrin M, Dias S, Gaddini A, Greacen T, Ioannidis E, Kluge U, Jensen NK, Lamkaddem M, Puigpinós I, Riera R, Kósa Z, Wihlman U, Stankunas M, Straßmayr C, Wahlbeck K, Welbel M, Priebe S. Experiences with treating immigrants: a qualitative study in mental health services across 16 European countries. Soc Psychiatry Psychiatr Epidemiol. 2013;48(1):105–16.
69. Pace P. The right to health of migrants in Europe. In: Rechel B, Mladovsky P, Devillé W, Rijks B, Petrova-Benedict R, McKee M, editors. Migration andhealth in the European Union. Maidenhead: Open University Press; 2011. p. 55–66.
70. Heinz A, Kluge U. Mental health in different groups of migrants and ethnic minority within Europe and beyond: regional and cross-national challenges and approaches in research, practice and training. Eur Psychiatry. 2012;27(2):S1–3.
71. Butow PN, Aldridge L, Bell ML, Sze M, Eisenbruch M, Jefford M, et al. Inferior health-related quality of life and psychological well-being in immigrant cancer survivors: a population-based study. Eur J Cancer. 2013;49(8):1948–56.
72. Chiarenza A, Robinson J, Spilker R, HPH TF MFCCH Task Force on Migrant Friendly, Culturally Competent Health Care. Developing standards for assessing equity of access, quality of health care for migrants, other vulnerable groups. Workshop of the Task Force MFCCH. Turku: International HPH Conference; 2011 June 1–3.
73. Kleinman A. Epilogue. Mental health in different groups of migrants and ethnic minority in Europe and beyond. Eur Psychiatry. 2012;27(2):S81–2.
74. Laban CJ, Komproe IH, Gernaat HB, JT DJ. The impact of a long asylum procedure on quality of life, disability and physical health in Iraqi asylum seekers in the Netherlands. Soc Psychiatry Psychiatr Epidemiol. 2008;43:507–15.
75. Wilson M, MacCarthy B. GP consultation as a factor in the low rate of mental health service use by Asians. Psychol Med. 1994;24:113–9.
76. Tarricone I, Atti AR, Salvatori F, Braca M, Ferrari S, Malmusi D, Berardi D. Psychotic symptoms and general health in a socially disadvantaged migrant community in Bologna. Int J Soc Psychiatry. 2009;55(3):203–13.
77. Tarricone I, Stivanello E, Ferrari S, Colombini N, Bolla E, Braca M, et al. Migrant pathways to community mental health centres in Italy. Int J Soc Psychiatry. 2012;58:505–11.
78. Tarricone I, Atti AR, Braca M, Pompei G, Morri M, Poggi F, et al. Migrants referring to the Bologna Transcultural Psychiatric Team: reasons for drop-out. Int J Soc Psychiatry. 2011;57:627–30.
79. Tarricone I, Braca M, Allegri F, Barrasso G, Bellomo A, Berlincioni V, Carpiniello B, Ceregato A, Conforti Donati M, Defilippi S, Del Vecchio V, De Rosa C, Ferrannini L, Ferrari S, Furio MA, Gramaglia C, La Cascia C, Luciano M, Mulè A, Nardini M, Podavini F, Primavera D, Reggianini C, Rigatelli M, Todarello O, Turella E, Ventriglio A, Zeppegno P, Fiorillo A, Berardi D. First-episode psychosis and migration in Italy

(PEP-Ita migration): a study in the Italian mental health services. BMC Psychiatry. 2014;14(1):186.
80. Husain N, Creed F, Tomenson B. Adverse social circumstances and depression in people of Pakistani origin in the UK. Br J Psychiatry. 1997;171:434–8.
81. Creed F, Winterbottom M, Tomenson B, Britt R, Anand IS, Wander GS, et al. Preliminary study of non-psychotic disorders in people fromthe Indian subcontinent living in the UK and India. Acta Psychiatr Scand. 1999;99:257–60.
82. Duddu V, Husain N, Dickens C. Medically unexplained presentations and quality of life: a study of a predominantly South Asian primary care population in England. J Psychosom Res. 2008;65:311–7.
83. Gater R, Tomenson B, Percival C, Chaudhry N, Waheed W, Dunn G, et al. Persistent depressive disorders and social stress in people of Pakistani origin and white Europeans in UK. Soc Psychiatry Psychiatr Epidemiol. 2009;44:198–207.
84. Ta TM, Neuhaus AH, Burian R, Schomerus G, von Poser A, Diefenbacher A, et al. Mental health care utilization of first generation Vietnamese migrants in Germany. Psychiatr Prax. 2015;42(5):267–73.
85. Griffiths G, Tarricone I, Berardi D, Donegani I, Fioritti A, Maisto R, Braca M, Menchetti M, Tonti L, Nolet M, Piazza A, Spigonardo V. The provision of mental health services to immigrants and refugees in Italy: the barriers and facilitating factors experienced by mental health workers. J Psychopathol. 2017;23(2):79–86.
86. Tarricone I, Mencacci E, Braca M, Salvatori F, Di Marco S, Nolet M, Storbini V, Berardi D. Work of the Bologna Transcultural Psychiatric Team (BoTPT) with refugees and asylum seekers: when remembering helps. J Psychopathol. 2013;19(3):234–41.
87. Conti, L., Dell'Osso, L. & Cassano, G.B. (1990) Il sistema AMDP. Manuale per la valutazione e la documentazione della psicopatologia. Milano: Edizioni Grafiche Mazzucchelli.
88. Arbeitsgemeinschaft fur Methodik und Dokumentation in der Psychiatrie. Das MDP-System (3 Auflage). Manual zur Dokumentation psychiatrischer Befunde. Berlin: Springer;1979.
89. Schedule for clinical assessment of neuropsychiatry, version 2.1. Geneva: World Health Organization, Division of Mental Health; 1998.
90. Pietzcker A, Gebhardt R. Depressive syndromes and scales in the AMDP-system. Acta Psychiatr Scand. 1983;310:65–84.
91. Pietzcker A, Gebhardt R, Strauss A, Stockel M, Langer C, Freudenthal K. The syndrome scales in the AMDP-system. Mod Probl Pharmacopsychiatry. 1983;20:88–99.
92. Diefenbacher A, Heim G. Somatic symptoms in Turkish and German depressed patients. Psychosom Med. 1994;56:551–6.
93. Mumford DB, Bavington JT, Bhatnagar KS, Hussain Y, Mirza S, Naraghi MM. The Bradford Somatic Inventory. A multi-ethnic inventory of somatic symptoms reported by anxious and depressed patients in Britain and the Indo-Pakistan subcontinent. Br J Psychiatry. 1991;158:379–86.
94. Mumford DB, Tareen IA, Bhatti MR, Bajwa MA, Ayub M, Pervaiz T. An investigation of 'functional' somatic symptoms among patients attending hospital medical clinics in Pakistan—II. Using somatic symptoms to identify patients with psychiatric disorders. J Psychosom Res. 1991;35(2–3):257–64.
95. Nicholls TL, Ronald R, Olley MC, Ogloff JRP, Hemphill F. Jail Screening Assessment Tool (JSAT), manuale e libretto intervista. Firenze: Giunti Editore; 2011.
96. Patton JH, Stanford MS, Barratt ES. Factor structure of the Barratt impulsiveness scale. J Clin Psychol. 1995;51(6):768–74.
97. Aragona M, Pucci D, Roma P, Aprigliano A, Camilo da Silva E, Urbinati S, Zakeri S, Frabotta P, Pisani R. Il LiMEs (List of Migration Experiences): Costruzione e validazione di uno strumento per valutare le esperienze traumatiche e le difficoltà di vita in contesti migratori. In: Aragona M, Geraci S, Mazzetti M, editors. Quando le ferite sono invisibili. Vittime di tortura e di violenza: strategie di cura. Bologna: Pendragon; 2014. p. 106–18.
98. Beusenberg M, Orley JH, World Health Organization, Division of Mental Health. A User's guide to the self reporting questionnaire (SRQ/compiled by M. Beusenberg and J. Orley). Geneva: World Health Organization; 1994.

99. Chaudhry N, Husain N, Tomenson B, Creed F. A prospective study of social difficulties, acculturation and persistent depression in Pakistani women living in the UK. Psychol Med. 2012;42(6):1217–26.
100. Wolf S, Hahn E, Dettling M, Nguyen MH, Wingenfeld K, Stingl M, Hanewald B, Ta TMT. Migration-related stressors and their effect on the severity level and symptom pattern of depression among vietnamese in Germany. Depress Res Treat. 2017;2017:8930432. Epub 2017 Aug 22.
101. Dreher A, Hahn E, Diefenbacher A, Burian H, Dettling M, Burian R, Ta TM. Cultural differences in symptom representation for depression and somatization measured by the PHQ between Vietnamese and German psychiatric outpatients. J Psychsom Res. 2017;(102):71–7.

Prevention in Psychosomatic Medical Care and Rehabilitation

8

Richard Fielding and Wendy Lam

Abstract

Addressing prevention of psychosomatic illness can approach the topic from the detailed study of proximal psychophysiological and brain sciences, or it can address the wider contextual factors and distal influences: This chapter addresses primarily the latter. In reviewing the impacts of social, developmental and environmental influences that have been associated with psychosomatic illness, it becomes apparent that political and economic contexts are major influences on psychosomatic processes that affect health, and it clearly indicates that this is the most powerful level that change can be instituted. The alternative of addressing individual-level interventions is feasible but reflects a primarily symptomatic approach rather than addressing the underlying causes. The chapter then looks at preventive options and briefly visits the question of rehabilitation before returning to the core conclusions.

8.1 Introduction

A psychosomatic illness is one having a distinct psychological component to its development. In the context of this chapter, we need to ask how can we best approach the question of what constitutes a psychosomatic illness and what factors are contributary. For several thousand years, traditional Chinese medicine (TCM) theory has warned that an excess of emotion can harm the body. The ancient Greeks linked personality and bodily processes, and more recently, Arab physicians in the tenth century proposed reciprocal interactions between body and mind. The late

R. Fielding (✉) · W. Lam
Division of Behavioural Sciences, School of Public Health, The University of Hong Kong, Sandy Bay, Hong Kong
e-mail: fielding@hku.hk

L. Grassi et al. (eds.), *Person Centered Approach to Recovery in Medicine*, Integrating Psychiatry and Primary Care, https://doi.org/10.1007/978-3-319-74736-1_8

nineteenth- and twentieth-century analysts and psychosomatic researchers have continued this tradition of assuming mechanisms of the body that are subtly affected by the emotions or other psychological processes. In the second half of the twentieth century, research on endocrinology and immunology began to document differences in hormonal and immune modulation as a result of various forms of "stress" [1, 2], and other studies claimed evidence for the impact of emotions on survival in common diseases, such as metastatic cancer, despite having serious methodological and interpretive flaws (e.g. [3]), and acute myocardial infarction, where the evidence has been much more robust but the effects of interventions remain quite modest [4]. The discovery of what became known as the gut-brain axis lead to an explosion of work, most recently on gut flora and how they might associate with specific diseases, including irritable bowel syndrome, autism, anorexia nervosa, Parkinson's disease, schizophrenia and anxiety and mood disorders (e.g. [5–7]). All of these theoretical models, from TCM to the gut-brain axis, have at their core one or more inferred subtle processes by which changes, often in in the emotional tone of the body as a result of psychological states or vice versa, result in developing, maintaining or inhibiting remediation of some pathological condition or state, currently emphasizing modification of immunity and inflammatory processes. However, unequivocal evidence of these mechanisms substantially influencing the trajectory of a major disease remains outstanding, despite many claims to the contrary and repeated and continuing attempts to identify robust mechanisms that translate to hard endpoints that respond significantly to therapeutic interventions [4, 8].

The alternative mechanism by which bodily state and psychological state might reciprocally influence one another is through the more indirect mechanisms of socio-economic contexts and behaviour. Here there is much more robust evidence for such associations and impacts in most diseases studied. The remainder of this chapter will therefore focus on these mechanisms. We will in turn look at social, economic and behavioural factors from the perspective of preventing ill health. Given the range of conditions and influences encompassed by these factors, it will be impossible to cover every condition in the space available for one chapter. Instead, we will focus on several key examples for each process as illustrating more general principles for exploring approaches to prevention relevant to psychosomatic disease and management.

8.2 Social Influences

The complexity and challenges to providing a succinct yet comprehensive picture of pathogenesis through behaviour are exemplified through a look at social influences and how they work. While we will attempt to look at different areas of behavioural influence in sequence, in reality the boundaries between them are arbitrary, and the different process are frequently acting concurrently.

Humans are quintessentially social creatures. We care very much what others think about us, spending significant amounts of time and money on ensuring we are well presented to signal relative social status and reproductive fitness to others of our species. This may be largely because social acceptance is so fundamental for both physical and psychological wellbeing. There are likely strong evolutionary roots for this. Primate species are predominantly social and hierarchical. Acceptance increases the likelihood of survival and reproduction; rejection, and more so exclusion, sharply diminishes survival. In contemporary human terms, the most direct equivalents to rejection range from ignoring someone through to discrimination, humiliation and bullying, both individually and institutionally and functionally and structurally. Exclusion may be a result of the actions of others or may result from other barriers, including emotional, such as fear, shame or embarrassment; physical, such as disability and impaired access; or economic, such as unaffordability. Often it is a combination of these. Such behaviours can be seen throughout childhood and into adulthood. Rejections by others intrinsically are most often acts by powerful—that is, influential and well-resourced individuals and groups—against powerless or relatively low power others, but not exclusively. Otherness, indicated by appearance, as in skin colour or clothing, language or behaviour, or by indicators of low social status (being poor) that does not conform to in-group expectations, is a well-recognized marker for targeting discriminatory behaviours within communities everywhere [9]. These behaviours when expressed by individuals are often held in check by disapproval from peers or the community majority. However, recent political developments in several Western countries show how quickly such community disapproval can, itself, become inhibited by the presence of an apparent upsurge in discriminatory attitudes, speech and behaviour, giving the appearance of a rapid shift in social norms of behaviour [10]. This seems to be most likely when there are perceived threats to social stability from any number of sources, but often economic. These shifts are rapid when initiated by key persons or groups, such as governments and media working in parallel, as has been witnessed in many Western countries with the introduction of austerity politics, but which for many communities who have faced long-term discrimination from the dominant social groups in societies remain transgenerational. African-Americans are one such group who exemplify long-standing lower status in US society. Where several low status markers converge, such as racial and economic indicators, being coloured and being poor or being disabled, the negative effects are particularly concentrated, markedly so for women and are exacerbated by the conflation of intrinsic and extrinsic factors into markers of personal worth. These, in turn translate into normative prejudicial attitudes. For example, studies indicate that viewing images of homeless people sleeping in doorways elicits almost no response in terms of empathy. However, such indifference is amenable to being deactivated by posing questions to observers about what the homeless person might like to eat, prompting them to empathize with the person to answer. This suggests that observers are more likely to view homeless people as of lower value, even sub-human [11]. This view is reinforced by the frequent targeting for abuse and often violence towards homeless people by groups.

8.2.1 Do These Social Effects Influence Health?

Multiple epidemiological studies of a significant range of health and behavioural dimensions show that ethnic minorities and economically disadvantaged groups within a given community have higher levels of sub- and ill-health and lower uptake of preventive health services. Even within communities, members who face rejection are more likely to suffer from poorer mental health, loneliness and isolation from peers—a factor particularly important for children and adolescents—have poorer-quality sleep and weaker immune responses, report more ill health and die sooner than peers not reporting isolation and loneliness [12, 13]. Social rejection is comparable to physical pain in several ways. Neuropsychological studies show that neurological activity in response to social rejection involves areas associated with processing physical pain, namely, the insula and dorsal anterior cingulate cortex, and giving people a simple centrally acting analgesic like aminocetaphen can effectively reduce the hurt associated with social rejection [14]. The health impacts of prolonged or chronic pain are well documented, including progressive disability, helplessness, depression, sexual health and impaired sleep quality, and can lead to long-term neurological modifications [15–17]. Recent work has shown that impaired motivation and depression seen in chronic pain may be attributable to increased galanin receptor-1 activity in the nucleus accumbens of mice subject to chronic pain [18]. Long-term social rejection may feasibly create similar detrimental health impacts to neurological function [19].

Social exclusion has more profound impacts and is particularly harmful to females [20]. During later childhood and early adolescence, social exclusion is common among girls (for whom closer intimate pair relationships are generally favoured), whereas in boys, physical aggression is a common tactic to exclude targeted individuals, often to demonstrate individual dominance to a wider group of same sex peers. Hormonal and mood impacts of exclusion are seen in both genders in experimental situations. Males and females show declines in testosterone levels and females increases in progesterone levels [21]. Progesterone release seems to be a marker of perceived social rejection [22]. The wider health impacts of exclusion are substantially documented. Exclusion is both a cause and a consequence of mental health problems [23], but because exclusion isolates people from potential sources of social support, it can also exacerbate other health problems and increase the risks associated with isolation, including substance abuse, anger and related antisocial behaviour and low self-esteem, poor self-care and chronic ill health. When accompanied by stigmatization and/or discrimination, health impacts are more severe [24]. Evidence has been reported for increased rates of depression, hypertension and heart disease and certain forms of cancer [25]. Perceived racism, for example, has been linked to hypertension [26]. However, it has proved difficult to disentangle these impacts. A large meta-analysis found consistent links between higher rates of perceived discrimination and more negative mental health generally ($r = -0.16$, 95%CIs −0.20 to −0.12), irrespective of gender or ethnicity, and poorer physical health ($r = -0.12$, 95%CI −0.16 to −0.10) [24].

8.2.2 What Mechanisms Might Underpin These Effects?

While social effects do not necessarily act as direct demands that tax the coping capacity of an individual, situations wherein the individual has lost control over their environment are intrinsically more threatening to that individual because they are not open to personal modification. When loss of control is intermittent or arbitrary, as in situations where an individual encounters episodic discrimination, predictability becomes difficult, and when a person cannot predict what responses are required in a given situation, this increases perceived coping demands. Such situations are particularly harmful to health. When these situations become chronic, the "wear and tear" hypothesis is frequently invoked to explain the link with ill health. However, many of these findings are inconsistent. A number of social-related factors also have been inconsistently linked to mediating the negative effects of discrimination, for example, strong group identity; it may be that we are still looking at partially social effects rather than fully psychophysiological ones. Pascoe and Richman's (2009) meta-analysis compared stress-based with behaviour-based models to account for their observed health ill effects associated with discrimination and found a relatively small effect ($r = -0.11$, 95%CI −0.18 to −0.05) for stress-based and a somewhat larger effect for behaviour-based explanations ($r = -0.179$, 95%CI −0.21 to −0.15). More females than males showed evidence of poorer behaviours ($r = -0.26$, 95%CI −0.33 to −0.20; −0.14, 95%CI −0.20 to −0.08, respectively) [24]. Social support was more likely to show a mediating effect for mental health outcomes. No support effects were seen for physical health outcomes. The effects of coping style and social identification were mixed and largely null for mental and physical health outcomes and stress responses and health behaviours.

Felt loneliness, often but not always a consequence of exclusion, is also implicated in ill health, with people who report greater loneliness experiencing higher morning peak cortisol responses [19]; poorer-quality sleep (particularly in older adults) after adjustment for a range of possible confounders, including self-rated health [17]; and impaired cognition, including self-regulatory responses associated with positive activities such as exercising [16], and has been linked to dementia onset [27], as well as ischaemic heart disease mortality [28] and overall mortality [29].

One potentially important mechanism for explaining why social rejection can impact health is that it can create a barrier for the uptake of health promotion and service delivery. There are examples from many places and times of how groups experienced significant explosions in ill health as a result of facing health-care utilization barriers. These include, for example, the outbreak of tuberculosis that occurred across America, particularly in New York in the 1980s and 1990s: The Reagan Administration's cuts to support for the homeless and the poor exacerbated by opposition to the federal TB programme lead to increase in those vulnerable to infection and yet unable to utilize what few health services were left for them [30]; discrimination against gay men in the early stages of the HIV epidemic in the USA which impaired help seeking among members of the gay community; the failure for non-native-speaking immigrants to be able to negotiate a health-care system which lacks facilities for translation when they cannot speak the dominant language; and the simple inability of disabled individuals to be able to physically access health-care services as needed.

Finally, the increasingly deliberate ideological identification of subgroups within society, the unemployed, the poor and the disabled for particular vilification in the mainstream media and by politicians via targeted policy decisions designed to withdraw social security from already marginalized groups under the name of austerity politics has pushed significant numbers of the general population into poverty. The impact of these moves inevitably impacts families and individuals socially by pricing them out of the social norms of success and material gain universally depicted in the media and advertising and thus marking them as not only "other" but also "under" (Untermenschen) people less worthy of respect from those less unfortunate and from themselves. This will be looked at in more detail in the following section.

8.3 Economic Influences

Economic status has long been recognized to be a major determinant of ill health and avoidable and premature mortality throughout the lifespan. Poverty, the most obvious manifestation of economic influence on health, has a corrosive and often lifetime effect. Impoverishment frequently arises from

1. Long-term national poverty where lack of employment or economic development limits the ability of families and communities to raise their standard of living beyond subsistence. This may be due to, in underdeveloped countries, overpopulation and migration to cities in search of work, misaligned economic policies including those dictated for receipt of loans by multilateral agencies such as the World Bank, forced procurement or theft of land or civil or national warfare. In more developed countries, regions with low economic productivity or population density, where there are high levels of unemployment beyond traditional agrarian practices, and inner city areas which concentrate low pay workers necessary for the service support of other activities.
2. In developed and relatively prosperous communities, where economic policies result in a loss of employment, for example, in England in the 1970s and 1980s when the coal mining industry was deliberately shut down with no replacement sources of work, or the progressive loss of traditional or manual-skilled jobs due to globalization, automation or manufacturing shifts. In the USA, globalization and free trade policies have seen manufacturing jobs in the US industrial heartlands exported to reduce costs, resulting in chronic loss of jobs in traditional industries.
3. Ill health, where medical costs and loss of earnings and high levels of existing debt, for example, a home mortgage, rapidly consume family savings and can result in eviction, inability to regain employment and a spiral into an inescapable poverty. (In the absence of ill-health, debt alone is a major problem that both reflects and causes economic hardship for a growing proportion of populations.)

Economic exclusion is associated with highly unequal societies. The Gini coefficient (GC) measures relative inequality within communities, where a GC of 0 indicates that everyone has the same level of wealth and a GC of 1 that a single individual has all the wealth. Higher values therefore indicate greater inequality. Since the early 1980s, there has been a sustained move to reduce the social gains in economic activity brought about by union and post-war economic policies, especially in North America and Western Europe, with the result that national Gini coefficients in those countries have been moving upwards, and this has accelerated particularly in the past decade in more economically developed countries particularly [31].

The growth of socioeconomic inequalities has quite profound impacts on health and in particular mental health at all levels of society [32]. Of the countries studied by Wilkinson and Pickett, those with the highest disparities between the top and bottom 20% of society, Singapore, the USA, Portugal and Great Britain, have far worse health outcomes than countries with the least disparities between the top and bottom 20% (Japan, Norway, Finland and Denmark). More equal societies tended to have higher levels of trust, social cohesion, community involvement and lower levels of violence [32]. At the levels in society where exclusion from what were seen as formerly universal acts of social participation is dictated by lack of money, these effects are most strongly felt. At the same time, there has been a growing pressure, particularly targeted at younger people and children to become consumers at younger and younger ages [33]. A combination of this consumer pressure in the context of a lack of spending power has been proposed as one reason why the levels of mental health problems in older children and adolescents, particularly girls, have rapidly increased during the early twenty-first century. Together with the Internet and a rise in social media, the perceived need to both meet peer expectations and at the same time being excluded from doing so shifts pressure to parents who may lack the means to provide the perceived necessities of modern childhood, such as up to date mobile phones, clothing and other things. This can have the effect of increasing parental consumer debt and under circumstances of precarious employment that currently exist creates further strain within households, which has detrimental impacts on adolescent mental health [34]. That children from lower socioeconomic status families have higher risk of mental health problems such as depression during adolescence is well established [35, 36]. However, while some researchers have questioned whether poverty inevitably causes mental health problems [37], citing, for example, teen pregnancy and low educational achievement which both increase the probability of raising children in poverty and that poor families tend to live in lower-quality neighbourhoods, attend underperforming schools and experience higher levels of nutritional deficiencies, poor parenting ability has also been blamed for these impacts, as have genetic factors. While the evidence is mixed, separating cause from correlation is needed, but the weight of accumulating evidence seems to support a causal association with evidence suggesting family income is an important determinant of mental health impacts. However this may in turn be modulated by how the poverty occurs. Impacts may be different for a family that was supportive and that had good relationships and higher educational backgrounds, who encounter unexpected poverty due to some change in external circumstances, such as unemployment or ill health, than for a family with long-standing poor relationships and where poverty comes as a result of behaviour such as substance abuse or gambling. Thus it is probably important to differentiate between short-term acute poverty and long-term institutionalized poverty. These effects can be modified by factors such as supportive school environment or even good peer relationships or exposure to violence given the right circumstances. Where parental function is effective, this can potentially help to ameliorate some of the worse effects of poverty. Conversely, stressed parents are likely to communicate that stress to their children. Economic difficulties affect parental mood and generate marital discord, which in young children can disrupt early attachment and lead to inconsistent discipline during childhood and adolescence [37]. Poor parental job opportunities with few opportunities for advancement can discourage school performance and help perpetuate the cycle of poverty, though not always. As family income increases, parents invest more resources in their child, and this enhances the child's cognitive and social skills. Family hardship and stress are also reduced resulting in more positive parenting. Reducing financial hardship improves management of children's problem behaviour while their academic achievement is enhanced by increased parental investment [38]. To achieve the latter, then, both removal of financial hardship and parental support are needed. Government policies, such as social safety nets and targeted support, investment in education and health care, can help to significantly moderate some of these deleterious effects [31].

8.4 Developmental Influences

Many developmental influences on mental health have already been touched on. Developmental influences can be thought of as beginning with intergenerational factors. A family may carry patterns of behaviour, such as teen pregnancy, substance abuse or abusive behaviour across several generations, being normative within a particular family group. As greater social awareness develops and more willingness to intervene on the part of, for example, schools, the more extreme of these trends are more likely to be disrupted, but some, such as sexual abuse, may be hidden from outside the family and persist. For example, women who are victims of childhood sexual abuse are more vulnerable to revictimization as adults. One US study found such women reporting twice the incidence of rape; 1.6 times the incidence of physical, particularly domestic, violence; 4 times as much self-harm; and more lifetime trauma than did a comparison group of women who were not victims in childhood [39]. More mundanely, generally poor parenting skills and low levels of education can be equally detrimental to mental health. However, probably the most prevalent (though not exclusively so) drivers of these factors are family, institutional and environmental poverty.

Beginning with poor nutrition, possibly compounded by substance use and higher levels of maternal stress during pregnancy, exposure to a poor nutritional environment in utero may programme the child's metabolism in ways that increase risk of adult health problems (Barker's or the foetal origins hypothesis) [40]. Barker's hypothesis implicates developmental plasticity as the key feature of embryonic adaptation to the anticipated environment signalled by the nature of the uterine environment. Developmental plasticity varies over the lifespan and may be of two types: immediate responses to current environmental circumstances and predictive adaptation to likely future circumstances. From the perspective of the present paper, predictive plasticity seems to offer most promise as a pathway setting the organism on a relatively fixed developmental trajectory designed to optimize reproductive fitness. This may be at cost to other developmental achievements, such as organ size, vascularization or other aspects of physical growth, some of which may increase psychological vulnerability. This may be enacted through modified hormonal or epigenetic programming influencing signalling sensitivity via altered receptor densities, for example [41].

However, as with many developmental issues, evidence for psychological effects in utero remains confounded by higher rates of maternal perinatal smoking, drinking and other lifestyle factors. These behaviours are well documented to have negative impacts on the foetus, from inter-uterine growth retardation through to foetal alcohol syndrome and tobacco-induced neurodevelopmental changes [42, 43]. This makes separating the underlying psychological state of the mother from the maladaptive coping impacts a difficult task. However, a number of studies have attempted to identify possible pathways for psychological impacts on embryonic and later postnatal infant development. While subjective maternal psychosocial stress during pregnancy is poorly correlated with amniotic cortisol, higher amniotic cortisol levels reportedly influence foetal growth and early childhood distress levels [44], though the mechanism is likely to be more complex than simple exposure [45]. In Australia, for example, approximately 9% of women experience depression in the antenatal period and 16% in the postnatal period [46], when bonding behaviour can be affected, and around 11% of women are affected by anxiety antenatally [47]. Such women may be more likely to have co-morbidities and take medication or self-medicate using a variety of agents, many of which have been shown to negatively influence aspects of foetal development, as has obesity, a growing problem in modern obstetrics [41], and also to smoke, which has long-term growth retardation effects [48]. Prenatal maternal anxiety has been associated with higher reported rates of inattention and hyperactivity in boys, but not girls at 5 years of age [49, 50].

Infant temperament is an important consideration and likely interacts with other perinatal factors. For example, immediately post-partum neonatal behaviour that is responsive to mother's efforts to interact with and calm the infant, easy feeding and an absence of mood disorder can facilitate maternal response to the neonate, building a positive initial experience. In contrast, a difficult delivery may leave the mother exhausted, she may experience disinterest and disappointment at lack of maternal feeling towards the baby, and the neonate may be a difficult feeder, cranky or difficult to calm, discouraging initial interaction which can alter later expectations and behaviour around interactions leading to poor patterning of sleep and feeding cycles and growing frustration with childcare. This in turn may influence the bonding between mother and baby and thereafter the nature of infant attachment to the mother. Whether the child's temperament is affected by maternal psychological state is relevant but is confounded in that mothers' ratings of their babies are influenced in turn by such factors as mother's personality, past experience of childcare and mood [41]. Nonetheless, studies using observers blinded to maternal neonatal status have reported correlation in indicators of neonatal temperament, such as fussiness, crying and sleep and higher maternal cortisol levels [51].

Where maternal anxiety or depression persists post-partum, the infant can be negatively affected [52]. Anxious parenting can negatively influence the behaviour of their offspring [53], while parental anxiety may mediate the impact of stressful events on children [54]. Evidence suggests an additive effect of parental anxiety irrespective of child's temperament, though this remains to be confirmed [53].

Persistent maternal or parental depression can have both intrusive and withdrawal effects on mother-baby dyad, interfering with the baby's exploratory play and generating hostile affect in the baby in the form of anger to discourage maternal intrusiveness, while withdrawal can contribute to negative affect in the baby, interfering with normal learning [55]. Behaviourally, depressed mothers are poor role models for problem solving and resilience, showing maladaptive functioning and impaired responsiveness, all of which can impact negatively on the child's behaviour. Little is known about the effects of paternal depression. Children of such parents are themselves at increased risk for affective disorders before the age of 30 [55]. However, many studies have noted that children of parents with psychopathology do not all demonstrate negative behaviours themselves. Contextual factors, such as family social class, levels of education, marital conflict and others, can modify children's behaviour. Having a caring and supportive father, and probably grandparents and older children, and to a lesser extent school, can significantly buffer impacts from maternal depression, while the characteristics of the child including sex differences, resilience and temperament also explain significant variance with boys being more vulnerable than girls to maternal depression [55]. Nonetheless, evidence is accumulating that childhood behavioural and conduct disorders are strong predictors of adult mental health and a major pathway through which social inequalities exert their effects [56].

By the time the child reaches adolescence, they have developed familial-driven coping behaviours often modelled on parental behaviours. At adolescence, young people become more responsive to peers and less responsive to parental drivers of behaviour, and if the adolescent has good social skills, peer support networks can be beneficial. However, in early adolescence, such networks are often unstable and changing and may be a source of significant stress for young people, particularly on social media.

This section has so far concentrated on mental health because most evidence indicates that somatic health problems in childhood frequently have strong psychological components, some directly arising from the child and some secondary from parental reaction to the child's health problems. However, unlike in adults, such conditions may manifest themselves differently in children and adolescent, usually as somatoform or behavioural disorders. Somatoform disorders are frequent reasons for medical consultation in many countries, accounting for up to 50% of medical outpatient visits. In 1991, a national prevalence study of mental disorders in the Finnish population indicated the prevalence of frequent headache at 2.8%, recurrent abdominal pain 2.4%, asthma 0.8%, enuresis at 1.5% and soiling in 0.3% of children in the general population [57].

Among youth, studies report prevalence rates of any depressive disorder at between 0.9 and 2.5% (point prevalence) in the UK and 2.1 and 3.4% (3–12 months' period prevalence) in the USA. For anxiety, equivalent figures are 3.3% (UK) and 2.2–9.5% (USA) [58]. These disorders are often co-morbid with other problems, including conduct disorder, low school performance, substance abuse, eating disorders and self-harm. Self-harm itself is often associated with trauma or sexual abuse [39]. Half of all mental health disorders start before age 14 years, but most go undetected [59].

Globally teen pregnancy remains a problem in many countries, complications of pregnancy and childbirth being the most common cause of death for females aged 15–19 years of age [59]. However, trends in teen pregnancy rates show substantial declines. In the USA a majority of these pregnancies (pregnancy rates, adolescent females aged 15–19: 1990—50.9/1000; 2014—24.2/1000) [60] occur outside of marriage and predominantly in the poorer southern and Midwestern states and among Hispanic and Black girls. Poor education achievement, having themselves been born during their mothers' teen years and living with other than their biological parents are risk factors [60]. A similar pattern of declines in teen pregnancy was seen in the UK. The provision of effective sex education and supportive teen sexual health advisory services, a change in social norms and the reduction of stigma associated with contraception, as well as the availability of emergency contraception, are believed to have played a major part in the observed declines. The example of teen pregnancy declines is illustrative of the multifactorial nature of many problems that straddle the psychological-somatic health domains. The message from this is that similar changes are needed to effect prevention in many of the other areas addressed in this chapter.

During early adulthood, among the most common health problems having strong behavioural components are unintentional injuries (many arising from higher rates of risk taking and occupations that include greater risk of injury and road accidents and drowning often in conjunction with drugs and alcohol use), tobacco, obesity and inactivity, HIV and violence. Males are disproportionately affected by these conditions, and in many cases, they are associated with broader contextual factors, including war, political and social instability, impoverished communities and low educational levels, coupled with higher risk taking in this age group and among males generally. Trauma in youth who have been exposed to violence and conflict is a growing problem that can contribute significantly to maladaption and psychosomatic behaviours generally. Where these occur in refugee and immigrant groups, the problems can be further compounded.

From early adulthood onwards throughout middle and later adulthood, growing numbers of young people are affected by chronic health problems arising from poor lifestyle, substance use and inactivity. These problems themselves generate collateral impacts on mental health, self-esteem and marital and intimate relationships and therefore also affect parent-child roles and behaviours. For example, cancer in younger adults impacts at a life stage where career and family may be closely interrelated. For a person in their 40s diagnosed with cancer, children are likely to still be dependent, may be in the more challenging teen years facing educational demands, and financial responsibilities mean that loss of work or impaired income can present significant additional stresses to families already struggling financially. If the patient had pre-existing coping difficulties, the additional demands of cancer can significantly compound these. For these and other reasons, it is well established that younger cancer patients report more difficulties and greater symptom impacts on average than do older cancer patients (e.g. [61]). The availability of sufficient coping resources, in many instances these are predominantly material and social, determines how well patients effectively cope with the demands of chronic illnesses such as cancer. Patients with limited coping or those with significantly constrained access to necessary resources are likely to face additional stress. Once primary treatments are concluded, the extent and persistence of residual symptoms and late effects of disease and treatments can themselves interfere considerably with return to normal life, and coupled with fear of recurrence, these factors can cast a significant shadow over family life and create substantial secondary difficulties. Difficulties in renormalizing bodily sensations after cancer can make it difficult for patients to put the experience of cancer behind them and helps to maintain, and be maintained by fear of disease recurrence. Residual symptoms such as fatigue and sleep disruption can limit return to work, and significant numbers of patients experiencing cancer report higher levels of anxiety, distress and depression, though in many cases these resolve without intervention.

In later adulthood, more frequent health challenges, accumulation of chronic diseases and gradually impaired activity and social roles, particularly following retirement or often worse after early redundancy or job loss, are associated with increased velocity of health deterioration, health-care utilization and increasing mental health challenges, particularly depression. These role, economic and other losses characterize this developmental stage. The deterioration of cognitive function that accompanies ageing can also further impair coping with health and other demands.

With the onset of chronic health problems, coping resilience is a critical function. Again, resource availability and coping capacity are factors that modify outcomes, in particular mental health [62]. People react differently depending on whether they view demands as losses, threats or challenges. Responding to a demand as a challenge tends to evoke more action-focussed coping to address the demand, whereas responding to demand as a threat or loss tends to evoke more passive, emotion control-oriented coping [63]. A similar emotion-focussed response is seen in relation to physical symptoms such as persistent pain in elderly adults [64]. With a rapid ageing of the global population, this demographic will form a growing and predominant pool of demand for health care. Effective preventive management is therefore imperative to avoid health-care systems from being overwhelmed.

Determinants of overall health perceptions interact with perceived coping capacity. In older adults better health status is associated with higher income. For example, among Canadian adults aged 45–64 and 65+, those in the highest income bracket were 4.65 and 1.94 times, respectively, to report better health than the lowest income bracket [65]. Given that Canada has a social insurance-based health-care system, access to care is less obviously a reason for such disparities than it might be in a country with private insurance-based health care such as the USA. Given that health perceptions are primary drivers of health-care utilization [66], the association between adequate resourcing and social support and the reduction of health-care demand in older adults are brought into sharp relief as important targets for prevention.

8.5 Environmental Influences

The role of environment in health can be construed in several ways, some of which have already been identified in the forgoing sections of this chapter. The direct effects of physical conditions can impact on health in a variety of ways, for example, the harms from living near a busy main road on child respiratory health [67]; the more indirect effects seen in impoverished communities, particularly in relation to living in poor-quality housing where effects can also be direct, such as from mould and damp [68]; psychological harms from having to live in circumstances that are both unpleasant and potential hazardous especially to children and in wider environments characterized by low social, cultural and financial capital [69]; and living in isolated or depopulated rural settings, some of which may be secure; others of which may be subject to violence, warfare or extreme disaster risks; and where health-care facilities may be at best distant and at worst degraded past use or completely absent.

There is a mixed causal picture with regard to the interactions between living in impoverished areas and poor health. In some cases, social housing acts as a safety net for the poor and ill [70], but such housing need not be of poor standard, though all too often it is. The functional capacity of families living in substandard housing is often compromised by low education, low income and opportunity occupations or unemployment and the stresses this produces, school underperformance in children, lack of access to positive activities and role models, substance misuse and poor diet all feeding in to limit coping resources and hence capacity.

These are compounded by the location of substandard housing in low-quality urban districts, adjacent to industrial sites or in flood-prone locations, disproportionately increasing exposure to and hence risks from natural and other disasters among poorer and more impoverished communities [71]. Witness the predominant impacts on poorer and mostly Black neighbourhoods in New Orleans and Houston, respectively, from Hurricanes Katrina in 2003 and Harvey in 2017. Following such episodes in the USA, for example, relief and rebuilding efforts tended to be slower and less extensive than those where predominantly white middle-class areas are affected [72].

8.6 Consequences for Prevention

8.6.1 Contextual Strategies

From the foregoing sections, it is obvious that multipronged and prolonged, probably multigenerational, approaches are needed to reduce and, whenever possible, prevent psychosomatic complications to health through the broad domains of behaviour and lifestyle. Because these processes are among the most important drivers of health overall, the payback from long-term investment in strategies such as infrastructure spending on building and maintaining to a high standard social and public housing, policing, education and other aspects of society that have been outlined above is extraordinary. Wilkinson and Pickett's 2013 summation of the evidence [32] (only one of several similar treatises reaching broadly comparable conclusions) of the health harms to all strata of society from high levels of inequalities provides powerful arguments for a societal-oriented economics based on strategies other than those of the free market which having been tried for almost 40 years have produced exactly the opposite outcomes to those needed to achieve prevention of exclusion by prevention of inequalities as a result of neoliberal political and economic policies. Governments frequently claim that reducing taxes on the upper income brackets and tightening spending on lower income "welfare" will stimulate economic growth. Despite being the basis for Western economic policy for over 40 years, however, evidence clearly indicates the opposite [31].

Key among these are policies designed to support and help families with significant social and educational needs. Programmes such as Sure Start can offer remarkably inexpensive and good value for money and high levels of effectiveness [73] when appropriately implemented. These programmes should involve other family members, in particular the mother, which can benefit both mother and child. Parents more involved with their children's education tend to have less conflict with the child, and the child in turn has better social skills [74]. However, the causal direction here is unclear. It may simply be that parents who are more involved also have greater personal resources and children who have benefitted developmentally from this. Similar early childhood intervention programmes have been tried in many developed countries. Longer-term findings are mixed, probably because of inconsistencies in implementation and a lack of further follow-up interventions designed to improve the wider community. What the few studies done tend to suggest is that the 0–3 age range is likely to be most cost-effective for interventions [75]. However, most existing studies have focused on programmes designed to reduce criminality and conduct disorder, and not necessarily health decrements from low-grade childhood environments. Interventions targeting post-partum [76] and later maternal depression [77] have been found to be effective in reducing child psychopathologies, but for logistical reasons, these studies are not sufficiently long term to look at outcomes into adolescence and beyond. The weight of evidence suggests such programmes to be very cost-effective [72]. More generally, enhancing positive parental interactions with their children overall is generally beneficial across a range of indicators [78].

Relatively uncontroversial programmes such as free playgroups and kindergarten education of all children can have quite profound effects in terms of exposing children to enriched learning environments and giving mothers relief from childminding. Engagement by parents in everyday activities in which parents model desirable behaviours benefits child learning of both behaviours and values [78], but this relies on the parent having the skills, opportunities and motivation to enact such modelling. For this reason, addressing the factors preventing access to and uptake of education; adequately salaried, secure work; and good standard housing with stable tenure is a crucial step in the longer-term prevention of psychosomatic contributions to health. Again we are brought back to the conclusion that to achieve this requires a move away from the economic policies that have been pursued since the mid-1970s that reflect political initiatives intended to reduce or remove social institutions developed to address these needs. The failure of deregulated banking in 2007–2008 leading to the subprime and wider banking crisis has served as a perfect opportunity for ideologically driven actions to reduce funding for social programmes put into place following the Second World War to aid recovery of European and other countries after that conflict. These actions coupled with globalized movement of manufacturing and promotion of consumption-based economics have reversed the steadily declining wealth inequalities arising in the first half of the twentieth century and the wider social achievements that had consequently accrued by the mid-1970s. There needs to be a sustained and evidence-based programme of investment into affordable good-quality housing, jobs and education as these three factors have been shown repeatedly and globally to accrue the largest gains in community wellbeing and individual health [31].

One notable trend has been a progressive loss of food skills in younger cohorts and a growing reliance on convenience foods that tend to have poor nutritional profiles and are also relatively expensive. In working families, time becomes a precious commodity, and avoiding spending large amounts of the buying, preparation and eating of food is something that in many places is now seen in terms of an opportunity cost. At the same time, marketing strategies and product ranges reliant on highly processed and refined carbohydrates and fats, demand for cheap foods and mass production of cheap meat have created a nutritional environment that is obesogenic. In settings of increasing social isolation partly as a result of exclusion and partly arising from greater urbanization and the associated barriers to easy social interactions, there is a need to help to regenerate ways that facilitate social interaction and engagement. This is dependent on the revitalization of community resources, including places such as well-designed public spaces, libraries and community centres that act as points of convergence for different threads of the community. These need to be sufficiently local that they enable people to recognize and repeatedly interact with one another to build relationships, mutual respect and support. City-level settings are too impersonal, and district-level settings are likely to be more effective. Traditionally, such functions were served by religious and other community institutions, such as, in the West, public houses, union and clubhouses and other groupings derived from mutual or common interests. Because many communication functions have been taken over by social media, this has allowed interaction in the absence of face-to-face exchange. This clearly has benefits in that it enables people to more easily keep in touch, particularly over longer distances, but it has probably contributed to a relative degree of isolationism as well.

In summary then, the main issues for primary prevention of psychosomatic overlay converge on maintaining good levels of mental health, and this is best achieved by national investments in education, social engagement and adequate material resources for individuals and families. In other words, building individual capacity through enhancing social and community capital is the critical context to address the foundations of community and individual wellbeing. This in turn relies on adequate, meaningful and fairly remunerated occupational opportunities, and these come from suitable population-oriented political and economic policies.

8.6.2 Rehabilitation Strategies

The importance of effective communication as a key plank in both the prevention of ill health and rehabilitation of people with existing health difficulties cannot be overemphasized. In the absence of adequate authoritative and evidence-based information from trusted sources, the primary, secondary and tertiary prevention of health problems becomes considerably more difficult. The ease with which belief-based rather than evidence-based information is promulgated both in the mainstream media (MSM) and the Wild West of the Internet is apparent in any number of areas of contemporary concern from vaccinations to climate change, from the reasons for the banking crisis to US presidential elections and the Brexit debate in the UK. The deliberate obfuscation of facts and the presentation of counter "evidence" through selective cherry picking, targeted lobbying and other means, to achieve the maintenance of doubt in the eyes of both the population and the policy makers, are highly effective strategies, developed by the public relations industry and used to devastating effect in delaying asbestos, lead and tobacco control, climate change action and tax reform, among other things [79]. Most of these "campaigns" have been with the aim of maintaining or boosting consumption or sales of products that are harmful or at best have little clear benefit. While robust evidence-based logic has probably never been the basis of much policy setting in the past 40 years, there has been a sustained effort to replace evidence-based policy making with belief or ideological policy making. The consequences of these policies, apparently misinformed by economic doctrine are that they have performed poorly for the majority but very well for a wealthy minority. That successive governments have failed to acknowledge, let alone addres these shortcomings, too often due to personal interest and ideological dogma, and those that have done are vilified in the mainstream media indicates a clear unwillingness to prioritize population wellbeing over ideology. It is of little surprise then that inequalities have expanded and become more entrenched with resulting impacts on the very community resources that help to maintain wellness [31, 32].

From an individual practitioner perspective, when focus is on those with existing illness, clear and effective communications enable a number of responses that facilitate recovery and help to avoid compounding physical health problems with additional psychological overlay. First, accurate preparatory information about ilness and symptom trajectories and outcomes, even when probabilistic, helps to enable more realistic expectations, and these in turn allow better prediction of coping demands. Uncertainty when there are anticipated threats, as we all experience from time to time, is a particularly uncomfortable state. In most instances, stress and the accompanying psychophysiological responses from increased arousal arise from appraising the outcome of a perceived demand as threatening in some way [80]. When demands can be better quantified, then it becomes easier to determine what resources are needed to meet those demands, and therefore good information about outcomes enables a person to reduce uncertainty and better plan to deal with what is coming. In some respects all information can be said to be either preparatory (about the future), when it can help to reduce uncertainty, or explanatory (about the present or past), when it can help account for experiences that are poorly understood. However, matching information provision to coping preference is important. People differ in their preference for information, with some preferring as much information as possible, and others less, and even none at all [81]. Most people fall somewhere between these two extremes. Miller's minimax theory indicates that predictability is not the only way that information reduces stress [81]. Predictability better enables control over the environment. However, if the person already perceives little control over their environment or the threat they face, such as in the case of a cancer diagnosis, for example, they can reduce stress by defaulting to a passive mode of coping that relies instead on managing their emotional state but also by engaging external agents (doctors) to act on their behalf. This in turn can enhance a sense of control for the patient, particularly when the doctor works closely with the patient and can build a sense of a shared task; in other words, if the doctor is able to give the patient a sense of their concern, support, attention and effort, the result is in effect the partial internalization of control for the patient, who may then be more motivated and positive about the outcomes. An engaged and supportive doctor helps to build a patients' sense of control. In most circumstances, therefore patients should seek to engage closer involvement with the doctor to increase their sense of control, a process called participatory control [82]. Under these circumstances the patient-doctor dyad works effectively to address the patient's health problem. From the doctor's perspective, this level of engaged working can be more emotionally demanding, requiring involvement at a more personal level that in effect needs relationship building. However, there may be a need to include more structured help, in the form of psychotherapeutic support such as cognitive behavioural therapies, particularly where threats are only partially controllable, as with cancer, for example.

A second way in which effective communications are crucial to the prevention of psychological compounding of physical health problems is that clear and effective information can improve decision-making. Frequently in health care, patients are given choices of treatments, but under these circumstances, a patient and their family may lack the background to feel confident in their choice. This can then have negative consequences for the patient that include doubt, regret and guilt over choices made if outcomes fail to meet expectations. For example, Lam and colleagues [83] have shown that women given the choice between breast cancer treatments often have higher levels of subsequent psychological distress up to 6 years later if they are given more or less responsibility for the treatment decision than their preferred level. Most women were given the choice to make themselves, but most preferred for the doctor to make the decision with their involvement, that is, in a joint manner [83]. Those women for whom their decision-involvement preference did not match their actual decision-making responsibility reported higher levels of distress 8 months later. It is therefore beneficial for doctors to optimize the degree of involvement patients have by matching their actual information requirement and decision-making with their actual preference. This is easily done by considering information need when meeting the patient for the first time when the doctor is ready to begin to give information to the patient by asking, for example, "How much information would you like about your condition? Do you want to told about everything that happens, like changes in your condition? If not, is there someone, a family member perhaps, who you would like to be kept informed and if necessary who can make decisions on your behalf? I also need to know how much you want to be involved in decisions about your care. Most people prefer to make these decisions with their doctor. But, if you prefer, you can make all the decisions, or I can make them on your behalf together with your designated family member". It is important to make statements such as these, particularly when working with ethnically diverse populations as cultural preferences for information vary considerably. In such circumstances, comprehension issues need to be considered and if needed a translator made available, often a bilingual second-generation family member. But it is important to explain to such family members the importance of not censoring the initial communication. For example, it is common in some Chinese communities for family members to try to protect elderly relatives by withholding information for fear they will suffer, give up hope and die more quickly. However, many elderly patients may want more information and be more able to exercise agency over decisions affecting them. Under such circumstances, it is important to ask the patient in the presence of the relatives so they hear the patient's preference for themselves. However, they must provide an honest translation in the first place about the request. Ideally, professional translators would be the best solution.

The effective control of and communication regarding symptoms and late effects of disease and treatments are also a crucial step in controlling the negative interactions between the physical aspects of the patient's health and their psychological state. It should be already apparent to the reader from the foregoing that the interplay between psychological state, behaviour and physical health is not really manageable by simply addressing only the physical aspects of an illness alone, though for many minor problems this may be sufficient. However, in the case of chronic or life-threatening illness, residual symptoms and late effects of treatments are probably major causes of psychological overlay to physical illness as well as major barriers to effective reintegration to normal life [84]. As such they are important targets for intervention. These symptoms can be classified in a number of ways. Reviews of early studies of symptom clusters in cancer consistently identified just one cluster, related to gastrointestinal symptoms, involving nausea and vomiting [85], and while more clusters were apparent in advanced cancer [86], these were not stable over time. This finding is partly due to methodological differences in reviewed studies as well and poor consistency of definitions of symptom clusters. More detailed studies suggest that symptoms are often related in a lagged or cascading fashion, with pain, for example, disturbing sleep, which in turn leads to fatigue and subsequently depression [87]. Sleep disturbances are prominent in a number of chronic diseases in addition to cancer, are particularly disruptive and in older adults appear to be secondary to co-morbidities, particularly depression, heart disease, bodily pain and memory disorders, rather than being a primary consequence of ageing [88, 89] affecting between 2.8 and 17% of the population aged over 50 in different countries [89], though reports from China suggest rates as high as 43% particularly among older females [90, 91] and that sleep difficulties are associated with alcohol use 5–7 days a week [90]. In turn, poor sleep is a major contributor to poor quality of life and may exacerbate fatigue and low mood [87], interfering with the ability to return to a normal life. Fatigued and tired people are more likely to have low activity levels, and this in turn can compound or perpetuate sleeping difficulties [92]. Conversely, increasing activity levels can help to improve sleep quality, though getting tired people to exercise sufficiently to have a noticeable effect needs good motivation. Motivational deficits are particularly prominent in depression, and the associations between impaired sleep and depression are well established [93], as both are with chronic pain [90]. Exercise has been shown to be an effective adjunct to treatment for depression [94, 95] though disagreement remains on the effect size.

Despite frequently being co-morbid in significant numbers of those reporting these problems, chronic pain and depression differentially impact on quality of life [91]. Around 34% (22–42%) of people in Hong Kong, for example, report some kind of chronic pain [96]; in the German population, ~20% report chronic non-disabling, non-malignant pain [97], while in the UK the prevalence in the general population is estimated at 43% (38–49%) [98], in Sweden 46% (25–57%) [99] and in the USA 30% (29.8–31.7%) [100]. While differences in prevalence are mostly due to different definitions and sample structures, these rates are high. The need for effective management of these high rates of pain raises significant concerns. The high rates of abuse of opioid-based prescription drugs in the USA have been blamed for contributing to a significant decline in the trend of gains in life expectancies for Americans, particularly white segments, among others, linked to an epidemic of chronic pain, increases in obesity and heart disease [101].

Conclusions

While much of the reported physical pain in the above prevalence studies is attributed to physical ill health associated with sedentary and ageing populations, it is also notable that we find ourselves back to the question that this chapter began with, namely, whether exclusion in the form of social isolation and alienation that is now so prevalent in developed countries, particularly among unemployed lower middle-class white industrial heartlands that have been most affected by economic policies of the past 40 years, might also account for much of the pain these communities experience [14–16, 20, 24]. The need to approach the psychosomatic health of communities from multiple levels is stark. A medical approach is only going to achieve limited success if the main sources of the distress overlaying physical health are addressed at the multiple levels they act on. Nonetheless, the physician needs to be aware of and prepared to act in ways that they can to achieve the best outcomes for the patient. At the most fundamental level, this requires relationships and good communications; at the most effective level, it requires a major change in the economic and social policies we are prepared to tolerate.

References

1. Keicolt-Glaser JK, Glaser R. Psychological stress and wound healing: Kiecolt-Glaser et al. (1995). Adv Mind Body Med. 2001;17:15–6.
2. Segerstrom SC, Miller GE. Psychological stress and the human immune system: a meta-analytic study of 30 years of inquiry. Psychol Bull. 2004;130:601–30. https://doi.org/10.1037/0033-2909.130.4.601.
3. Speigel D Kraemer HC, Bloom J, Gottheil E. The effect of psychosocial treatment on survival of patients with metastatic breast cancer. Lancet. 1989;2(8668):887–91.
4. Carney RM, Freedland KE. Depression and coronary heart disease. Nat Rev Cardiol. 2017;14:145–55. https://doi.org/10.1038/nrcardio.2016.181.
5. Wang Y, Kasper LH. The role of microbiome in central nervous system disorders. Brain Behav Immun. 2014;38:1–12. https://doi.org/10.1016/j.bbi.2013.12.015.
6. Saxena R, Sharma VK. A metagenomic insight into the human microbiome: its implications in health and disease. In: Kumar D, Antonarakis S, editors. Medical and health genomics. Rotterdam: Elsevier Science; 2016. p. 117. https://doi.org/10.1016/B978-0-12-420196-5.00009-5.
7. Foster JA, McVey Neufelt KA. Gut-brain axis: how the microbiome influences anxiety and depression. Trends Neurosci. 2013;36:305–12. https://doi.org/10.1016/j.tins.2013.01.005.
8. Dhabha FS. Effects of stress on immune function: the good, the bad, and the beautiful. Immunol Res. 2014;58:193–210. https://doi.org/10.1007/s12026-014-8517-0.
9. Fassin D. The biopolitics of otherness: undocumented foreigners and racial discrimination in French public debate. Anthropol Today. 2001;17:3–7.
10. Ahmed D. Racist hate crime is so out of control that even white British people are being attacked. The Independent. 2016. http://www.independent.co.uk/voices/brexit-racism-hate-crime-figures-rise-white-british-being-attacked-a7360836.html
11. Fiske ST. From dehumanization and objectification, to rehumanization: neuroimaging studies on the building blocks of empathy. Ann N Y Acad Sci. 2009;1167:31–4. https://doi.org/10.1111/j.1749-6632.2009.04544.x.
12. DeWaal CN, Bushman BJ. Social acceptance and rejection: the sweet and the bitter. Curr Dir Psychol Sci. 2011;20:256–60. https://doi.org/10.1177/0963721411417545.
13. Masi CM, Chen HY, Hawkley LC, Cacioppo JT. A meta-analysis of interventions to reduce loneliness. Personal Soc Psychol Rev. 2011;15(3) https://doi.org/10.1177/1088868310377394.
14. DeWall CN, MacDonald G, Webster GD, Masten C, Baumeister RF, Powell C. Acetaminophen reduces social pain: behavioral and neural evidence. Psychol Sci. 2010;21:931–7.
15. Fine PG. Long-term consequences of chronic pain: mounting evidence for pain as a neurological disease and parallels with other chronic disease states. Pain Med. 2011;12:996–1004. https://doi.org/10.1111/j.1526-4637.2011.01187.x.

16. Hawkley LC, Thisted RA, Cacioppo JT. Loneliness predicts reduced physical activity: cross-sectional and longitudinal analyses. Health Psychol. 2009;28:354–63. https://doi.org/10.1037/a0014400.
17. Jacobs JM, Cohen A, Hammerman-Rozenberg R, Stressman J. Global sleep satisfaction of older people: the Jerusalem cohort study. J Am Geriatr Soc. 2006;54:325–9.
18. Schwartz N, Tamkin P, Jurado S, Lim BK, Helfets BD, Polepalli JS, Malenka RC. Decreased motivation in chronic pain requires long-term depression in the nucleus accumbens. Science. 2011;345(6196):535–42. https://doi.org/10.1126/science.1253994.
19. Hawkley LC, Cacioppo JT. Perceived social isolation: social threat vigilance and its implication for health. In: Decety J, Cacioppo JT, editors. The Oxford textbook of social neuroscience. New York: OUP; 2011.
20. Benenson JF, Markovits H, Hulfgren B, Nguyen T, Bullock G, Wrangham R. Social exclusion: more important to human females than males. PLoS One. 2013;8(2):e55851. https://doi.org/10.1371/journal.pone.0055851.
21. Seidel EM, Silani G, Metzler H, Thaler H, Lamm C, Gur RC, Kriypin-Exner I, Habel U, Derntl B. The impact of social exclusion vs inclusion on subjective and hormonal reactions in females and males. Psychoneuroendocrinology. 2013;38:2925–32. https://doi.org/10.1016/j.psyneuen.2013.07.021.
22. Maner JK, Miller SL, Schmidt MB, Eckle LA. The endocrinology of exclusion: rejection elicits motivationally tuned changes in progesterone. Psychol Sci. 2010;21:581–8. https://doi.org/10.1177/0956797610362676.
23. Horowiz AV, Schied TL, editors. A handbook for the study of mental health: social contexts, theories and systems. Cambridge: Cambridge University Press; 1999.
24. Pascoe EA, Richman LS. Perceived discrimination and ill health: a meta-analytic review. Psychol Bull. 2009;135:531–54.
25. Taylor TR, Williams CD, Makhambi KH, Mouton C, Harrel JP, Cozier Y, Palmer JR, Rosenberg L, Adams-Cambell LL. Racial discrimination and breast cancer incidence in US Black women: the Black Women's Health Study. Am J Epidemiol. 2007;166:46–54. https://doi.org/10.1093/aje/kwm056.
26. Steffen PR, McNeilly M, Anderson N, Sherwood A. Effects of perceived racism and anger inhibition on blood pressure in African Americans. Psychosom Med. 2003;65:746–50.
27. Wilson RS, Kreuger KR, Arnold SE, Schneider JA, Kelly JF, Barnes LL, et al. Loneliness and risk of Alzheimer's disease. Arch Gen Psychiatry. 2007;64:234–40.
28. Valtorta NK, Kanaan M, Gilbody S, Ronzi S, Hanratty B. Loneliness and social isolation as risk factors for coronary heart disease and stroke: systematic review and meta-analysis of longitudinal observational studies. Heart. 2016;102:1109–16.
29. Holt-Lundstad J, Smith TB, Baker M, Harris T, Stevenson D. Loneliness and social isolation as risk factors for mortality: a meta-analytic review. Perspect Psychol Sci. 2015;10:227–37. https://doi.org/10.1177/1745691614568352.
30. Specter M. Neglected for years, TB is back with strains that are deadlier. New York Times, October 11, 1992. http://www.nytimes.com/1992/10/11/nyregion/neglected-for-years-tb-is-back-with-strains-that-are-deadlier.html?pagewanted=all. Accessed 25 Jan 2017.
31. Dabla-Norris E., Kochar K, Ricar S, Supharphiphat N, Sounta E. Causes and consequences of income inequality: a global perspective. International Monetary Fund; 2015. https://www.imf.org/external/pubs/ft/sdn/2015/sdn1513.pdf. Accessed 11 Sept 2017.
32. Wilkinson R, Pickett K. The spirit level: why more equal societies almost always do better. London: Allen Lane; 2009.
33. Beder S. This little Kiiddie went to market: the corporate capture on childhood. London: Pluto Press; 2009.
34. Saxena S, Saraceno B. Social determinants of mental health. Geneva: World Health Organization; 2014.

35. Gilman SE, Kawachi I, Fitzmaurice GM, Buka SL. Family disruption in childhood and risk of adult depression. Am J Psychiatry. 2003a;160:939–46. https://doi.org/10.1176/appi.ajp.160.5.939.
36. Gilman SE, Kawachi I, Fitzmaurice GM, Buka SL. Socio-economic status, family disruption and residential stability in childhood: relation to onset, recurrence and remission of major depression. Psychol Med. 2003b;33:1341–55. https://doi.org/10.1017/S0033291703008377.
37. Yoshikawa H, Aber LJ, Beardslee WR. The effect of poverty on the mental, emotional and behavioural health of children and youth. Am Psychol. 2012;67:272–84.
38. Gershoff ET, Aber JL, Raver CC, Lennon MC. Income is not enough: incorporating material hardship into models of income associations with parenting and child development. Child Dev. 2007;78:70–95. https://doi.org/10.1111/j.1467-8624.2007.00986.x.
39. Noll JG, Horowitz LA, Bonnano G, Trickett PK, Putnam FW. Revictimization and self harm in females who experienced childhood sexual abuse. J Interpers Violence. 2003;18:1452–71.
40. Barker DJP. The Wellcome Foundation Lecture, 1994. The fetal origins of adult disease. Proc Biol Sci. 1995;262:37–43.
41. Lewis AJ, Austin A, Knapp R, Vaiano T, Galbally M. Perinatal maternal health, foetal programming and child development. Healthcare (Basel). 2015;3:1212–27. https://doi.org/10.3390/healthcare3041212.
42. Hofhuis W, de Jongste JC, Merkus PJFM. Adverse health effects of prenatal and postnatal tobacco smoke exposure on children. Arch Dis Child. 2003;88:1086–90.
43. Andrews-Espy K, Fang H, Johnson C, Stoppe C, Weiber SA, Respass J. Prenatal tobacco exposure: developmental outcomes in the neonatal period. Dev Psychol. 2011;47:153–6. https://doi.org/10.1037/a0020724.
44. Balbazarova E, van de Beek C, Cohen-Kettenis PT, Buitellar J, Shelton KH, van Goozen SHM. Influence of prenatal maternal stress, maternal plasma cortisol and cortisol in the amniotic fluid on birth outcomes and child temperament at 3 months. Psychoneuro. 2013;38:907–15. https://doi.org/10.1016/j.psyneuen.2012.09.015.
45. Zijlmans MAC, Riksen-Walraven JM, de Weerth C. Associations between maternal prenatal cortisol concentrations and child outcomes: a systematic review. Neurosci Biobehav Rev. 2015;53:1–24.
46. Buist A, Bilszta J. The beyondblue National Postnatal Screening Program, Prevention and Early Intervention 2001–2005, Final Report Volume I: National Screening Program; Melbourne, Australia: Beyondblue; 2006.
47. Gotlib IH, Whiffen VE, Mount JH, Milne K, Cordy NI. Prevalence rates and demographic characteristics associated with depression in pregnancy and the postpartum. J Consult Clin Psychol. 1989;57:269–74.
48. Muraro AP, Gonçalves-Silva SMV, Moreira NF, Gonçalves-Fareirra M, Nunes-Freitas NL, Abreu-Villaça Y, Sichieri R. Effect of tobacco smoke exposure during pregnancy and preschool age on growth from birth to adolescence: a cohort study. BMC Pediatr. 2014;14:99. https://doi.org/10.1186/1471-2431-14-99.
49. Loomans EM, van der Stelt O, van Eijsden M, Gemke RJBJ, Vrijkotte T, van den Bergh BR. Antenatal maternal anxiety is associated with problem behaviour at age five. Early Hum Dev. 2011;87:565–70.
50. O'Connor TG, Heron J, Golding J, Glover V, the ALSPAC Study Team. Maternal antenatal anxiety and behavioural/emotional problems in children: a test of a programming hypothesis. J Child Psychol Psychiatry. 2003;44:1025–36.
51. Davis EP, Glynn LM, Schetter CD, Hobel C, Chicz-Demet A, Sandman CA. Prenatal exposure to maternal depression and cortisol influences infant temperament. J Am Acad Child Adolesc Psychiatry. 2007;46:737–46.
52. Lewis AJ. Depression in pregnancy and child development: understanding the mechanisms of transmission. Berlin, Germany: Springer; 2014.
53. Hudson J. Parent child relationship in early childhood and development of anxiety and depression. In: RE Tremblay, M Bovin, R DeV Peters, editors, Encyclopedia on early childhood development. Centre of excellence on early childhood development. Universite De

Montreal; 2013. http://www.child-encyclopedia.com/anxiety-and-depression/according-experts/parent-child-relationships-early-childhood-and-development. Accessed 6 Sept 2017.
54. Platt R, Williams SR, Ginsberg GS. Stressful life events and child anxiety. Examining parent and child mediators. Child Psychiatry Hum Dev. 2016;47:23–34. https://doi.org/10.1007/s10578-015-0540-4.
55. Bernard-Bonin AC. Maternal depression and child development. Paediatr Child Health. 2004;9:575–83.
56. Friedli L. Mental health, resilience and inequalities: World Health Organisation; 2009.
57. Linna SL, Mollanen I, Keistenen H, Ernvall MN, Karpinen MN. Prevalence of psychosomatic symptoms in children. Psychother Psychosom. 1991;56:85–7. https://doi.org/10.1159/000288535.
58. Merikangas KR, Nakamura EF, Kessler RC. Epidemiology of mental disorders in children and adolescents. Dialogues Clin Neurosci. 2009;11(1):7–20.
59. World Health Organization. Adolescents: health risks and solutions. Fact Sheet. 2017. http://www.who.int/mediacentre/factsheets/fs345/en/. Accessed 6 Sept 2017.
60. United States Government Department of Health & Human Services (USHHS). Trends in teen pregnancy and childbearing. https://www.hhs.gov/ash/oah/adolescent-development/reproductive-health-and-teen-pregnancy/teen-pregnancy-and-childbearing/trends/index.html. Accessed 6 Sept 2017.
61. Papachristou N, Barnarghi P, Cooper BA, Hu X, Maguire R, Apostolidis K, Armes J, Conley YP, Hammer M, Katsaragakis S, Kober KM, Levine JD, McCann L, Patiraki E, Paul SM, Ream E, Wright F, Miaskowski C. Congruence between latent class and K-modes analysis in the identification of oncology patients with distinct symptom experiences. J Pain Symptom Manage. 2018;55(2):318–333.e4. https://doi.org/10.1016/j.jpainsymman.2017.08.020.
62. Borklof JH, Engedal K, Selbaek G, Kouwenhoven SG, Helvik AS. Coping and depression in old age: a literature review. Dement Geriatr Cogn Disord. 2013;35:121–54. https://doi.org/10.1159/000346633.
63. McCrae RR. Situational determinants of coping responses: loss, threat, and challenge. J Pers Soc Psychol. 1984;46:919–28. https://doi.org/10.1037/0022-3514.46.4.919.
64. Andrusczkiewicz A, Basinska MA, Felsman M, Banaszkiewicz M, Marzec A, Kedziora-Kornatoska K. The determinants of coping in geriatric patients with chronic pain—the role of a sense of coherence. Clin Interv Aging. 2017;12:315–23. https://doi.org/10.2147/CIA.S118136.
65. Bonner WIA, Weiler R, Orisatoki R, Lu XY, Andkhoie M, Ramsey AD, Yaghoubi M, Steeves M, Szafron M, Farag M. Determinants of self-perceived health for Canadians aged 40 and older and policy implications. Int J Equity Health. 2017;16:94. https://doi.org/10.1186/s12939-017-0595-x.
66. Connely JE, Philbrick JT, Smith GR, Kaiser DL, Wymer A. Health perceptions of primary care patients and influence on health care utilization. Med Care. 1989;27:S99.
67. Sonnappa S, Bastardo CM, Aurora P, Whyatt D, Kelley FJ, Beevers SD, Grigg J. Residential proximity to main roads and lung health in young children. Eur Respir J. 2011;37:1525–6. https://doi.org/10.1183/09031936.00181910.
68. Hynes HP, Brugge D, Osgood D, Snell J, Vallarino J, Spengler J. "Where does the damp come from?" Investigations into the indoor environment and respiratory health in Boston public housing. J Public Health Policy. 2003;24:401–26.
69. Cutrona C, Wallace G, Wesner KA. Neighbourhood characteristics and depression: an examination of stress characteristics. Curr Dir Psychol Sci. 2006;15:188–92. https://doi.org/10.1111/j.1467-8721.2006.00433.x.
70. Ruel E, Oakley D, Elton-Wilson G, Maddox R. Is public housing the cause of poor health or a safety net for the unhealthy poor? J Urban Health. 2010;87:827–38. https://doi.org/10.1007/s11524-010-9484-y.
71. Crouse Quinn S. Hurricane Katrina: a social and public health disaster. Am J Public Health. 2006;96:204. https://doi.org/10.2105/AJPH.2005.080119.

72. Fussell E, Sastry N, van Landingham M. Race, socioeconomic status, and return migration to New Orleans after Hurricane Katrina. Popul Environ. 2010;31:20–42. https://doi.org/10.1007/s11111-009-0092-2.
73. Edwards RT, Ceilleachair A, Bywater ET, Hughes DA, Hutchins J. Parenting programme for parents of children at risk of developing conduct disorder: cost effectiveness analysis. BMJ. 2007;334(7595):682. https://doi.org/10.1136/bmj.39126.699421.55.
74. El Nokali LE, Bachman HJ, Votruba-Drzal E. Parent involvement and children's academic and social development in elementary school. Child Dev. 2010;81:988–1005. https://doi.org/10.1111/j.1467-8624.2010.01447.x.
75. Stevens M. The costs and benefits of early interventions for vulnerable children and families to promote social and emotional wellbeing: economics briefing. UK National Institute for Clinical Excellence. 2011. Expert report 32. https://www.nice.org.uk/. Accessed 7 Sept 2017.
76. Dennis CL, Hodnett ED. Psychosocial and psychological interventions for treating postpartum depression. Cochrane database of systematic reviews. Chichester, UK: Wiley; 2007.
77. Gunlicks ML, Weissman MM. Change in child psychopathology with improvement in parental depression: a systematic review. J Am Acad Child Adolesc Psychiatry. 2008;47:379–89.
78. Berkowitz T, Schaeffer CS, Rozek S, Beilock SL, Levine SC. The parent connection. Psychologist. 2017;30(9):28–32.
79. Michaels D. Doubt is their product: how industry's assault on science threatens your health. New York: OUP; 2008. ISBN: 9780195300673.
80. Lazarus RA, Folkman S. Stress, appraisal and coping. New York: Springer; 1984. ISBN 9780826141910.
81. Miller SM. Controllability and human stress: method, evidence and theory. Behav Res Ther. 1979;17:280–304.
82. Lefcourt HM. Research with the locus of control construct: extensions and limitations, vol. 3. Toronto: Elsevier; 2013.
83. Lam WWT, Chan M, Ka HW, Fielding R. Treatment decision difficulties and post-operative distress predict persistence of psychological morbidity in Chinese women following breast cancer surgery. Psychooncology. 2007;16(10):904–12.
84. Jim HS, Andryowski MA, Munster PN, Jacobson PB. Physical symptoms/side effects during breast cancer treatment predict posttreatment distress. Ann Behav Med. 2007;34:200–8.
85. Fan G, Filipczak L, Chow E. Symptom clusters in cancer patients: a review of the literature. Curr Oncol. 2007;14:173–9.
86. Dong ST, Butow PN, Costa DSJ, Lovell MR. Symptom clusters in patients with advanced cancer: a systematic review of observational studies. J Pain Symptom Manage. 2014;48:411–50.
87. Jim HSL, Jacobsen PB, Phillips KM, Wenham RM, Roberts W, Small BJ. Lagged relationships among sleep disturbance, fatigue, and depressed mood during chemotherapy. Health Psychol. 2013;32:768–75.
88. Foley D, Ancoli-Israel S, Brinz P, Walsh J. Sleep disturbances and chronic disease in older adults: results of the 2003 National Sleep Foundation Sleep in America Survey. J Psychosom Res. 2004;56:497–502.
89. Koyanagi A, Garin N, Olaya B, Asuyo-Mateos JL, Chaterjee S, Leonardi M, Koskinen S, Tobiasz-Adamczyk B, Haro JM. Chronic conditions and sleep problems among adults aged 50 years or over in nine countries: a multi-country study. PLoS One. 2014;9(12):e114742. https://doi.org/10.1371/journal.pone.0114742.
90. Wong WS, Fielding R. Prevalence of insomnia among Chinese adults in Hong Kong: a population-based study. J Sleep Res. 2011;20:117–26. https://doi.org/10.1111/j.1365-2869.2010.00822.x.
91. Luo JF, Zhu GX, Zhao QH, Guo QH, Hong Z, Meng HJ, Ding D. Prevalence and risk factors of poor sleep quality among Chinese elderly in an urban community: results from the shanghai aging study. PLoS One. 2013;8(11):e81261. https://doi.org/10.1371/journal.pone.0081261.
92. Kline CE. The bidirectional relationship between exercise and sleep: implications for exercise adherence and sleep improvement. Am J Lifestyle Med. 2014;8:375–9. https://doi.org/10.1177/1559827614544437.

93. Nutt D, Wilson S, Paterson L. Sleep disorders as core symptoms of depression. Dialogues Clin Neurosci. 2008;10:329–36.
94. Kvam S, Kleppe CL, Nordhus IH, Hovland A. Exercise as a treatment for depression: a meta-analysis. J Affect Disord. 2016;202:67–86. https://doi.org/10.1016/j.jad.2016.03.063.
95. Schuch FB, Vancampfort D, Richards J, Rosembaum S, Ward PB, Stubbs B. Exercise as a treatment for depression: a meta-analysis adjusting for publication bias. J Psychiatr Res. 2016;77:42–51. https://doi.org/10.1016/j.jpsychires.2016.02.023.
96. Fielding R, Wong WS. Prevalence of chronic pain, insomnia, and fatigue in Hong Kong. Hong Kong Med J. 2012;18(S3):9–12.
97. Hauser W, Wolfe F, Henningsen P, Schmutzer G, Brahler E, Hinz A. Untying chronic pain: prevalence and societal burden of chronic pain stages in the general population—a cross-sectional survey. BMC Public Health. 2014;14:352. https://doi.org/10.1186/1471-2458-14-352.
98. Fayaz A, Croft P, Langford RM, Donaldson LJ, Jones GT. Prevalence of chronic pain in the UK: a systematic review and meta-analysis of population studies. BMJ Open. 2016;6:6. https://doi.org/10.1136/bmjopen-2015-010364.
99. Jakobsson U. The epidemiology of chronic pain in a general population: results of a survey in southern Sweden. Scand J Rheumatol. 2010;39(5):421–9. https://doi.org/10.3109/03009741003685616.
100. Johannes CB, Lu TK, Zhao X, Johnson JA, Dworkin H. The prevalence of chronic pain in United States adults: results of an internet-based survey. J Pain. 2010;11:1230–9. https://doi.org/10.1016/j.jpain.2010.07.002.
101. Rogers K. Life Expectancy in U.S. Declines Slightly, and Researchers Are Puzzled. https://www.nytimes.com/2016/12/08/health/life-expectancy-us-declines.html?mcubz=0.

Communication and Relational Skills in Medicine

9

Carmel Loughland, Philippa Ditton-Phare, and David W. Kissane

Abstract

Effective clinical communication is key to high-quality person-centered health care, but this can be challenging for medical professionals, especially when the news is unwelcome, distressing, or complex to deliver. Despite inherent challenges, effective communication can be taught. Two advanced communication training programs are discussed. The Comskil model teaches advanced modules to cancer clinicians about how to communicate distressing diagnostic and prognostic news to oncology patients and families. The program has matured into a comprehensive curriculum and utilizes highly trained simulated patients and small group role-plays that allow trainees to learn, practice, and evaluate communication skills in a safe learning environment. Digital recordings along with facilitator and peer group discussions are used to provide immediate feedback to trainees about their performance. The validity and utility of the Comskil program have been demonstrated, applied to over 1000 clinicians, as has the use of facilitator-led small group role-play sessions. This framework provided a useful model from which to develop a communication skills training program specific to psychiatry. The ComPsych model focuses on schizophrenia and management approaches aligned to a recovery-orientated framework and has demonstrated acceptability, utility, and efficacy for psychiatry. A greater understanding is

C. Loughland · P. Ditton-Phare
Department of Psychiatry, Centre for Brain and Mental Health Research, University of Newcastle, Newcastle, NSW, Australia

Hunter New England Mental Health Service, Newcastle, NSW, Australia

D. W. Kissane (✉)
Department of Psychiatry, Monash University, Melbourne, VIC, Australia

Szalmuk Family Psycho-Oncology Research Unit, Cabrini Health, Malvern, VIC, Australia
e-mail: david.kissane@monash.edu

L. Grassi et al. (eds.), *Person Centered Approach to Recovery in Medicine*, Integrating Psychiatry and Primary Care, https://doi.org/10.1007/978-3-319-74736-1_9

needed of how medical professionals use a reflective process to make sense of their communication with patients, how training impacts communication style, and how communication style is further developed in practice.

9.1 Introduction

The very essence of high-quality person-centered care in the twenty-first century is grounded in effective communication between the clinician and the person receiving care. This is a complex task subject to a mutual understanding of needs, preferences, and expectations, with appropriate cultural sensitivity and insight into health literacy, and built upon a trusting relationship. When communication is truly patient-centered, it has the potential to promote healing and ameliorate suffering [1].

The reasons to enhance physician-patient communication are several and relate to optimizing the quality of care, the resultant satisfaction with care, and importantly enhancing the optimal take-up of evidence-based recommendations, when treatment is crucial to enhanced health and well-being. Such care delivery is nevertheless challenging, especially when unwelcome news about poor health needs to be shared and prognosis discussed, treatment choices are complex, and a threat to life (or quality of life) exists for the recipient of such information. Despite these inherent challenges, communication can be taught as a skill, such that clinicians may employ sensible strategies, choose language wisely, behave compassionately, and clarify understanding, so that essential information can be not only transmitted to but integrated by the patient, who can then utilize it for health-promoting benefits [2].

Three decades of research and endeavors to teach communication have resulted in the irrefutable finding that effective communication can be taught—basic models are employed by medical and nursing undergraduate schools, while advanced models have been applied to specialty training [3]. Clinicians can be taught to respond empathically to human distress because they can learn to recognize emotional cues, rehearse verbal utterances that they can make in response, and cultivate the ability to prioritize such behaviors in settings that benefit clinically from such responses.

9.2 Models of Communication Skills Training

In its early origins, communication skills training (CST) developed tasks to solve certain perceived problems in medical communication [4, 5]. Examples included "how to ask a question?" or "how to increase empathic responsiveness?" Work matured with simulated patients creating safe environments for clinicians in small groups to test awkward scenarios in a creative endeavor to find ways to improve their communication [6]. Such development was a little random and haphazard, being facilitated by a trainer who asked clinicians to nominate the major predicaments that challenged them and then sought collectively with each small group to build a more adaptive response [7]. As medical schools took up the gauntlet, their focus was initially on assessment techniques for optimal history taking, and they developed classifications like open, closed, and focused questions to respond to their need. As others researched specific encounters that led to frameworks for shared decision-making, the movement from a paternalistic medical model to deeper patient-centeredness matured. Gradually researchers questioned the theory, objectives, and techniques that were being employed in search of a more integrated approach [8].

Given the prospect at Memorial Sloan Kettering Cancer Center (MSKCC) of developing a dedicated Communications Skills Training and Research Laboratory, which became known as the Comskil laboratory, we sought to better define what should be taught so that it could in turn be measured, with outcomes assessed [9]. Drawing on goals, plans, and actions as a theoretical model [10, 11], we built the Comskil model that defined for each training module a communication goal, a set of sequential strategies to follow to achieve that goal, and in turn behavioral tasks and verbal skills that ensured accomplishment of each strategy (see Fig. 9.1) [12]. This quickly evolved into a reproducible and learner-centered facilitation model, which had the aim of training learners undertaking CST to develop a language to describe the strategies and skills they used, which empowered individual reflection about what the clinician was doing at any time. Such a reflective function, exactly what the psychotherapist uses in seeking to develop mentalization in the mind of a patient, proves invaluable to the clinician. This could be thought of as building a communication literacy, because by naming strategies, skills, and processes that advance patient-centered communication, we empower the clinician with the ability to choose requisite strategies and skills at recognizable predicaments.

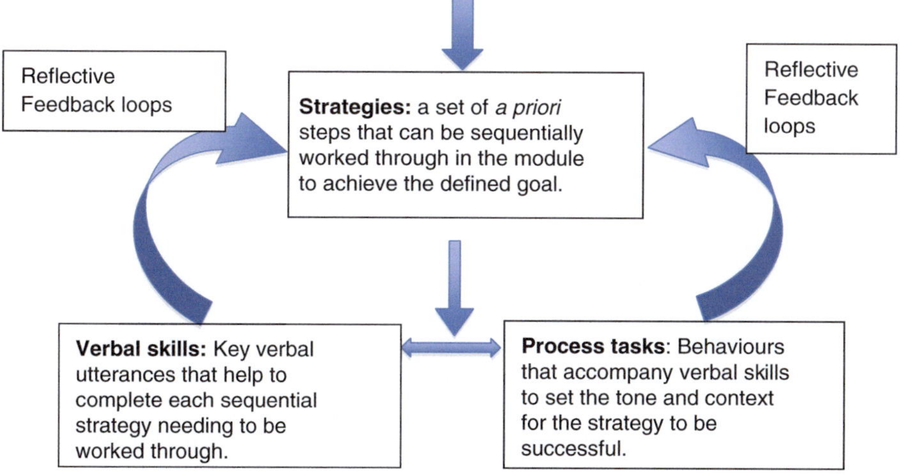

Fig. 9.1 Comskil model as a framework for communication skill training

An example might illustrate this theoretical notion. When a topic has been well discussed, the clinician may be ready to move on to the next concern. But is the patient aligned with this clinician's perspective? The skill of "taking stock" checks to see if the timing is right to move on. Here the clinician offers a brief summary of what has been discussed and asks directly if the patient has understood all of this, such that they give permission to move on. To put a name to this skill, and to identify its place among an array of communication options, is what we mean by building a communication literacy in the armamentarium of the clinician. Thus, when confronted with a difficult predicament, the clinician can reflect to him- or herself on what strategies will be needed to resolve the predicament and in turn consider what skills will optimally accomplish each strategy. The accompanying process tasks are usually more basic and include behaviors like maintaining eye contact with the patient, offering tissues when tears occur, or choosing a private space for a consultation that delivers the results of key investigations.

Our result was the Comskil model, which clustered teachable skills into six higher-ordered categories, within which we could define each skill and illustrate its application [13]. Examples of these categories of skill clusters included (1) agenda setting and framework, (2) questioning, (3) information organization, (4) checking preferences and level of desire for knowledge, (5) empathic skills, and (6) shared decision-making communication skills. We will illustrate and define these shortly (see Table 9.1).

In addition, a curriculum was readily established as we recognized the series of predicaments that clinicians identified as moments of challenge that can occur across any consultation. Each reproducible predicament was termed a module, as it had a focused goal to achieve its resolution, often unique strategies to fulfill this, and different skills and tasks proved relevant to particular modules. Working initially in the oncology setting, this modular curriculum followed the journey of the cancer illness: breaking diagnostic news, discussing prognosis, achieving a shared treatment decision, responding to difficult emotions, dealing with denial, responding to spouses/carers in the consultation, working with interpreters, preparing for survivorship, dealing with unexpected surgical events, supporting disease recurrence, transitioning to palliative care, running a family meeting, and talking about death and dying [14]. While these modules originated in the oncology setting, they carried broad applicability to many other challenges in dealing with complex medical and surgical illnesses.

We only needed to validate a coding schema to confirm the uptake of learning goals [15], standardize facilitation techniques to optimize learner-centered needs in experiential training [16], and comparably develop a coding schema to confirm the fidelity of our educational approach [17], and we then had a comprehensive approach to communication skills training with broad applicability to all of medicine.

9.2.1 Definitions of Key Skills to Build a Literacy of Communication Skills Training

Let us take time to define and illustrate the common skills within the broad six clusters of skills that we recognized. These are set out in Table 9.1.

Table 9.1 The verbal utterances forming the common communication skills used in medical practice with illustrative examples

Broad skill category	Name of specific skill	Example of verbal utterance
1. *Agenda setting and framework skills*:		
	(a) Invite patient's agenda	"Tell me what issues or concerns you have come with today?"
	(b) Declare clinician's agenda	"I note it is also time to review your blood pressure and order some annual health checks."
	(c) Negotiate shared agenda	"So let's learn about these new symptoms first and then see what examination and tests we need."
	(d) Take stock of progress	'Thus far, I have a good sense of your history. Are you ready for me to conduct a physical examination?"
	(e) Summarize progress	"The history and examination point to the need for three sorts of tests we should plan for to complete this assessment. These are…"
2. *Questioning skills*		
	(a) Open-ended, linear questions	"Tell me the story of this symptom that you developed?"
	(b) Focused questions	"How would you describe this pain?"
	(c) Structured systematic questions	"Let me ask you what aggravates and also what improves this pain?"
	(d) Closed questions	"Do you ever think that life is not worth it anymore?"
	(e) Circular questions	"How do your children communicate with one another?"
	(f) Strategic or therapeutic questions	"What are the benefits and burdens of caring for your sick parent at home?"
3. *Information organization skills*		
	(a) Previewing	"There are four potential side-effects from this medication that I want to review with you."
	(b) Categorizing	"Treatments for your condition can be grouped into (1) surgical; (2) radiotherapy; and (3) active surveillance. Let's discuss each in turn."
	(c) Information provision	"Let me explain this operation as I draw here to illustrate what I would do."
	(d) Summarizing	"So there are benefits and risks associated with each potential treatment, all of what can deliver a satisfactory outcome. Your preferences matter a lot here, and we need to discuss together what appeals to you and why."
	(e) Educational brochures	"I want to send you home with some more reading material about these options and give you some time to think through your preference and discuss it with your close relatives."
4. *Checking skills*		
	(a) Checking patient understanding	"What I presented is a complex concept. Please explain it back to me to help me understand what level of detail you have grasped?"
	(b) Checking patient preference for detail	"Some prefer a lot of detail, including statistics; others prefer more of an overview. Please guide me as to how much detail you want to grasp about this illness."
	(c) Checking interest in prognosis	"Some people ask directly about their prognosis; others say they are not ready to know. Guide me with your level of interest."
	(d) Patient summarizing	"I've shared a lot of detail with you today. Summarize for me the key points that you are taking away with you?"

(continued)

Table 9.1 (continued)

Broad skill category	Name of specific skill	Example of verbal utterance
5. *Empathic skills*		
	(a) Emotional acknowledgement	"I can see a lot of grief as a result of these results."
	(b) Emotional normalization	"The sadness you feel now is quite a normal response that many others experience in these circumstances."
	(c) Emotional validation	"Your anger at this outcome is both comprehensible and almost inescapable given the tough hand you have been dealt."
	(d) Silence	"I see the tears. I feel your pain. There are no easy words for what you are being asked to cope with."
	(e) Foster spousal or caregiver support	"I sense your partner has been hit hard by this news. What words would you use to describe what is being felt?"
6. *Shared decision-making skills*		
	(a) Priority of personal choice	"Are you the sort of person who really likes to make an independent choice about their body?"
	(b) Medical recommendation preferred	"Some people do like their doctor to recommend what is best."
	(c) Partnership statement	"Let's try together to work out what might be the best treatment choice for you."

9.2.2 Standardization of Coding Communication in Research Endeavors

Once programs establish which skills they want to teach and what role-play scenarios they will use to help learners develop mastery of these skills, it becomes important to be able to demonstrate success resultant upon any educational process. We have created standardized patient assessments (SPAs) to do this in the laboratory or in vitro setting, wherein actors are trained to offer reproducible responses across a range of encounters with different learners [18]. The reliability and discriminant validity of the SPA have been demonstrated previously [19–21]. With adequate rehearsal and clear direction, actors can effectively simulate realistic encounters and do so in a manner than can be graded in an objective and structured manner. This has been used for medical student exams for many years (OCSE = Objective Clinical Structured Examination) and can similarly be used as a pre- and post-training assessment to generate competency as a result of CST.

9.2.3 Standardization of Facilitation of Role-Play Learning

In like manner, it becomes possible to adopt a strengths-based and learner-centered approach to facilitation of role-play exercises with simulated patients in small groups by following a series of guidelines that help facilitators to optimize these learning sessions. We have found the following principles for providing feedback most beneficial:

1. Identify what worked in the role-play encounter (offer praise first).
2. Invite the learner to self-reflect about what proved challenging and why.
3. Seek constructive feedback from observers.
4. Observe the interaction through immediate playback of a video recording of the encounter.
5. Determine that the goal was achieved, or select an alternative strategy that may overcome any perceived difficulty.
6. Rerun the encounter to explore the benefits of using alternative skills or strategies.
7. Re-discuss what worked well and what proved challenging.

Occasionally learners find it stressful to expose their skills in front of peers. The facilitator carries responsibility for maintaining safety in the small group [22].

As we built experience, we quickly learnt that respected specialists from the discipline of any learner prove important for the modeling they can provide and accurate interpretation of technical treatment issues that are met by that specialty. Nevertheless, psychosocial experts did best when it came to recognition and modeling of empathic opportunities that could be easily missed by a specialist from an unrelated discipline. We therefore developed a co-facilitation model, wherein the specialist from the learner's discipline took responsibility for the discipline-specific content under discussion, while the psychosocial co-facilitator took responsibility for adherence to the model of training and the empathic skill development that occurred. Thus a blended model of facilitation proved optimal to accomplish the complex goals that we aimed to achieve [2].

9.2.4 Evidence for Comskil Effectiveness in Oncology Training

In mounting CST for over 1000 faculty and trainees progressing through the Comskil laboratory at MSKCC, we undertook a formal evaluation under the auspices of an R25 grant mechanism from the National Cancer Institute (CA134252, Principal Investigator, D.W. Kissane). Over 4 academic years, a total of 85 oncology faculty formed interdisciplinary pairs to co-facilitate experiential learning for 262 postgraduate trainees, who took part in some 536 small group CST role-plays. Fidelity of CST facilitation was confirmed though application of the Comskil facilitator competence coding schema [17]. Participants reported high satisfaction with the CST experience [2] and revealed significant skill growth through pre- and post-training SPAs in the laboratory (mean increase of 1.19 new skills, effect size $d = 0.60$), but transfer of these skills into the clinic was incomplete [23]. Some 803 outpatients gave feedback and permitted consultation recordings. The important finding was that participants with lower baseline scores had the largest improvements in their use of communication skills with both SPAs and in clinic recording of real patients.

In this MSK program, many attending physicians restricted the role that their trainee fellows could play with patients in the clinic, as the institution was a private one. The fellows often took histories but did not engage in shared decision-making discussions with the patients, waiting instead for the oncologists to have these with their private patients. This restricted considerably the observations that we could record and assess to ascertain how much the skills taught in the laboratory could be transferred into the real clinical setting.

Nevertheless, it was our experience at MSKCC that trainees learnt to be able to reflect on their communication, enhance their use of empathic comments, and better structure the content of their conversations so that efficiency was increased, while message delivery was enhanced for the benefit of all. It is a universal challenge the world over to show the transfer of communication skills learnt in the in vitro setting of the laboratory to the in vivo real clinic with patients. This is as much a methodological challenge for research, as it is clear to many of us who have facilitated communication training through the years that our own clinical skills have increased as a result of the teaching we have done.

9.3 The Psychiatry Model of Communication Skills Training

There are few formal postgraduate educational programs specific to psychiatry involving the experiential use of CST. The ComPsych program was developed based on the Comskil model. ComPsych teaches advanced modules to psychiatrists about how to communicate distressing diagnostic, prognostic, and treatment-related news to mental health patients and their families and carers. ComPsych, likewise, has strong theoretical underpinnings that draw on experiential, interpersonal, and culturally sensitive role-play from sociolinguistic theory and goals, plans, and actions theory [24]. Communication is viewed as a goal-driven process, which ultimately may modify the behavior of the recipient [25]. According to the model, communication consists of five components: goals, strategies, skills, process tasks, and cognitive appraisals [12]. This is not a prescriptive but rather a flexible model that aims to further develop participants' communication skills by allowing them to choose those that are necessary and appropriate for an individual situation. ComPsych teaches learners a reflective language about their communication skills and strategies through which they can self-evaluate future communication and continuously seek improvement.

Current practices within psychiatry were examined using a brief e-list survey of clinicians about the communication of diagnostic information, particularly for severe psychotic illnesses (e.g., schizophrenia) [26]. Findings identified broad endorsement for the complexity of communicating a schizophrenia diagnosis, the challenge it presents to clinicians, and acknowledgement of the impact of the illness on communication (e.g., patients' cognitive disorganization and impaired insight). Dilemmas around the uncertainty about diagnosis and the use of explanatory models (e.g., a stress-diathesis model) that promoted an optimistic therapeutic framework were also identified.

A parallel series of qualitative studies were also conducted with both clinicians and patients. Mental health patients reported unmet information needs. They described difficulties obtaining information about their diagnosis, prognosis, and treatment and discussed the long and difficult road to being told a diagnosis, the haphazard means of finding out the diagnosis, and exclusion from the medical care process [27]. Patients highlighted poor clinician communication and engagement as a major concern [28].

Mental health clinicians discussed the dilemmas they face in communicating this information. In one study [29], slightly more than half of clinicians interviewed supported the need to inform people with schizophrenia of their diagnosis yet listed several reasons for not doing so, including concerns about diagnostic uncertainty, patient distress, loss of hope, and risk of suicide. In a second study [30], the vital role of clinical context and environment was examined in promoting or inhibiting optimal communication around a schizophrenia diagnosis. Clinicians articulated their frustrations about team functioning and leadership and identified contextual and environmental barriers to discussing a schizophrenia diagnosis with patients, including poorly functioning multidisciplinary teams, differing models of leadership, and lack of planning resulting in ad hoc communication and tensions between team members.

The strong themes identified in the research provided the foundation for the development of the ComPsych advanced communication skills training program for psychiatry and construction of our detailed modules.

9.3.1 The ComPsych Program

The ComPsych program is deliverable within existing psychiatry development programs. To date, the program has focused on schizophrenia, primarily because it is identified by clinicians as presenting a more challenging set of communication tasks than other mental health problems and the illness is frequently encountered within mental health services.

The program consists of four modules based on best practice techniques: *Discussing Diagnosis* focuses on key skills in agenda setting, empathic responding, and checking understanding [12]; *Discussing Illness Prognosis* utilizes a "best/worst/most likely" case scenario model [31, 32]; and *Discussing Treatment* utilizes principles of patient-centered, shared decision-making that promotes adherence to recommended medications and counseling approaches [33, 34], while *Conducting Family Meetings* makes use of communication skills unique to the family setting to foster mutual empathic support within the family [35, 36]. ComPsych consists of educational resources, presentation slides, exemplary videos, and facilitation guidelines for each module. Didactic sessions provide a theoretical and empirical introduction to the topic and an overview of communication goals, strategies, skills, and process tasks and present specific examples of gold-standard communication behaviors. These management approaches are aligned to a recovery-orientated framework to promote hope and rehabilitation as conversations happen.

A key innovation in ComPsych is the use of small group role-play sessions led by trained facilitators using simulated patients (SP) specifically trained for the session and digital feedback during sessions [16, 37]. An SP pool and SP resources (i.e., training manuals, scenarios, assessment tools, etc.) specific to psychiatric care have been developed. Role-play sessions are learner-centered allowing trainees to identify key communication challenges, safely practice new communication skills with an SP, and receive immediate feedback about performance using digital playback and facilitator-led peer discussion.

9.3.2 Evidence for ComPsych Effectiveness in Psychiatry Training

Kirkpatrick's training evaluation triangle [38] was selected to evaluate the ComPsych program with respect to its acceptability and utility and its efficacy as a program. Kirkpatrick's framework has four levels of evaluation: Level 1 utilizes learner self-report. Level 2 uses observations and objective simulated patient assessments (SPAs) to evaluate skill development. Level 3 examines the translation of training into "real-world" practice. Level 4 evaluates the impact of such training and skill development on patient outcomes.

9.3.3 ComPsych Evaluation Level 1: Acceptability and Learner-Reported Outcomes

To evaluate the utility and feasibility of the ComPsych training, self-reported confidence in a range of communication tasks was obtained pre-post training, along with trainees' views of the training methods and resources. Thirty-eight psychiatry trainees completed training. Significant improvements (effect sizes from $d = -0.98$ to -1.68) in confidence were observed post-training for discussing schizophrenia prognosis and working with simulated patients and in the ability to critically evaluate ones' own communication skills. Trainees also reported high levels of satisfaction with the training program, especially the use of small group workshops, role-plays, and the digital feedback. The findings support the translation to psychiatry of the well-established Comskil oncology educational model to address core clinical communication tasks in psychiatry [39].

9.3.4 ComPsych Evaluation Level 2: Skills Demonstrated in a Simulated Setting

To objectively assess communication skills acquisition, 22 psychiatry trainees completed a standardized patient assessment (SPA) pre-post training. Each SPA was conducted with a trained SP using a standardized patient scenario. SPAs lasted 15 min each and were digitally recorded. Pre-post-SPA performances for each trainee were coded using a standardized instrument to score frequency, breadth of skills, and processes [2, 15, 40]. Coders were independent and blind to pre-post SPA order. A significant improvement in agenda setting skills ($d = -0.97$) was observed, with a corresponding decrease in questioning skills, suggesting early agenda setting diminished the volume of questioning required to conduct the meeting. A dose effect was also observed, with trainees attending two or more training sessions outperforming those attending only one. The findings provided preliminary evidence that training can successfully improve the frequency of specific patient-centered communication behaviors [41].

9.3.5 ComPsych Evaluation Levels 3 and 4: Translation of Skills to Practice and Impact on Patients

A systematic review of current evidence [42] revealed a significant gap in knowledge about how communication training is translated into practice and the impact on patients' experiences of care. Also identified were a variety of barriers to undertaking this research, including the significant resources and high-level expertise required to conduct translational research; inadequate sample sizes due to regular rotation of trainees through clinical placements impacting follow-up; busy, dynamic workplaces not conducive to objective assessment methods; and significant health service governance support requirements. Undertaking translational research in mental health care settings necessitates strong partnerships with and between mental health clinicians, researchers, educators, and regulatory bodies if it is to be successful.

Since this review was published, a cluster randomized controlled trial was conducted by McCabe et al. [43], with the intervention group showing an increase post-training in self-repair ($d = 0.91$), an increase in psychiatrist confidence ($p < 0.01$), as well as a significantly improved therapeutic relationship on both psychiatrist ratings ($p = 0.022$) and patient ratings ($p = 0.043$). Patient ratings of the therapeutic relationship between themselves and the psychiatrist are the first reported level 4 outcome [44] of psychiatry CST. This budding research in psychiatry CST is the foundation from which further higher-level evaluations need to occur for a greater understanding of how CST translates into clinical practice.

9.4 Methodological Limitations

Previous research on communication skills training [45–49] has shown that transfer of learning into the workplace is hampered by context-specific issues such as a supportive work environment, supervisors' availability, dose of training, and time constraints, as well as trainee-specific factors such as fatigue, and existing beliefs and attitudes toward communication and communication skills. Exactly how this complex interaction of factors seems to be influencing transfer remains unclear. There is a need for more clarification research [50] to gain insight into these underlying mechanisms [51] and their measurement, specifically how to foster lasting improvements of communication skills following the ComPsych intervention, and how to integrate these in participants' continuous development, rather than a onetime improvement in "off-site" training and assessment.

9.5 Summary

This chapter outlined two communication skills training programs, namely, Comskil and ComPsych, and subsequent assessments of their efficacy in oncology and psychiatry. Studies demonstrate the utility and feasibility of the Comskil and ComPsych models as a framework for advanced experiential CST in medical training. The next step for future research is to utilize both qualitative and quantitative methodology to determine the barriers and enablers to translation of these programs to clinical practice and the effect of CST on patient outcomes. It will be important to understand how medical professionals use reflective thinking to make sense of how they communicate with patients, how CST programs affect their communication style, and how they further develop their communication style in practice.

References

1. Epstein RM, Street RL Jr. Patient-centered communication in cancer care: promoting healing and reducing suffering. Bethesda: National Cancer Institute; 2007.
2. Kissane DW, Bylund CL, Banerjee SC, Bialer PA, Levin TT, Maloney EK, et al. Communication skills training for oncology professionals. J Clin Oncol. 2012;30(11):1242–7.
3. Barth J, Lannen P. Efficacy of communication skills training courses in oncology: a systematic review and meta-analysis. Ann Oncol. 2011;22(5):1030–40.
4. Lipkin M Jr, Quill TE, Napodano RJ. The medical interview: a core curriculum for residencies in internal medicine. Ann Intern Med. 1984;100(2):277–84.
5. Maguire P, Fairbairn S, Fletcher C. Consultation skills of young doctors—benefits of feedback training in interviewing as students persist. Br Med J. 1986;292:1573–8.
6. Maguire P, Pitceathly C. Key communication skills and how to acquire them. Br Med J. 2002;325(7366):697–700.
7. Fallowfield L, Jenkins V. Effective communication skills are the key to good cancer care. Eur J Cancer. 1999;35(11):1592–7.
8. Cegala DJ, Lenzmeier Broz S. Physician communication skills training: a review of theoretical backgrounds, objectives and skills. Med Educ. 2002;36(11):1004–16.
9. Brown RF, Bylund CL, Kissane DW. Principles of communication skills training in cancer care. In: Holland JC, Breitbart WS, Jacobsen PB, Lederberg MS, Loscalzo MJ, McCorkle R, editors. Psycho-oncology. 2nd ed. Oxford: Oxford University Press; 2010.
10. Miller K. Communication theories: perspectives, processes, and contexts: McGraw-Hill Humanities/Social Sciences/Languages; 2005.
11. Wilson SR, Morgan WM. Goals-plans-action theories: theories of goals plans and planning processes in families. In: Braithwaite DO, Baxter LA, editors. Engaging theories in family communication: multiple perspectives. Boston, MA: McGraw-Hill; 2006.
12. Brown RF, Bylund CL. Communication skills training: describing a new conceptual model. Acad Med. 2008;83(1):37–44.

13. Brown R, Bylund CL. Theoretical models of communication skills training. In: Kissane DW, Bultz BD, Butow P, Finlay I, editors. Handbook of communication in oncology and palliative care. Oxford: Oxford University Press; 2010.
14. Kissane DW, Bultz BD, Butow PN, Bylund CL, Noble S, Wilkinson S, editors. Oxford textbook of communication in oncology and palliative care. 2nd ed. Oxford: Oxford University Press; 2017.
15. Bylund CL, Brown R, Gueguen JA, Diamond C, Bianculli J, Kissane DW. The implementation and assessment of a comprehensive communication skills training curriculum for oncologists. Psycho-Oncology. 2010;19(6):583–93.
16. Bylund CL, Brown RF, di Ciccone BL, Levin TT, Gueguen JA, Hill C, et al. Training faculty to facilitate communication skills training: development and evaluation of a workshop. Patient Educ Couns. 2008;70(3):430–6.
17. Bylund CL, Brown RF, Lubrano di Ciccone B, Diamond C, Eddington J, Kissane DW. Assessing facilitator competence in a comprehensive communication skills training programme. Med Educ. 2009;43(4):342–9.
18. Heinrich P. The role of the actor in medical education. In: Kissane DW, Bultz BD, Butow PN, Bylund CL, Noble S, Wilkinson S, editors. Oxford textbook of communication in oncology and palliative care. 2nd ed. Oxford: Oxford University Press; 2017. p. 357–62.
19. Joorabchi B. Objective structured clinical examination in a pediatric residency program. Am J Dis Child. 1991;145(7):757–62.
20. Sloan DA, Donnelly MB, Johnson SB, Schwartz RW, Strodel WE, Browne BJ, et al. Use of an Objective Structured Clinical Examination (OSCE) to measure improvement in clinical competence during the surgical internship. Surgery. 1993;114(2):343–51.
21. Sloan DA, Donnelly MB, Schwartz RW, Strodel WE. The Objective Structured Clinical Examination. The new gold standard for evaluating postgraduate clinical performance. Ann Surg. 1995;222(6):735–42.
22. Levin T, Horner J, Bylund C, Kissane D. Averting adverse events in communication skills training: a case series. Patient Educ Couns. 2010;81(1):126–30.
23. Bylund CL, Banerjee SC, Bialer PA, Manna R, Levin TL, Parker PA, et al. The impact of a cancer communication skills program on trainees and patients. Cancer. 2017.
24. Dillard JP. Goals-plans-action theory of message production: making influence messages. In: Baxter LA, Braithwaite DO, editors. Engaging theories in interpersonal communication: multiple perspectives. Thousand Oaks, CA: Sage; 2008. p. 65–76.
25. Bylund CL, Peterson EB, Cameron KA. A practitioner's guide to interpersonal communication theory: an overview and exploration of selected theories. Patient Educ Couns. 2012;87(3):261–7.
26. Levin TT, Kelly BJ, Cohen M, Vamos M, Landa Y, Bylund CL. Case studies in public-sector leadership: using a psychiatry e-list to develop a model for discussing a schizophrenia diagnosis. Psychiatr Serv. 2011;62(3):244–6.
27. Outram S, Harris G, Kelly B, Bylund CL, Cohen M, Landa Y, et al. We didn't have a clue': family caregivers' experiences of the communication of a diagnosis of schizophrenia. Int J Soc Psychiatry. 2015;61(1):10–6.
28. Loughland C, Cheng K, Harris G, Kelly B, Cohen M, Sandhu H, et al. Communication of a schizophrenia diagnosis: a qualitative study of patients' perspectives. Int J Soc Psychiatry. 2015;61(8):729–34.
29. Outram S, Harris G, Kelly B, Cohen M, Sandhu H, Vamos M, et al. Communicating a schizophrenia diagnosis to patients and families: a qualitative study of mental health clinicians. Psychiatr Serv. 2014;65(4):551–4.
30. Outram S, Harris G, Kelly B, Cohen M, Bylund CL, Landa Y, et al. Contextual barriers to discussing a schizophrenia diagnosis with patients and families: need for leadership and teamwork training in psychiatry. Acad Psychiatry. 2015;39(2):174–80.
31. Kiely BE, Tattersall MH, Stockler MR. Certain death in uncertain time: informing hope by quantifying a best case scenario. J Clin Oncol. 2010;28(16):2802–4.

32. Kiely BE, Soon YY, Tattersall MH, Stockler MR. How long have I got? Estimating typical, best-case, and worst-case scenarios for patients starting first-line chemotherapy for metastatic breast cancer: a systematic review of recent randomized trials. J Clin Oncol. 2011;29(4):456–63.
33. Tattersall MH. Clinical perspectives on shared decision-making. In: Kissane DW, Bultz BD, Butow P, Finlay I, editors. Handbook of communication in oncology and palliative care. Oxford: Oxford University Press; 2010. p. 339–50.
34. Kissane DW. Communication training to achieve shared decision making. In: Kissane DW, Bultz BD, Butow P, Finlay I, editors. Handbook of communication in oncology and palliative care. Oxford: Oxford University Press; 2010. p. 127–34.
35. Gueguen JA, Bylund CL, Brown RF, Levin TT, Kissane DW. Conducting family meetings in palliative care: themes, techniques, and preliminary evaluation of a communication skills module. Palliat Support Care. 2009;7(2):171–9.
36. Coyle N, Kissane DW. Conducting a family meeting. In: Kissane DW, Bultz BD, Butow PM, Finaly IG, editors. Handbook of communication in oncology and palliative care. New York, NY: Oxford University Press; 2010. p. 165–75.
37. Ditton-Phare P, Halpin S, Sandhu H, Kelly B, Vamos M, Outram S, et al. Communication skills in psychiatry training. Australas Psychiatry. 2015;23(4):429–31.
38. Bates R. A critical analysis of evaluation practice: the Kirkpatrick model and the principle of beneficence. Eval Program Plann. 2004;27(3):341–7.
39. Loughland C, Kelly B, Ditton-Phare P, Sandhu H, Vamos M, Outram S, et al. Improving clinician competency in communication about schizophrenia: a pilot educational program for psychiatry trainees. Acad Psychiatry. 2015;39(2):160–4.
40. Bylund CL, Brown RF, Bialer PA, Levin TT, Lubrano di Ciccone B, Kissane DW. Developing and implementing an advanced communication training program in oncology at a comprehensive cancer center. J Cancer Educ. 2011;26(4):604–11.
41. Ditton-Phare P, Sandhu H, Kelly B, Kissane D, Loughland C. Pilot evaluation of a communication skills training program for psychiatry residents using standardized patient assessment. Acad Psychiatry. 2016;40(5):768–75.
42. Ditton-Phare P, Loughland C, Duvivier R, Kelly B. Communication skills in the training of psychiatrists: a systematic review of current approaches. Aust N Z J Psychiatry. 2017;51(7):675–92.
43. McCabe R, John P, Dooley J, Healey P, Cushing A, Kingdon D, et al. Training to enhance psychiatrist communication with patients with psychosis (TEMPO): cluster randomised controlled trial. Br J Psychiatry. 2016;209(6):517–24.
44. Kirkpatrick DL. Great ideas revisited: revisiting Kirkpatrick's four-level model. Train Dev J. 1996;50(1):54–9.
45. Fallowfield L, Jenkins V, Farewell V, Solis-Trapala I. Enduring impact of communication skills training: results of a 12-month follow-up. Br J Cancer. 2003;89(8):1445–9.
46. Lienard A, Merckaert I, Libert Y, Bragard I, Delvaux N, Etienne AM, et al. Transfer of communication skills to the workplace during clinical rounds: impact of a program for residents. PLoS One. 2010;5(8):e12426.
47. Hulsman RL, Ros WJ, Winnubst JA, Bensing JM. Teaching clinically experienced physicians communication skills. A review of evaluation studies. Med Educ. 1999;33(9):655–68.
48. Henwood PG, Altmaier EM. Evaluating the effectiveness of communication skills training: a review of research. Clin Perform Qual Health Care. 1996;4(3):154–8.
49. Heaven C, Clegg J, Maguire P. Transfer of communication skills training from workshop to workplace: the impact of clinical supervision. Patient Educ Couns. 2006;60(3):313–25.
50. Cook DA, Bordage G, Schmidt HG. Description, justification and clarification: a framework for classifying the purposes of research in medical education. Med Educ. 2008;42(2):128–33.
51. van den Eertwegh V, van Dulmen S, van Dalen J, Scherpbier AJ, van der Vleuten CP. Learning in context: identifying gaps in research on the transfer of medical communication skills to the clinical workplace. Patient Educ Couns. 2013;90(2):184–92.

Somatic Health Issues in Trauma-Related Disorders: Effects on Psychobiological Axes Affecting Mental and Physical Health

10

Anthony P. King

Abstract

Psychological trauma is common and can have long-lasting deleterious effects on mental and physical health. Childhood adversity and maltreatment, as well as adult exposures to interpersonal violence, accidents and disasters, and other life-threatening medical events, such as myocardial infarcts can all be associated with psychological trauma, as can even lifesaving medical procedures such as surgeries and intensive care unit stays. Exposure to trauma in childhood and as adults is associated with increased risk for psychiatric morbidity, in particular posttraumatic stress disorder (PTSD), but also increased rates of depression and anxiety disorders. It has long been appreciated that PTSD has substantial comorbidity with other psychiatric disorders, including in depression and substance use disorders, and there is also accumulating evidence that childhood adversity, adult trauma exposure, and PTSD all have considerable somatic health consequences and are associated with increased disease risk and increased medical morbidity and mortality. These include conditions often associated with somatization and psychiatric morbidity, such as irritable bowel disorder, fibromyalgia, and other chronic pain disorders, but also more common medical disorders such as coronary artery disorder, atherosclerosis, cancer, and stroke. Trauma exposure and PTSD are associated with increased levels of health risk behaviors, such as smoking, alcohol and drug use, poor diet, and physical activity, as well as increased body mass index (BMI) and rates of obesity; PTSD is also associated with poorer medical compliance and healthcare utilization. All of these at-risk health behaviors likely contribute to the increased morbidity and mortality associated with trauma exposure and PTSD. It is possible that, in addition, specific

A. P. King
Department of Psychiatry, University of Michigan, Ann Arbor, MI, USA
e-mail: samadhi@med.umich.edu

L. Grassi et al. (eds.), *Person Centered Approach to Recovery in Medicine*, Integrating Psychiatry and Primary Care, https://doi.org/10.1007/978-3-319-74736-1_10

physiological processes related to trauma exposure and PTSD may also contribute to disease processes and increase morbidity. This chapter will review evidence linking trauma and PTSD to several psychobiological processes or "axes" that may contribute and/or mediate increased morbidity. Long-term effects of trauma and PTSD are presumably mediated and maintained by alterations on the brain/central nervous system (CNS) that then lead to alterations in output and activity of peripheral nervous system and autonomic as well as neuroendocrine systems that then effect changes on peripheral physiological processes such as cardiovascular function, immune function, and metabolism that lead to increased pathophysiological processes and disease risk. This chapter will review evidence of effects of trauma and PTSD on specific CNS functions that may be associated with "downstream" pathological processes, as well as evidence of effects of trauma and PTSD on the sympathetic autonomic system, the hypothalamic-pituitary-adrenal (HPA) axis, and immune function (in particular, inflammatory processes), all of which could contribute and/or mediate effects of trauma and PTSD on medical morbidity.

10.1 Trauma and Trauma-Related Psychiatric Syndromes

Psychological trauma is highly prevalent: estimates of lifetime exposure have ranged from 62% in a nationally representative sample [1] to over 90% in a Detroit-area cohort [2]. However, lifetime prevalence of posttraumatic stress disorder (PTSD) is much lower, indicating that the majority of trauma-exposed individuals do not develop PTSD and that exposure to a potentially traumatizing event per se is not sufficient to cause PTSD. [1–3]. Epidemiological studies point toward specific environmental events, particularly early life adversity such as child abuse or other childhood trauma, as risk factors for PTSD [4–7], suggesting that childhood adversity and maltreatment may mold psychological and physiological processes toward greater psychiatric vulnerability, and this may also have important repercussions for somatic health. A number of other environmental factors, including the nature and severity of the index trauma, previous trauma exposure, age at time of the trauma, and sociodemographic factors such as poverty and social support, all influence risk for PTSD, as do pre-existing or family history of depression and anxiety [1, 2, 8]. Currently those neurobiological factors that lead to increased vulnerability to PTSD in some and increased resilience in others are still an area of active research.

In general, psychological trauma is often associated with transient psychological reactions, which can include many of the core intrusive, avoidant, hyperarousal, and emotional negativity symptoms of PTSD. For most people, these transient reactions are followed by a period of recovery and a return to baseline functioning; however, for a significant minority, trauma can precipitate the development of PTSD [9]. Some people who do not develop PTSD following a trauma develop major depressive disorder (MDD), and some develop a combination of PTSD and MDD. Even when the experience of trauma does not directly precipitate an immediate psychiatric disorder, it may lead to greater risk for development of psychiatric problems later, perhaps many years later. A developmental perspective of PTSD risk factors could suggest that experience of trauma in early life could lead to disruption of neurodevelopmental processes or specific alterations in key neural systems that lead to long-term changes in adult patterns of emotional processing and/or physiological alterations in stress-responsive systems, leading to vulnerability to PTSD when the individual experiences additional trauma. Presumably, the experience of trauma also leads to alterations in neurobiological and physiological functions that may also impinge on a number of behavioral and pathophysiological systems that also may increase risk for somatic health disorders, and these pathophysiological processes may in some cases become further exacerbated by the syndrome of PTSD, further increasing health risks.

PTSD is highly prevalent and is associated with considerable human suffering, disability, and economic costs. The National Comorbidity Survey Replication study [10], a nationally representative sample of over 10,000 adults in the USA, found the lifetime prevalence of PTSD was over 7%, and the 12-month prevalence (percent of people who had met criteria for PTSD over the past year) was 4%. Thus PTSD is the third most prevalent disorder in the USA, after major depression (17% lifetime) and social anxiety disorder (12% lifetime), and worldwide prevalence appears similar. Furthermore, PTSD is twice as common in women (11% lifetime) than in men (5%). PTSD risk is higher in some subpopulations (e.g., 15–30% in combat veterans [11–13] and up to 45% in low SES people living in urban areas [14]. Over 20% of all Desert Storm combat-exposed veterans were diagnosed with PTSD 6 years after deployment [13] and up to 20% of all military veterans deployed to Iraq (OIF) and Afghanistan (OEF). PTSD has high levels of disability and family disruption that can last for decades [1, 3, 12, 13], often leading to significant loss of productivity, unemployment, and high economic costs to patients and to society [15]. Chronic PTSD is highly comorbid with major depressive disorder (MDD) . Chronic depression is a leading cause of disability, associated with notoriously high levels of relapse [16], and is often associated with trauma, and the combination of chronic PTSD and chronic depression can be particularly difficult to treat.

Definition of Trauma and PTSD Severe psychological disruptions associated with the experience of psychological trauma have been documented since ancient times, and descriptions of maladies similar to PTSD can be found in Homer, *The Book of Job*, the Mahabharata, Herodotus, and Shakespeare. However, the formal diagnostic category of "posttraumatic stress disorder" did not appear in the modern medical nosological system until the publication of the third edition of the Diagnostic and Statistical Manual of Mental Disorders (DSM-III-R) by the American Psychiatric Association in 1980. The specific definition of what constitutes a "trauma" and the diagnostic criteria of PTSD have continued to be refined since that time. The latest edition of the American Psychiatric Association's DSM-5 defines "trauma" as an aversive event in which a person experienced, witnessed, or was confronted with an event or events that involved actual or threatened death or serious injury, or a threat to the physical integrity of self or others, such as through sexual assault. (The previous requirement from DSM-IV of a reaction of fear, helplessness, or horror occurring right after the trauma has been removed from the trauma criteria definition, as it did not improve diagnostic accuracy for the disorder). In addition to the experience of a traumatic event, a specific constellation of symptoms must be present for at least 1 month. DSM-5 has four clusters of PTSD symptoms: **(A) intrusion** (e.g., intrusive, upsetting memories, getting upset to reminders of the trauma, nightmares, etc.), **(B) alterations in arousal and reactivity avoidance** (e.g., hypervigilance, exaggerated startle, concentration problems, irritability, sleep disturbance), **(C) avoidance** (e.g., avoiding trauma reminders), and **(D) negative alterations in cognitions and mood** (e.g., negative affect, anhedonia, feelings of isolation, overly negative thoughts about oneself or the world, exaggerated blame of self or others for causing the trauma)

PTSD can develop following a variety of traumas such as combat or exposure to wartime hostilities, physical and sexual assault, kidnapping, torture, and injuries from accidents, fires, and major disasters. PTSD can also develop from other very difficult but relatively "routine" and relatively common life events such as death of a loved one, miscarriage, abortion, and stressful medical procedures [1–3, 17]. Depression and PTSD can develop following stressful life events, including medical illnesses. Medical conditions requiring intensive care, such as myocardial infarctions and major surgeries, produce particularly high rates of psychiatric morbidity in several forms, including depression, anxiety, and posttraumatic stress disorder (PTSD). Elevated depressive symptoms are seen in as many as 65% of patients following myocardial infarction (MI), with up to 20% developing major depressive disorder [18]. Depression following cardiac artery bypass graft (CABG), and the relationship between depression and post-surgery cardiac outcomes, has been examined in a number of studies [19–21] with rates of depression following major surgery documented at 20–30%.

PTSD symptoms are also common in acute cardiac syndromes (ACS) which are clearly life-threatening [17]—a PTSD rate of 12% was reported in a large meta-analysis of ACS [22, 23]. Interestingly, elevated rates of PTSD have also been reported following surgical procedures [24–27]. Cardiac events represent extreme stressors both psychologically and physiologically, posing sudden grave threats to life and function, but cardiac and vascular surgeries, even when undertaken electively, are also associated with substantial rates of psychiatric morbidity. PTSD rates following bypass surgery or heart transplant can be as high as 20% [28–30], likely because even scheduled surgery of this type carries significant morbidity, threat of mortality, physiological trauma, and exposure to intensive care units (ICU), where fear of dying, helplessness, and loss of control are common. We have shown retrospectively that elective abdominal vascular surgery is associated with substantially elevated levels of postoperative depression, anxiety, and PTSD [31] overall, about a fourfold risk in new psychiatric syndromes following the surgery, although of course, retrospective report may be biased by presence of current psychopathology. We recently replicated a greater than fourfold increase in risk for development of de novo psychiatric disorders (depression, PTSD, GAD) in AAA patients who had open surgeries compared to those who had nonsurgical treatment followed over 18 months in a prospective study ([32]; all patients did not have a psychiatric diagnosis at the time of intake).

Early Life Trauma and PTSD Childhood adversity has long been theorized as an important component of psychiatric diathesis in psychodynamic as well as biopsychosocial models of adult clinical psychiatry. As reviewed in Briere and Jordan [33], child abuse and neglect, especially sexual abuse, is associated with PTSD both in children (e.g., [34]) and later in adults (e.g., [35, 36]). Child abuse and neglect has also been associated with a number of other psychiatric problems in adulthood, including mood and anxiety disorders [33] and chronic interpersonal difficulties [33]. Childhood sexual abuse is a particularly psychological challenging form of developmental insult. Women with a history of childhood sexual abuse are at increased risk for major depressive disorder (MDD) in adulthood [37], and there is work which suggests that the effects of CSA on MDD are causal [38]. Childhood sexual abuse can be associated with severe PTSD and a range of psychopathological disorders. Childhood adversity is also associated with increased risk for adult PTSD, even controlling for type of adult index trauma. There is now clear evidence that developmental insults including childhood traumas, such as physical and sexual abuse, or witnessing violence directed against the child's mother, are associated with much higher rates of development of PTSD after trauma exposure in adulthood. The effect of childhood trauma and adversity on adult PTSD risk is pronounced, with two- to fourfold increased risk in studies of male and female general medical patients [39] in an urban community to samples from epidemiological studies of males and females in inner-city Detroit [2, 40] and primarily females in inner-city Atlanta [41], to primarily male combat veterans deployed to Vietnam [5] and deployed to Iraq or Afghanistan [4]. Similar to the findings of Felitti et al. [42], not only childhood traumas per se but also other forms of childhood adversity such as loss of a parent and having a substance-dependent adult or seriously mentally ill adult residing in the childhood home are associated with substantially increased risk for PTSD in adult combat veterans (primarily men) deployed to Iraq [4]. Furthermore, the cumulative effects of the number of categories of ACE experienced had a pronounced and graded effect on risk for PTSD in this study of (primarily male) Iraq combat veterans (~8% incidence in soldiers with no childhood adversity following deployment to Iraq, compared to 30% incidence of PTSD in soldiers with four or more categories of ACE following deployment to Iraq; [4]).

10.2 Somatic Health Risks Associated with Trauma and Trauma-Related Psychiatric Syndromes

There is considerable epidemiological evidence that exposure to trauma as children and as adults and development of PTSD are all associated with poorer health outcomes and increased risk for several diseases and that development of the syndrome of PTSD further increases risk in terms of adult trauma exposures. Experiences of adversity and trauma during childhood appear to be particularly harmful to health outcomes. The Adverse Childhood Experiences (ACE) Study [42] was one of the first large-scale epidemiological studies of risks of childhood adversity to mental health and physical health. It examined seven categories of adverse childhood experiences in 9508 adults who were aged 19–34 years. The categories of ACE included psychological, physical, or sexual abuse, witnessing violence against one's mother, and living with adult household members who were substance abusers or seriously mentally ill. This study found 18% of respondents reported sexual abuse, 25% experienced at least one category of childhood adversity, and 38% experienced two or more categories. Having high levels of childhood adversity (exposure to four or more "ACEs") was associated with 4–5-fold increase in risk for major depression in the past year and a 12-fold increased risk for lifetime suicide attempt, controlling for SES and other risk factors. This study also found that having high levels of childhood adversity was associated with higher incidence of a number of health risk behaviors, including a five- to tenfold increase in alcoholism, illicit drug use, and intravenous drug use, approximately threefold increase in having a high number (>50) of lifetime sexual partners and lifetime risk for sexually transmitted disease, as well as approximately twofold increased risks for current smoking, severe obesity (BMI >35), and physical inactivity [42]. Epidemiological studies also find high levels of childhood adversity are significantly associated with higher risk for a number of serious somatic health disorders and diseases in these 19–39-year-old people [42–45], including approximately fourfold increased risk for chronic bronchitis or emphysema; two- to threefold increased risk for ischemic heart disease, any form of cancer, and stroke; approximately twofold increased risk for lifetime incidence of broken bones, hepatitis, and an overall self-rating of one's health as "fair or poor"; and significantly elevated risk for diabetes. Subsequent analyses have confirmed increased adult risk for several somatic diseases in people with high childhood adversity, including liver disease [46], chronic obstructive pulmonary disease (COPD, [43]), ischemic heart disease [44], and autoimmune disorders [45]. A retrospective study of relationship of the number of adverse childhood experiences ("ACE score") and selected mental health and physical health outcomes looked at >17,000 patients across four successive birth cohorts (1900–1931, 1932–1946, 1947–1961, and 1962–1978) and found statistically significant elevation of risks in all birth cohorts among people reporting the highest levels of childhood adversity, with 3–4-fold increased risk for depression, 10–20-fold increased risk for suicide attempts, and 1.5–3-fold risks for multiple sexual partners, smoking, and alcoholism, suggesting that somatic health risks associated with childhood adversity have remained relatively stable across the past century [45].

Epidemiological evidence also finds that adult trauma exposures and PTSD are also associated with substantially increased health risks in a wide range of diseases, including rheumatoid arthritis, stroke, heart disease and cancer, and cardiovascular and cardiometabolic diseases [5, 47–49]. In an epidemiological study of $N = 2490$ US military veterans of the conflict in Vietnam (1965–1976), Boscarino et al. [50] found significantly elevated levels of several autoimmune disorders among veterans with PTSD, in models adjusting for age, education, race, IQ, income, geographic region, Army volunteer status, number of times married, and history of antisocial personality, alcohol abuse, drug abuse, and cigarette smoking. There was a 3.3-fold increased risk for having any of the 20 autoimmune disorders tested and 3–8-fold increased risk for rheumatoid arthritis, psoriasis, insulin-dependent (type II) diabetes, Graves' disease, and hypothyroidism. This study also found significant derangements in several immune and neuroendocrine system laboratory measures, including three- to fivefold increased risk for elevated total and T-lymphocyte counts, elevated cell-mediated immunity response, elevated IgM, and lower levels of DHEA-S [47].

Perhaps the strongest evidence to date for the association of PTSD with health risks is in cardiovascular and metabolic diseases. Several large, methodologically rigorous, and well-controlled prospective population-based studies have now examined the association of PTSD with a number of cardiovascular outcomes in both veteran and civilian populations; the follow-up time has ranged from 3 to nearly 20 years, and several studies now have followed populations with tens to hundreds of thousands of people; and meta-analyses show ca. 1.5–2.0 hazard ratio for PTSD [48]. A study of 4000 US Vietnam veterans also found PTSD associated with about a twofold increase in overall heart disease mortality, after controlling for smoking, BMI, and intelligence, as well as history of major depression [47]. Several other large studies of US military veterans have also found PTSD associated with increases in incident cardiovascular disease. PTSD was associated with a 1.5-fold increased risk for heart failure in a study of 8248 veterans followed for 7 years and controlling for age, BMI, smoking, and demographic and metabolic measures, as well as depression [51]. Another well-controlled study of over 130,000 military veterans followed for 10 years reported PTSD associated with about a 1.5-fold increase in myocardial infarct (MI), peripheral vascular disease, congestive heart failure, and cerebrovascular disease [52], and the largest study to date of military veterans (over 350,000) found slightly lower but statistically significant hazard ratio of 1.39 controlling for age, race, smoking, substances, hypertension, etc. [53] and a smaller but still significant HR of 1.16 when also controlling for depression, which is commonly comorbid with PTSD. Population-based prospective studies in civilians found PTSD associated with an approximately 1.5- to 2-fold increase in MI and stroke in an 8-year follow-up of a 4000 person Danish population [54], and a recent study found an over 3-fold increase in risk for stroke in PTSD in a 26,000 person sample of Taiwanese [55]. Large and well-controlled prospective studies have also reported PTSD associated with a 2-fold increase in type 2 diabetes in over 44,000 US military members [56] and approximately 1.3- to 1.5-fold risk in a study of over 50,000 US nurses exposed to trauma and with varying levels of PTSD symptoms [57], controlling BMI, smoking, family genetic loading, and history of major depression.

In addition to distal childhood maltreatment and adult traumas associated with interpersonal violence and disasters, psychiatric symptoms that are associated with medical illnesses and invasive medical procedures can also contribute to medical morbidity [58, 59] and mortality [28], undermining outcomes and adding substantially to costs of care. For example, PTSD symptoms following MI double the risk of death or a second heart attack [22]. Even when physical recovery occurs, depression, posttraumatic stress, and anxiety symptoms [17, 26, 28, 31] can impair functional outcomes and raise costs [60, 61].

10.3 Potential Biological Pathways Related to PTSD and Somatic Health

Thus both early life adversity and trauma exposure and PTSD are associated with substantially elevated risk behaviors, including smoking, alcohol and substance use, risky sexual behaviors, poor diet, and inactivity, that are all likely to convey substantial health risks on affected people. Each of these behaviors/exposures has deleterious effects on specific organ systems, physiological axes, and metabolic processes. In addition to (and potentially in combination with) these specific health behavior-mediated risks, long-term alterations in the brain and peripheral physiological processes caused by trauma and/or PTSD are also likely to lead to additional health risks. This chapter will consider several physiological systems that have evidence of being altered by childhood trauma, adult trauma, and/or PTSD and that may contribute to health risk effects. Long-term effects of trauma and PTSD are presumably mediated by alterations on the brain and central nervous system (CNS) that lead to a new "steady state" or allostasis in affected brain systems that also may maintain the syndrome of PTSD symptoms. Specific brain alterations affected by trauma and PSTD may lead to alterations in output and activity of peripheral autonomic nervous system and neuroendocrine systems that then effect changes on peripheral physiological processes such as cardiovascular function, immune function, and metabolism that lead to increased pathophysiological processes and disease risk. This chapter will therefore review existing evidence of effects of trauma and PTSD on specific brain system functions that may be linked to "downstream" pathological processes, as well as existing evidence of effects of trauma and PTSD on the sympathetic nervous system (SNS) and parasympathetic nervous system (PNS), cardiovascular and hemodynamic/endothelial function, the hypothalamic-pituitary-adrenal (HPA) axis, and immune function (in particular, inflammatory processes), all of which could contribute and/or mediate effects of trauma and PTSD on medical morbidity. Figure 10.1 shows a simple schematic linking effects of childhood and adult trauma and PTSD

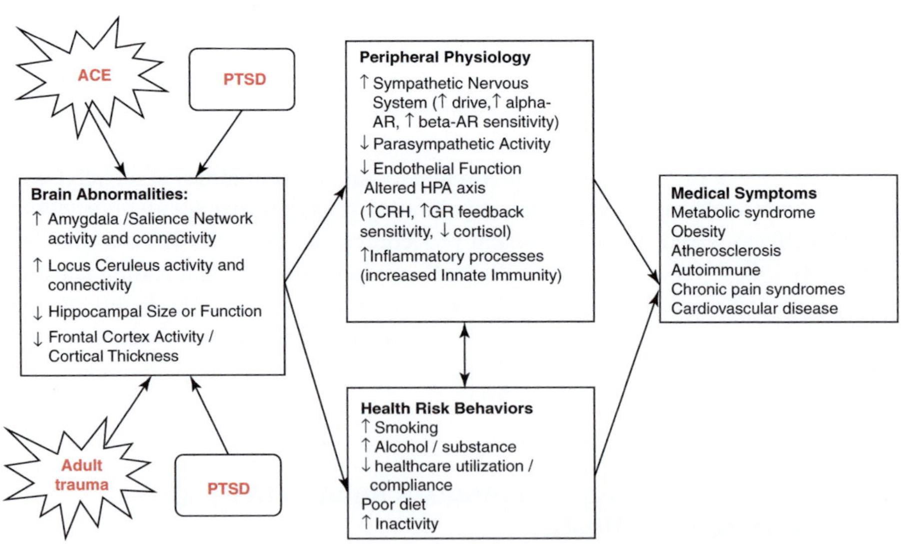

Fig. 10.1 Schematic diagram of effects of childhood and adult trauma and PTSD on brain and peripheral physiological systems, health risk behaviors, and medical symptoms. (*ACE* adverse childhood events; *AR* adrenergic receptor; *CRH* corticotropin releasing hormone; *GR* glucocorticoid receptor; *HPA* hypothalamic pituitary adrenal)

on selected brain systems, which are thought to be "driving" or linked in various ways to both peripheral physiological systems and to altered health risk behavior patterns, both of which contribute to increased health risks and medical symptoms.

10.4 Central Nervous System Effects of Trauma and PTSD

The effects of childhood and adult traumas on brain/CNS function have been an active area of research in humans and animal models for several decades, and recent advances in knowledge from human neuroimaging techniques (e.g., fMRI and PET) over the past 20 years have begun to elucidate a large number of alterations in processes that might be relevant for understanding symptoms of PTSD as well as effects of trauma and PTSD on physical health. A comprehensive review of the effects of trauma and PTSD on brain/CNS function is beyond the scope of this chapter, but meta-analyses find reliable alterations in the functional activity of amygdala, insula, dmPFC, vmPFC, dorsal ACC, and hippocampus [62–64]; effects of trauma and PTSD on a few selected brain systems that may be particularly relevant to "downstream" physiology and pathological processes will be briefly discussed. It is possible that specific trauma- and PTSD-related brain alterations may be associated with maladaptations or exaggerated activity of the autonomic (e.g., SNS), neuroendocrine (e.g., HPA axis), and/or neuroimmunological (e.g., inflammatory) responses that contribute to pathophysiological processes and increased health risks. In particular, potential trauma- and PTSD-related alterations will be discussed in the *amygdala* (and limbic system and "salience network") and the *locus ceruleus*, which appear important in generating and upregulating fear responses, and the *prefrontal cortex* and the *hippocampus*, which appear to be important in the successful downregulation and healthy modulation of fear responses.

For example, chronically altered amygdala, limbic, and salience network reactivity and connectivity associated with PTSD could lead to increased locus ceruleus (LC) activity and central noradrenergic signaling and associated functions, which can lead to exaggerated autonomic SNS responses and thus long-term effects on cardiac output and mean arterial pressure. Exaggerated or increased SNS output can also have effects on stimulating pro-inflammatory immune responses and complex effects on both the innate and adaptive immune system, all of which if dysregulated could have deleterious pathophysiological effects on cardiovascular and other systems. Similarly, chronically altered amygdala/limbic reactivity could lead to altered activity of the HPA axis and circulating cortisol levels, via modulation of corticotropin-releasing factor (CRF) output from the parvocellular cells of the periventricular nucleus (PVN) of the hypothalamus (PVH) onto the median eminence, which triggers the release of adrenocorticotropic hormone (ACTH) from the pituitary and thus HPA axis peripheral physiological responses. Cortisol has wide-ranging effects across multiple tissue and organ systems, and thus chronically altered circulating cortisol levels could affect a large number of organ systems, including multiple complex effects on immune function. Altered cortisol levels can also lead to feedback adaptations at the level of the pituitary and also at the level of the brain that could contribute to the long-term stabilization and maintenance of the syndrome of PTSD and associated pathophysiology. Both high-affinity glucocorticoid receptors (GR) and low-affinity mineralocorticoid (MR) receptors are found in the hippocampus and the prefrontal cortex, which, as described below, are major regulators of fear- and stress-responsive circuits. Increased amygdala activity is also linked to stimulation of CRH in brain region areas outside the PVN, in particular from the bed nucleus of the stria terminalis (BNST) [65]. Increased levels of CRF in the brain (as measured in cerebrospinal fluid, CSF) are associated with increased fear and startle responses in animals [66] as well as in humans with PTSD [67, 68], providing another mechanism that dysregulated amygdala activity can lead to peripheral pathophysiological phenomena.

The amygdala, ventromedial prefrontal cortex (vmPFC), and hippocampus are all involved in fear-associated learning "fear conditioning" [69]. PTSD patients show increased amygdala activity [70], suggesting enhanced fear signal processing and decreased vmPFC activity [71]. Decreased vmPFC activity potentially reflects deficits in fear inhibition [72] and/or emotion regulation [73] that might contribute to both amygdala hyperactivity and extinction recall deficits [74]. The amygdala plays crucial roles in fear conditioning and extinction. PTSD is often conceptualized as a disorder of conditioned fear responses, and successful treatment and remission are thought to involve successful extinction of these conditioned fear responses, such as through trauma exposure-based psychotherapies (e.g., prolonged exposure psychotherapy). The neural mechanisms of both fear conditioning and extinction have been elucidated over the past 30 years in animal models [75–77] and in humans [70, 78], and recent work has been focused on PTSD [74, 79]. Fear conditioning appears to involve creation of new specific neural connections ("traces") between neurons in the basolateral and central nuclei of the amygdala. Extinction of fear conditioning appears to involve creation of new neural connections from inputs from the prefrontal cortex (infralimbic [IL] cortex in rats and ventromedial prefrontal cortex [vmPFC] in humans) with GABAergic inhibitory interneurons in intercalated layer of the amygdala that are able to inhibit conditioned fear response circuits under certain circumstances. This process is further regulated by hippocampal circuits, which provide further contextual information to moderate conditioned fear responses vs inhibition of fear responses (e.g., extinction via vmPFC inputs) within the appropriate contexts (e.g., danger or safety contexts, respectively). Hippocampus also appears abnormal in PTSD, with evidence of reduced volume [80], reduced hippocampal neuronal integrity [81], and aberrant activity [82]. Thus both the frontal cortex/vmPFC and the hippocampus are crucial for healthy regulation of fear responses, and effects of trauma or PTSD on the function of these brain circuits could lead to dysregulation and exaggerated fear responses and downstream pathophysiology.

Amygdala Activity and PTSD The amygdala plays crucial roles in threat detection of threat, fear expression, and fear conditioning. A number of fMRI studies in humans have reported that PTSD is associated with greater amygdala activation compared to trauma-exposed healthy controls in response to general threat-related stimuli, such as and fearful facial expressions [70, 83–85], and also in response to combat trauma-related sounds or smells [86–88], trauma-related photographs or words [89, 90], and autobiographical trauma memories [84, 91]; however other studies have not shown exaggerated amygdala activation in PTSD [92–95] (Phan et al, 2006). Deficits in fear conditioning extinction recall have been hypothesized as a central process underlying PTSD. Extinction memory or extinction recall refers to a long-term form or learning that a stimulus that once was learned to be dangerous is then learned to be safe; for example, when a stimulus that has been previously fear conditioned (paired to a noxious stimulus like electric shock) and also has been "extinguished" (repeatedly presented in a manner not paired to electric shock) and thus has been learned to now be "safe" is presented on the following day. Increased amygdala activation has been reported in PTSD during fear conditioning [96]. Importantly, increased amygdala activity is also seen in PTSD during "extinction recall" [79].

Large-Scale Neural Connectivity Networks and PTSD Mounting evidence from basic, translational, and treatment research converges on the view that neural underpinnings of psychiatric disorders like PTSD may be better understood by dysfunctions in relationships between large-scale neural "connectivity networks" [97–100] rather than micro-circuit "locationist" approaches such as looking at activity in amygdala alone. Multiple large-scale distributed brain networks or "intrinsic connectivity networks (ICNs)" have been identified at rest that correspond to task-related connectivity patterns [101, 102]. A comprehensive description is not possible here, but the ICNs particularly relevant to the nature and treatment of PTSD include the **salience network** (SN), with nodes in amygdala, insula, and dorsal anterior cingulate (dACC), associated with detection of salience and threat and integration of interoceptive, autonomic, and emotional information, and "task-negative" **default mode network** (DMN), with nodes in the posterior cingulate cortex (PCC), ventromedial PFC (vmPFC), and subgenual PFC (sgPFC) associated with social cognition, self-referential processing, autobiographical memory, and "mind wandering." Several research groups, including our own lab, report that individuals with PTSD evidence hyper-connectivity within salience network (e.g., amygdala-insula) [103–106] and aberrantly increased DMN-SN (e.g., DMN-amygdala and insula) cross-network connectivity/desegregation [94, 106, 107].

Locus Ceruleus (LC) Central Noradrenergic System and PTSD The locus ceruleus (LC) is a small midbrain nucleus in the pons that is the primary source of noradrenergic neurons in the brain. The LC noradrenergic system has widespread reciprocal projections to many other brainstem and neocortical areas. Increased LC activity leads to the release of NA at target neurons that has neuromodulatory effects associated with enhancement of sympathetic autonomic responses, including increasing alertness and heightening sensory processing acuity and motor responses

[108, 109]. Several lines of evidence from animal studies have implicated hyperactivity in the LC noradrenergic system as related to various forms of behavioral hyper-responsiveness, including in animal models of PTSD. Early studies of inescapable shock paradigms in rodents found behavior effects that resembled some aspects of PTSD and were also associated with hyperactivity in LC and noradrenergic functioning (reviewed in [110]). Studies in monkeys found that electrical and pharmacological activation of the LC led to an increase in behaviors that resembled some aspects of PTSD in humans [111] and that exposure to fear-inducing stimuli increased LC activity. A recent multimodal study of LC activity in rats measured LC tyrosine hydroxylase (TH) mRNA levels as an index of norepinephrine utilization, as well as electrophysiological recordings of LC neurons and spontaneous and evoked responses to a noxious event (paw compression) in a validated rodent model of PTSD, the single prolonged stress (SPS) paradigm of the research group of Israel Liberzon [112]. Rats who were exposed to the SPS PTSD model showed lower spontaneous LC activity but higher evoked responses, leading to an enhanced signal-to-noise ratio of LC neurons, and also showed impaired recovery from post-stimulus inhibition. SPS rats also had lower LC TH mRNA expression at baseline but exaggerated TH expression following restraint stress.

There has been less direct evidence of the role of LC noradrenergic system in PTSD in humans, but research to date is generally supportive of the idea of increased LC output in PTSD. As discussed below, several studies have reported evidence of increased noradrenaline levels in cerebrospinal fluid (CSF) in PTSD patients, suggesting exaggerated LC activity in PTSD [113, 114]. Furthermore, pharmacological challenge studies in PTSD patients with yohimbine, an antagonist of the inhibitory α2-adrenergic "autoreceptor" that disinhibits and increases the activity of the LC and leads to increased secretion of noradrenaline into the bloodstream, suggest exaggerated LC activity plays a role in PTSD. Yohimbine caused greater increases in plasma noradrenaline in PTSD patients [115], and also led to exacerbation of PTSD symptoms, as well as triggering panic attacks and trauma flashbacks only in PTSD patients [115]. In contrast to effects of blockading α2-adrenergic receptors, blockade of the stimulatory postsynaptic α1-adrenergic receptor with α1 antagonist prazosin (a hypertension medication) leads to improvement in PTSD symptoms, in particular, decreases in PTSD nightmares. Several RCTs have demonstrated the efficacy of prazosin for decreasing PTSD nightmares and sleep disruption and improving PTSD symptoms overall [116].

In terms of human neuroimaging work, a positron emission tomography (PET) study with the radioligand [^{11}C]methylreboxetine reported lower levels of the noradrenaline transporter in the LC PTSD patients [117], which may result in exaggerated synaptic availability of noradrenaline in projection areas, such as the cortex. A very recent fMRI study compared reactions of PTSD patients and trauma-exposed people who did not develop PTSD to blasts of loud noise using pupillometry, and peripheral psychophysiology to compare brain activity in the LC with the peripheral responses in the LC adrenergic sympathetic nervous system [118] provides the first direct evidence of LC hyperactivity in humans with PTSD. Patients with PTSD had increased sympathetic autonomic arousal compared to trauma controls, as reflected by tachycardia, increased skin conductance, and pupillary dilation and an exaggerated startle response. In the fMRI scans, PTSD patients also showed a hyperactivation of the LC as well as several structures that receive dense input from the LC, including the caudal dorsal premotor cortex and supplementary motor area (SMA). Although both PTSD and trauma-control participants reported the noises had similar intensity and unpleasantness, only the PTSD patients responded with increased LC activity in the scans. Interestingly, the level of activity in the regions "downstream" of LC correlated with both autonomic reactivity and PTSD symptom severity, but activity in the LC per se did not [118], suggesting that LC activity may be "permissive" but not sufficient for symptoms of PTSD; it is also possible that the small size of the LC and lack of power in this initial study were not able to resolve.

Structural Neuroimaging Studies of Hippocampus in Childhood and Adult Trauma and PTSD The hippocampus is a bilateral subcortical structure located in the mesial temporal lobe that appears to be critically involved in a number of basic brain functions. While the most widely appreciated roles played by the hippocampus are in memory acquisition and consolidation, some of which are hippocampal dependent [119, 120]; the hippocampus also appears to play important role in psychophysiological aspects of stress regulation, including dampening of amygdala and neuroendocrine HPA axis fear responses [121–124]. The hippocampus is a major site of both type I (high-affinity mineralocorticoid, MR) and type II (low-affinity glucocorticoid receptors, GR) and is an important brain site in stress-response feedback inhibition loops [125].

The hippocampus exerts inhibitory regulatory control on the stress axis in animal models, and, thus, findings of smaller hippocampal volume in adult PTSD patients could suggest the possibility that environmental stressors such as childhood trauma could lead to smaller hippocampal volume that, in turn, leads to deficits in hippocampal stress regulation function and thus higher PTSD risk. Animal studies have shown that high cortisol levels can cause specific damage to hippocampal neurons [126]. There have also been suggestions that the smaller hippocampal volume in PTSD may result from excessive cortisol secretion and subsequent neurotoxicity leading to hippocampal damage in humans [92]. Support for this idea in humans comes from studies which have found smaller hippocampal volumes in patients with Cushing's disorder [127]. However, an alternate possibility is that the hippocampal abnormalities in PTSD are unrelated to cortisol secretion and actually predate the development of clinical syndrome. Such preexisting neurobiological abnormality may predispose individuals to develop PTSD.

Given the centrality of the hippocampus in both memory and regulation of stress responses, it has been an area of intense interest in neurobiological studies of trauma and PTSD. Hippocampal volume, as determined by anatomical tracing of structural T1 MRI scan slices, has been extensively studied in survivors of trauma and in persons with PTSD over the past 15 years, with over 40 independent published studies comparing the size (volume) of right and left hippocampi among trauma-exposed persons with and without PTSD and/or non-trauma-exposed healthy controls. As will be described, the most common finding reported in these studies has been decreased hippocampal volume (ca. 8–13% reduction) in subjects with PTSD compared to either trauma-exposed or non-exposed healthy controls.

Several studies have now examined hippocampal volume associated with PTSD in military combat veterans and in civilian populations; while most have found evidence of decreased hippocampal size in PTSD, other studies have not. Given the mixed findings reported on hippocampal size and PTSD, and the potential confounds due to heterogeneity of studies, meta-analyses that adjust for multiple factors are important. Several meta-analyses reported to date have more consistently reported PTSD-associated reductions in hippocampal volume [63, 128–130]. One meta-analysis found an association between PTSD and lower hippocampal volume (15 studies, $n = 562$), and smaller-sample meta-analyses found smaller volumes for the amygdala (7 studies, $n = 320$) [128], and a more recent meta-analysis found smaller volumes in the hippocampus (36 studies, $n = 1623$) [63]. However, these meta-analyses are still potentially confounded by differences in structural MRI processing/analysis methodologies and potential publication bias. A recent and largest meta-analysis to date (16 cohorts and $N = 1868$ subjects) attempted to overcome these issues by processing all of the MRI scans using the same analytic platform, a standardized image-analysis and quality-control pipeline established by the ENIGMA consortium [131]. This meta-analysis found significantly smaller hippocampi in subjects with current PTSD compared with trauma-exposed control subjects (Cohen's $d = 20.17$, $p = .00054$) that was significant after Bonferroni correction. Thus taken together, it appears that both childhood trauma and adult PTSD are associated with decreased hippocampal volume. It is possible that smaller hippocampi lead to dysregulated hippocampal activity and thus dysregulation of neuroendocrine and autonomic resting and stress-responsive activity.

Medial Prefrontal Cortex A large number of neuroimaging studies have also reported decreased activation or failure to activate the mPFC (including the medial frontal gyrus and rostral and subgenual ACC) in PTSD. This includes decreased mPFC activation during autobiographical trauma recall [92, 93, 132–134] (Lanius et al, 2001; 2004a), in response to trauma-related stimuli [92, 135, 136], as well as general negative emotional stimuli [84, 85, 95, 137]. PTSD patients have been reported to have decreased activity of mPFC in general cognitive tasks [138, 139] as well as emotional tasks [140]. Decreased activity of mPFC in PTSD also has been shown during fear extinction [96] and during fear extinction recall [74, 79]. There has also been intriguing evidence from several PTSD treatment studies that successful treatment of PTSD leads to increased mPFC activation and/or that the degree of increase in mPFC activity following treatment is positively associated with improvement in PTSD symptoms [141–144].

There is accumulating evidence linking PTSD avoidance symptoms to alterations in large-scale neural networks involving vmPFC and hippocampus. PTSD patients show decreased within-network DMN connectivity (PCC-vmPFC and PCC-hippocampus) [94, 106, 145] and decreased vmPFC-hippocampus connectivity [103, 106, 146]. We have previously hypothesized that increased DMN-SN connectivity at rest underlie PTSD hyperarousal symptoms, associated with intrusive, automatic distress reactions to both external cues and internal physiological states. A recent seed-based functional connectivity study of 113 OEF/OIF combat veterans (69 with PTSD) found differences in DMN (PCC-seed) connectivity with the hippocampus [147]. Intriguingly this altered DMN connectivity was correlated with avoidance/numbing symptoms in the veterans with PTSD, but not correlated with intrusive and hyperarousal symptoms [147].

10.5 Effects of Stress and Trauma on Sympathetic Autonomic Nervous System

The sympathetic nervous system (SNS) underlies the "fight, flight, or freeze response" and has long been implicated in responses to trauma and the pathology of PTSD. The stress-responsive adrenergic SNS is activated by amygdala and locus ceruleus (the source of central noradrenergic neurons) inputs into brainstem nuclei. These inputs activate descending sympathetic pathways in the spinal cord which innervate multiple areas of the body and multiple organ systems, including the heart, lungs, gut, vasculature, and immune system, leading to the classic sympathetic responses. Given that multiple core symptoms of PTSD involve what appear to be hyper-adrenergic states (e.g., physiological and emotional responses to triggers and other re-experiencing symptoms, increased heart rate/tachycardia, increased blood pressure, anxiety, hypervigilance/hyperarousal, exaggerated startle, etc.), the noradrenergic SNS has been a central target of PTSD research for many years (for review see [115, 148–150]).

Combat-related psychosomatic conditions marked by a rapid pulse, anxiety, and trouble breathing during the US Civil War (1861–1865)—known as "soldier's heart" or "irritable heart"—appear likely to be coextensive with what is now known as combat PTSD, and conceptualizations of these disorders focused on cardiac and cardiovascular function. A US military physician Jones [151] concluded this was due to overstimulation of the heart's nervous system and described what came to be known as "Da Costa's syndrome." Clinical and laboratory studies over the past 30 years have provided strong evidence that PTSD is associated with increased peripheral nervous noradrenergic system/sympathetic nervous system (SNS) activity. Clinical and psychophysiological measures of SNS activity are well documented in PTSD, with findings of increased blood pressure, heart rate, and skin conductance at baseline and in response to trauma recall having been reported in a large number of studies comparing PTSD patients to normal and psychiatric controls [152–157].

In addition to increased SNS baseline activity and stress-related responses, several studies also report decreased activity of the parasympathetic nervous system (PNS) in PTSD, including decreased baroreceptor reflex sensitivity [158]and various heart rate variability (HRV)/respiratory sinus arrhythmia (RSA) measures of parasympathetic tone at rest [159, 160] and in response to psychological stressor [161]. Another peripheral indicator of noradrenergic activity is pupil diameter: increased pupil diameter appears to be correlated with LC activity and central noradrenergic function [162]. Studies have reported increased pupil diameter in PTSD compared to controls, in particular in response to threat stimuli [163, 164].

In addition to peripheral cardiovascular and psychophysiological measures, there is also peripheral neurochemical evidence of increased adrenergic outflow, including increased 24-h urinary excretion of catecholamines (adrenaline, noradrenaline, and metabolites) in PTSD patients compared to healthy and psychiatric controls [165] and other studies found increased urinary noradrenaline in women with current PTSD but not those with history of PTSD or trauma exposure without PTSD [166, 167]. Increased circulating levels of catecholamines (adrenaline and noradrenaline) in plasma have also been shown in PTSD patients compared to controls, at baseline [86] and following exposure to stress (Blanchard et al., 1991), including trauma recall [86]. PTSD has also been associated with increased levels of salivary alpha-amylase, considered to be an index of SNS activation and PNS, at baseline and in response to stressors [168] and in circadian measures [169], indicative of excessive noradrenergic SNS activity.

Evidence of excessive central nervous system noradrenergic tone has also been reported in PTSD. In studies measuring catecholamines in cerebrospinal fluid (CSF), PTSD patients were reported to have significantly increased levels of noradrenaline. One study found elevated CSF noradrenaline levels in PTSD patients and that noradrenaline levels positively correlated with levels of PTSD symptoms as measured by the CAPS [113]. Another study reported that heart rate and noradrenaline levels increased in combat PTSD patients when they watched a video containing combat footage but not a neutral video, and heart rate responses correlated with the levels of CSF noradrenaline increase [114]. Furthermore, CSF noradrenaline remained elevated for several hours following the combat video, and the level of increase in CSF noradrenaline strongly correlated with subjective reports of worsening of mood in the PTSD patients [114].

Pharmacological challenge studies with adrenergic agents also suggest exaggerated responses in the LC-sympathetic system. Yohimbine is an antagonist of the inhibitory α2-adrenergic "autoreceptor" that is expected to disinhibit (and thus increase the activity) the LC. A yohimbine challenge leads to increased secretion of overall noradrenaline into the bloodstream (as assessed by a metabolite MHPG) of both PTSD patients and controls. Although baseline resting plasma MHPG levels were not different between PTSD patients and controls, yohimbine caused greater increases in plasma noradrenaline in PTSD patients [115]. Interestingly they also found that yohimbine led to profound subjective emotional and physiological responses in only PTSD patients. The majority of PTSD patients experienced panic attacks and nearly half had trauma flashbacks, and furthermore overall PTSD symptoms of emotional numbing, trauma memories, and grief all increased in PTSD patients, as did heart rate and blood pressure. In contrast, none of these effects were seen in healthy controls [115]. Blockade of the stimulatory postsynaptic $\alpha 1$-adrenergic receptor with $\alpha 1$-antagonist prazosin (a hypertension medication) leads to improvement in PTSD symptoms, and prazosin is now commonly used for PTSD, in particular, for improving PTSD-related nightmares and sleep disturbances. Several RCTs have examined the efficacy of prazosin for decreasing PTSD nightmares and sleep disruption and improving PTSD symptoms overall, compared to pill placebo and in crossover designs [116] and compared to placebo as well as behavioral sleep interventions

A longitudinal study on trauma survivors suggests that a higher peri-traumatic heart rate (measured in the emergency room) predicted PTSD diagnosis at follow-up [170]. Furthermore, an intriguing pilot study suggested that peri-traumatic treatment of survivors with the beta-adrenergic antagonist (beta-blocker) propranolol in the emergency room may prevent the development of PTSD [171]; however subsequent studies of propranolol on combat veterans and burn victims have shown mixed results [172–175], and more research is needed. For example, examining genetic factors and early childhood experiences in such a longitudinal design of peri-traumatic SNS function and subsequent development of PTSD could shed important light on PTSD pathogenesis.

10.6 Effects of Stress and Trauma on HPA Axis Neuroendocrine System

The hypothalamic-pituitary-adrenal (HPA) axis is a major stress-responsive neuroendocrine system that is crucial for survival. Like the SNS, the HPA axis is also activated in response to stressors and traumas in humans and in animals, but with a different timecourse; whereas the SNS responds within seconds, HPA axis responses peak at about 15–30 min and usually resolve at 60–90 min. This neuroendocrine axis functions as a hormone "cascade," which involves secretion of corticotropin-releasing hormone (CRH) from specialized neurons of the paraventricular nucleus (PVN) of the hypothalamus into the hypophyseal "portal circulation," in which it travels to the anterior pituitary and then binds to specific CRH receptors on the surface of adrenocorticotropic cells. These specialized pituitary cells in turn release another protein hormone, adrenocorticotropic hormone (ACTH) , into the peripheral bloodstream. ACTH then travels through the bloodstream to the adrenal gland, where it binds cell surface receptors on cells in the adrenal cortex, which leads to synthesis and release of glucocorticoid steroid hormones (cortisol in humans and corticosterone in many animals).

Glucocorticoid hormones have multiple effects on a large number of physiological systems, including glucose utilization and metabolism, lipolysis, immune function, and hemodynamics. They also appear to have important physiological effects on the brain. The receptors for glucocorticoid receptors are nearly ubiquitously expressed in peripheral tissues, as well as cortical and subcortical brain structures [176]. The widespread actions of cortisol on metabolism and immune function have led many to hypothesize that the stress-responsive HPA axis may mediate the deleterious effects of psychological stress on health. Glucocorticoid effects on the brain are consistent with significant roles for these steroids in shaping behavioral adaptations to changing and/or challenging environments [176].

Several factors suggest the HPA as a potential site that could mediate effects of childhood and adult trauma and PTSD on physical health. The adult functioning of the HPA axis is shaped, in animals and humans, by early life stressors [177–179], and these early life stressors also contribute to risk for adult psychopathology and poor health outcomes/disease risk [180, 181]. The HPA axis changes also mediate behavioral changes relevant to psychopathology in the animal early stress models (Ladd, Thrivikraman, Huot, & Plotsky, 2005) [182–185]).

Models of early life trauma in rodents and primates suggest that manipulation of the early developmental environment can lead to long-term, sometimes lifelong, alterations in behavior, brain gene expression, and patterns of stress hormone and neurophysiological responses to stress. Prolonged maternal separation is a well-characterized model of early life adversity that leads to profound changes in neuroendocrine stress responses and behavior (for review see [184]). The maternal separation model examines the effects of separating neonate rat pups (2–14 days old) from their mothers for either 3 h/day for 10 days (maternal separation) or for only 15 min a day ("handled control"). After separation from their pups for 3 h, rat mothers show decreases in important maternal behaviors, such as pup retrieval, licking, grooming, and nursing, compared to rat mothers not separated from their pups or those who were separated for only 15 min [185]. Maternal separation appears to have long-term effects on multiple behavioral and neurobiological systems of the separated rat pups. Behaviorally, rats who are separated from their mothers for 3 h a day as neonates show increased anxiety-like behaviors, hypervigilance, and development of a depression-like syndrome as adults, including anhedonia and a proclivity for increased ethanol intake. They also show exaggerated and prolonged HPA axis responses to the mild psychological stressor of an airpuff as adults. Interestingly, these exaggerated HPA axis responses persist throughout the adult life of the animal. Furthermore, a number of other pronounced neurobiological alterations have now been demonstrated in adult rats who experienced maternal separation as neonates. These include decreased gene expression of glucocorticoid receptors (GR) in the hippocampus and medial prefrontal cortex. This decrease in brain GR is thought to lead to decreased glucocorticoid feedback sensitivity, and to drive the exaggerated and prolonged corticosterone stress responses, since HPA axis activation now come under much reduced inhibitory negative feedback. These findings indicate that early life experiences can lead to lifelong behavioral and neurobiological alterations. It would also appear that differences in responses to stressors and traumas seen in adult rats exposed to neonatal maternal separation may translate to an increase in psychological vulnerability. This may be a valuable model to elucidate the effects of childhood trauma and other adversity on psychological vulnerability in humans. An animal model of adult PTSD, the single prolonged stress (SPS) model, developed by the research group of Israel Liberzon, results in a number of HPA neuroendocrine abnormalities which have also been observed in PTSD patients, including enhanced glucocorticoid negative feedback (i.e., increased dexamethasone fast feedback) in response to psychosocial stressors [186], and relative increases in GR gene expression in the hippocampus [187]. These findings are in stark contrast to the decreased hippocampal GR gene expression seen in adult rats who were exposed to prolonged maternal separation as neonates [188] or who had mothers who exhibited low levels of maternal care ("licking and grooming") [189] (Meaney et al., 1996). These differential findings between various rodent models of early life adversity and adult trauma are still a matter of study, although it is interesting that the SPS model is the only rodent model that has yet shown the pattern of GR feedback hypersensitivity that has been observed in adult human PTSD. At least at the level of glucocorticoid negative feedback sensitivity, the maternal separation model appears more similar to the patterns of HPA axis function found in major depression in humans.

Potential alterations in the HPA axis neuroendocrine system in humans in the context of trauma exposure and PTSD have been an area of considerable study over the past 20 years, and there is evidence that the HPA axis is dysregulated in patients with PTSD as well as major depression [190–193]. Early stress exposure can create lasting HPA axis dysregulation in humans that parallels those seen in the animal models and which is often best seen in adulthood in the context of challenge studies [194, 195]. However, the exact role that HPA axis dysregulation plays in the etiology development and expression of PTSD symptoms has not been fully elucidated.

There is evidence of alterations in stress hormone responses to social stressors and trauma recall in adult survivors of childhood traumas, such as childhood sexual assault. Heim and colleagues found that women with a history of childhood abuse exhibited greatly increased HPA axis and autonomic responses to a social stressor (the "Trier Social Stress Test" or TSST) compared with women without childhood abuse [194]. The exaggerated responses were particularly robust in women with current symptoms of depression and anxiety. Women with a history of childhood abuse and a current major depression diagnosis exhibited a more than sixfold greater ACTH response to stress than age-matched controls. The authors concluded that that exaggerated HPA axis and autonomic nervous system responses are a persistent consequence of childhood abuse that may contribute to the diathesis vulnerability for adulthood psychopathological conditions. They further hypothesized that this HPA and sympathetic hyper-reactivity was related to CRH hypersecretion in women with childhood trauma exposures, suggesting that CRH hypersecretion may mediate the effects of childhood trauma on the risk of adult psychopathology in response to stress. However, other studies with individuals with abuse-related PTSD (i.e., history of childhood physical or sexual abuse) that examined cortisol responses to psychosocial stressors have shown more subtle differences in HPA axis reactivity. A study of 23 women with childhood abuse-related PTSD and 18 matched healthy controls exposed to a 20-min cognitive challenge (e.g., arithmetic and problem-solving tasks) found elevated cortisol levels before the task was begun (potentially reflecting elevated anticipatory anxiety) but cortisol response in PTSD patients that were not different than healthy controls [196]. Another study exposed women with childhood abuse-related PTSD to personalized trauma scripts and again found that PTSD patients had significantly higher cortisol levels before and during script exposure, but did not have exaggerated "responses" to the trauma scripts [197]. There was however a correlation between PTSD symptom severity and cortisol levels during exposure.

There has been mixed evidence that the basal or resting activity of the HPA axis is altered in adults with PTSD who experienced trauma during adulthood. Several studies have shown evidence of elevated levels of the hormone CRH in the cerebrospinal fluid of PTSD patients, consistent with the notion of increased activation of the system. Higher levels of CRH have been found in cerebrospinal fluid (CSF) in PTSD patients (obtain from lumbar punctures) [67, 68]. A study found both increased CRH and cortisol levels in CSF over a 6-h sampling period, with CRH and cortisol levels were positively correlated [198]. Studies examining downstream effects of CRH-mediated central drive in PTSD patients have also provided mixed results. Blunted ACTH response to CRH was reported in patients with combat-related PTSD, but only in patients with a comorbid diagnosis of MDD (Smith et al., 1989). One study found women with PTSD (exposed to physical or sexual abuse) had higher CRH-induced ACTH and cortisol responses [199], but another study of men and women with PTSD related to assault or a motor vehicle accident found no significant differences in basal or total CRH-stimulated ACTH or cortisol responses [200].

Assessment of peripheral cortisol across the day (i.e., "circadian cortisol") in PTSD patients has produced considerably varying results, with studies showing peripheral cortisol levels in PTSD patients to be significantly lower than [201], and significantly higher than [202, 203], and no different from [67, 199], healthy control subjects. In a large longitudinal epidemiological study, saliva [204] and urine [167] cortisol measures were obtained from patients with PTSD, patients with trauma exposure but no PTSD, and healthy controls. PTSD was associated with elevated evening saliva cortisol levels but only in individuals with a comorbid diagnosis of MDD. In contrast, patients with PTSD alone showed normal evening saliva and urine cortisol levels. A negative correlation has been observed between 24-h urinary cortisol levels and PTSD symptoms in combat veterans [67], but the same study failed to find group differences in circulating cortisol between veterans with and without a PTSD diagnosis. A study examining 2490 Vietnam veterans found 8:00 A.M. cortisol levels were significantly lower (by 4%) in PTSD patients compared to healthy controls. Interestingly, lower awakening cortisol has been associated with current or lifetime PTSD or a past diagnosis of depression in women who were recently (i.e., 6 months) diagnosed with breast cancer [205].

As well, a civilian PTSD group showed substantially reduced cortisol response to awakening (i.e., in the first 60 min after awakening) compared to control groups [206], and PTSD symptoms were found correlated with dampened cortisol response to awakening in active duty police officers [207]. However, another recent report found cortisol response to awakening did not predict PTSD symptom severity and was only nonsignificantly lower among firefighters with high PTSD risk [208]. Taken together, these data suggest evidence for some link between PTSD and reduced levels of circulating cortisol, but the nature of that linkage, and the clinical relevance of potential group differences, remains unclear.

In addition to the basal level of cortisol "output," trauma and PTSD could be associated with altered sensitivity to effects of stress-induced cortisol. Cortisol negative feedback sensitivity can be assessed in human using the dexamethasone suppression test (DST). The use of this test in patients with major depression, which found a significant proportion of MDD patients showed substantially blunted DEX suppression, was a finding that greatly stimulated the field of biological psychiatry. The use of the DST in PTSD has yielded somewhat more consistent results. However, the pattern found in trauma exposure and PTSD is the opposite to that found in MDD. Several studies have shown a significantly greater reduction in ACTH and/or cortisol in PTSD patients following dexamethasone treatment, suggesting sensitized inhibitory feedback mechanisms in PTSD [201, 209, 210]. PTSD patients with early childhood abuse also showed hypersuppression of ACTH following dexamethasone treatment [211]. However, a correlation between DST response and PTSD symptom severity is only been reported in some studies [201, 212]. Thus, studies examining differences in circadian cortisol levels have also been inconsistent, although some studies have suggested a potential relationship between low cortisol levels and trauma exposure and with especially high PTSD symptom severity. However, it remains unclear whether the dysregulations documented reflect a consequence of trauma exposure, pre-existing alterations that constitute traumatic vulnerability, or a more specific correlate of the disease process.

Only a few studies have examined the effects of psychological challenges on neuroendocrine responses in PTSD patients with adult trauma. Our group observed higher autonomic (i.e., skin conductance and heart rate) and catecholamine responses to white noise and combat-related sounds in Vietnam military veterans with PTSD, but the acute (immediate postexposure) ACTH and cortisol responses to these challenges were not different from that of controls [86]. In a separate study, our group recently examined acute plasma ACTH responses to trauma-specific (autobiographical trauma script-driven imagery) and non-specific (IAPS pictures) aversive emotional stimuli over 20 min in Vietnam combat PTSD patients ($n = 16$), Vietnam combat veterans without a history of PTSD symptoms ($n = 15$), and noncombat healthy controls ($n = 15$). We found acute plasma ACTH responses to trauma recall, but not to other emotional stimuli. Both groups of combat veterans (with or without PTSD) showed significant acute ACTH responses to the trauma scripts, but not to aversive IAPS pictures, suggesting that sensitized HPA axis responses observed in this paradigm were related to trauma exposure rather than PTSD, per se. However, the magnitude of ACTH response was positively correlated with the severity of symptoms in PTSD subjects. In contrast, noncombat-exposed controls did not have ACTH responses to aversive autobiographical scripts or IAPS pictures. While the general and trauma-specific aversive challenges elicited strong subjective emotional responses among all participants, acute ACTH responses were seen only to personalized trauma scripts in combat-exposed groups, supporting the notion that the human HPA axis responds to specific psychological stimuli (in this case, memories of personal threat) rather than to general emotional distress.

In summary, these mixed data suggest that abnormalities in circadian cortisol levels in PTSD patients may exist in certain conditions. There does seem to be some evidence for a link between PTSD and low 24-h cortisol levels in some patients, which contrasts with the hypercortisolemia seen in depression. The degree to which changes in cortisol levels might result from trauma exposure itself, rather than PTSD per se, requires further investigation. As well, whether different circadian levels represent consequences of PTSD or vulnerability factors that are present at the time of trauma and increase the risk of developing PTSD also remains unresolved. A possibility suggested by animal models is that the psychopathology of PTSD in adults is associated with altered HPA axis stress responses, and while the available data are limited, there has been some evidence for such differences in adults with PTSD from childhood abuse [196, 197] (Bremner et al., 2003). However a study of combat veterans with adult trauma found ACTH responses to trauma recall were a function of adult trauma exposure rather than PTSD status. An additional intriguing possibility suggested by animal models is that the experience of childhood trauma itself, with or without subsequent psychopathology, may lead to exaggerated HPA axis stress hormone responses later in life and that these may lead to greater PTSD vulnerability to subsequent trauma. There has been evidence of differences in acute HPA axis responses to psychosocial stressors and trauma recall in adults with childhood trauma exposures with or without depression compared to non-trauma-exposed adults [194].

10.7 Effects of Trauma and PTSD on Immune System and Inflammatory Processes

There is accumulating evidence that trauma exposure and PTSD are associated with several abnormalities in immune system function that may contribute to pathophysiological processes and diseases. In particular, PTSD appears to be associated with increased pro-inflammatory signaling and the innate immunity system; these immune abnormalities could be linked to aberrations in both the sympathetic noradrenergic system and the glucocorticoid system described above. There is currently accumulating data suggesting PTSD may be associated with elevated levels of autoimmunity and that in addition, while there is as yet still some mixed findings and heterogeneity in the reports in the literature, PTSD patients without autoimmune disorders may also exhibit a low-grade systemic pro-inflammatory state. Such a chronically elevated inflammatory state could be one mechanism by which PTSD could contribute to atherosclerosis and cardiovascular disease. For example, an epidemiological study of $N = 2490$ US military veterans deployed to Vietnam that found significantly elevated risk for autoimmune disorders among veterans with PTSD [50] also found significant derangements in several immune and neuroendocrine system laboratory measures, including three- to fivefold increased risk for elevated total and T-lymphocyte counts, elevated cell-mediated immunity response, elevated IgM, and lower levels of DHEA-S [50].

Evidence of altered immune function in PTSD in humans also comes from a number of studies examining alterations in basal or "resting" levels of immune signaling molecules such as pro-inflammatory cytokines in plasms and saliva, alterations in secretagogue stimulation of cytokines from isolated leukocytes, and altered levels of leukocyte gene expression in inflammatory and glucocorticoid gene networks. Cytokines are immune system protein molecules secreted by a large number of immune cells, including lymphocytes and monocytes, that have specialized functions to regulate host responses to infection, immune responses, inflammation, and trauma. "Pro-inflammatory" cytokines such as interferon gamma (IFN-γ); interleukins 1, 2, 6, 12, etc. (IL-1, IL-2, IL-6, IL-12); and tumor necrosis factor alpha (TNF-a) stimulate inflammation by triggering cascades of gene expression of inflammatory mediators in immune cells such as B lymphocytes and the endothelium. In contrast, "inhibitory cytokines" such as IL-4, IL-10, and IL-13 have effects to decrease inflammation by blocking or suppressing gene expression of inflammatory mediators. There have been over 20 studies reported comparing pro-inflammatory cytokines in people with PTSD to healthy trauma- or non-trauma-exposed controls, and most have found evidence of increased levels of pro-inflammatory cytokines. Several studies of combat veterans or active duty military personnel compared to healthy controls report higher levels of plasma or serum TNF-α in combat veterans with PTSD [213–216], including two studies that found increased TNF-α when also controlling for BMI and smoking [217]. However, other studies of combat veterans did not find elevations in TNF-α in PTSD [218–221]. Several studies of PTSD from noncombat trauma also report increased plasma or serum TNF-α [222, 223]; one study that did not find elevated TNF-α also had low levels of detection [224]. Similarly, several studies find elevated levels of plasma or serum IL-6 in combat PTSD [213, 215, 217, 225] and civilian PTSD [223]. There are more limited data reporting PTSD-related elevations in IL-1β [222, 223] and INF-γ [217, 225], but again there are also negative studies that did not find significant differences in IL-1β or INF-γ, and furthermore, only few studies have statistically controlled for effects of smoking, BMI, and other factors that could confound measurement of PTSD effects.

Thus while the data reported to date generally support the notion of increased resting levels of plasma or serum pro-inflammatory cytokine levels, clarification of the exact role of cytokines in the syndrome of PTSD will be helped by additional better-controlled studies and meta-analyses. A recent meta-analysis of cytokine levels from 2015 in 20 studies of PTSD found higher levels of IL-6, IL-1β, and INF-γ in PTSD overall compared to healthy controls and elevated TNF-α in a subgroup analysis of unmedicated PTSD patients [226]. A subgroup meta-analysis of studies that excluded comorbid major depressive disorder also found significant elevations in TNF-α, IL-1β, and IL-6 in PTSD patients compared to controls. As might be expected, the meta-analysis found high levels of between-study heterogeneity for most cytokine variables measured (I(2) > 75%) and furthermore found a potential publication bias for interleukin 1β. This study also conducted meta-regression analyses and fitted a model composed of several variables (e.g., major depressive disorder comorbidity, psychotropic medications, assay type, and time of blood draw) that explained heterogeneity in interleukin 1β, interleukin 6, and C-reactive protein studies.

Another recent "transdiagnostic" meta-analysis was reported of the effects of trauma exposures on plasma or serum levels of several cytokines and pro-inflammatory marker in 36 independent samples and >14,000 participants [227]. This study used strict definitions of trauma exposure (e.g., PTSD criteria A) and included several studies that focused on PTSD diagnosis, but also included population studies that contain participants with other (or no) psychiatric diagnoses, as well as studies with cohorts of people with major depression, cardiovascular disease, schizophrenia, etc.

This meta-analysis also found significant effects of trauma exposure predicting elevations in several cytokines and inflammatory markers, including C-reactive protein (CRP), IL-1β, IL-6, and TNF-α. The effects of trauma on inflammatory markers appeared to positively correlate with severity of trauma exposures. Furthermore, the severity of psychiatric symptoms (PTSD as well as non-PTSD) significantly predicted increased effect sizes for IL-1β and IL-6 in meta-regression models. However, no significant relationships with trauma were seen with fibrinogen, IL-2, IL-4, IL-8, or IL-10.

In addition to resting circulating levels of pro-inflammatory cytokines in serum or plasma, a smaller number of studies have also compared in vitro stimulation cytokine production from specific leukocytes between people with PTSD (military combat, civilian trauma, refugees) and controls. This approach seeks whether the syndrome of PTSD may alter the capacity to produce and secrete pro-inflammatory cytokines by specific immune cells. One study of whole blood leukocyte stimulation with bacterial lipopolysaccharide (LPS) compared male combat veterans with and without PTSD, and noncombat controls [228, 229], and reported PTSD patients had reduced production of LPS-stimulated TNF-α compared to healthy controls but not combat controls (and the control groups were also not different), and IL-10 secretion was not different among the groups. Another more recent study of LPS stimulation of peripheral blood mononuclear cells (PBMCs) in Croatian combat PTSD patients and healthy non-veterans did not find a difference between PTSD and controls in LPS-stimulated production of TNF-α, INF-γ, IL-2, or IL-4, but did find a reduction of IL-2 and INF-γ in unstimulated PBMC from PTSD patients. A study of LPS stimulation of whole blood in Bosnian refugees reported increased secretion of IL-6 but not TNF-α [230], and another study of refugees also found evidence of increase in both

IL-6 and TNF-α secretion from LPS-stimulated PBMCs [224]. A study of women with PTSD and female trauma and non-trauma controls also found increased in LPS+PHA stimulation of secretion of IL-6 and TNF-α in PTSD patients greater than both trauma and non-trauma controls, but no differences in IL-1β secretion between groups (Gill et al., 2008). While data are mixed and not sufficient to make strong conclusions, three studies have found increased stimulated IL-6 in civilians with PTSD.

Several studies of gene expression in blood leukocytes have also found intriguing evidence suggestive of increased expression of genes contributing to inflammatory activity, and decreased expression of genes involved in regulation of inflammation contributes to the pathophysiology and development of PTSD. In candidate gene expression studies, PTSD has been associated with increased expression of IGF-2 and decreased expression of IL-16, IL-18, and CSF [231] and decreased expression of FKBP5, STAT5B, and MHC class II in people exposed to the 2001 WTC attack with PTSD compared to without PTSD [232]. Genome-wide gene expression studies have reported PTSD is associated with a decreased expression of STAT5B and nuclear factor I/A [233] and decreased expression in 32 genes within the IL-18 and STAT pathway in PTSD patients who also had "risk-associated" SNPs in the FKBP5 gene [234]. Another recent genome-wide gene expression study used RNA sequencing of whole blood leukocytes in $N = 188$ US Marines before and after deployment to combat zones in Iraq and Afghanistan [235]. This study used a gene network approach to identify high-order properties of PTSD symptoms on gene co-expression levels rather than individual gene expression. This study found increased co-expression of gene network "modules" involved in immune system functioning, interferon signaling (INF-a, b, g), and cytokine signaling pathways at both pre- and post-deployment, and this module was overexpressed in Marines who developed PTSD, suggesting innate immune system and interferon gene networks as involved in the pathophysiology of PTSD vulnerability and development [235]. Intriguingly, this study also found increased expression of a separate gene network module of genes involved in hemostasis, platelet activation, and clotting cascade at the post-deployment time-point only, which showed greater expression in Marines who did not develop PTSD, suggesting a potential resilience profile.

Thus taken together, there is accumulating evidence that trauma and PTSD are associated with increased circulating levels of pro-inflammatory cytokines IL-1β, IL-6, and TNF-α and the inflammatory marker CRP, and PTSD may also be associated with increased stimulated expression of IL-6 from leukocytes, increased expression of genes involved in stimulation inflammatory processes, and decreased expression of genes involved in regulating inflammation. This suggests that part of the syndrome of PTSD pathophysiology may include the prolonged maintenance of a low-grade systemic pro-inflammatory state, which could be a mechanism mediating the effects of PTSD on atherosclerosis and cardiovascular disease

10.8 Summary and Conclusions

In this chapter we have reviewed evidence that both childhood traumas, e.g., from adversity and/or maltreatment, and adult trauma and PTSD are associated with considerable negative effects on mental and somatic health. In addition to psychiatric comorbidities, childhood trauma and adult PTSD are associated with considerably increased risk disorders thought to have a strong psychosomatic component, such as IBS and fibromyalgia, as well as for a broad range of somatic diseases, including autoimmune disorders, cancer, diabetes and other metabolic disorders, stroke, and cardiovascular disease. Epidemiological data finds childhood trauma exposure and PTSD associated with increased levels of health risk behaviors, such as smoking, alcohol and drug use, poor diet, and physical activity, as well as increased body mass index (BMI) and rates of obesity, and also with poorer medical compliance and healthcare utilization. However, we also review epidemiological evidence that trauma PTSD-related health risks are apparent even when controlling for a number of risky health behaviors. We further reviewed neurobiological and physiological evidence that trauma and PTSD are also associated with a number of changes in the brain activity and structure, including increased activity and altered connectivity in the amygdala, insula, and the "salience network," increased activation of the locus ceruleus central noradrenergic system, and decreased activity in hippocampus and frontal cortex regulatory circuits. We also reviewed evidence of trauma- and PTSD-related changes in the peripheral sympathetic autonomic nervous system, the HPA axis, and the immune system, all of which have implications for health risks including effects potentially moderating autoimmune, metabolic, cardiovascular, and cerebrovascular disease processes. While the exact nature and degree of relationships of these brain effects on peripheral physiological alterations have yet to be fully delineated, the emerging picture is that early trauma in particular, as well as adult PTSD, may lead to long-term changes in brain function that are driving derangements in several neurobiological axes that impinge on somatic health.

References

1. Kessler RC, Sonnega A, Bromet E, Hughes M, Nelson CB. Posttraumatic stress disorder in the National Comorbidity Survey. Arch Gen Psychiatry. 1995;52(12):1048–60.
2. Breslau N, Davis GC, Andreski P, et al. Traumatic events and posttraumatic stress disorder in an urban population of young adults. Arch Gen Psychiatry. 1991;48:216–22.
3. Kulka RA, Schlenger WE, Fairbanks JA, Hough RL, Jordan BK, Marmar CR, Weiss DS. Trauma and the Vietnam War generation: report of findings from the National Vietnam veterans readjustment study. New York: Brunner/Mazel; 1990.
4. Cabrera OA, Hoge CW, Bliese PD, Castro CA, Messer SC. Childhood adversity and combat as predictors of depression and post-traumatic stress in deployed troops. Am J Prev Med. 2007;33(2):77–82. https://doi.org/10.1016/j.amepre.2007.03.019.
5. Koenen KC, Moffitt TE, Poulton R, Martin J, Caspi A. Early childhood factors associated with the development of post-traumatic stress disorder: results from a longitudinal birth cohort. Psychol Med. 2007;37(2):181–92.
6. Shalev AY, Peri T, Canetti L, Schreiber S. Predictors of PTSD in injured trauma survivors: a prospective study. Am J Psychiatry. 1996;153(2):219–25.

7. Widom CS. Posttraumatic stress disorder in abused and neglected children grown up. Am J Psychiatry. 1999;156(8):1223–9.
8. Koenen KC, Harley R, Lyons MJ, Wolfe J, Simpson JC, Goldberg J, et al. A twin registry study of familial and individual risk factors for trauma exposure and posttraumatic stress disorder. J Nerv Ment Dis. 2002;190(4):209–18.
9. Rothbaum BO, Foa EB, Riggs DS, Murdock T, Walsh W. A prospective examination of post-traumatic stress disorder in rape victims. J Trauma Stress. 1992;5(3) https://doi.org/10.1002/jts.2490050309.
10. Kessler RC, Berglund P, Demler O, Jin R, Koretz D, Merikangas KR, et al. The epidemiology of major depressive disorder: results from the National Comorbidity Survey Replication (NCS-R). JAMA. 2003;289(23):3095–105. https://doi.org/10.1001/jama.289.23.3095.
11. Fulton JJ, Calhoun PS, Wagner HR, Schry AR, Hair LP, Feeling N, et al. The prevalence of posttraumatic stress disorder in Operation Enduring Freedom/Operation Iraqi Freedom (OEF/OIF) Veterans: a meta-analysis. J Anxiety Disord. 2015;31:98–107. https://doi.org/10.1016/j.janxdis.2015.02.003.
12. Hoge CW, Castro CA, Messer SC, McGurk D, Cotting DI, Koffman RL. Combat duty in Iraq and Afghanistan, mental health problems, and barriers to care. N Engl J Med. 2004;351(1):13–22.
13. Kang HK, Natelson BH, Mahan CM, Lee KY, Murphy FM. Post-traumatic stress disorder and chronic fatigue syndrome-like illness among Gulf War veterans: a population-based survey of 30,000 veterans. Am J Epidemiol. 2003;157(2):141–8.
14. Gillespie CF, Bradley B, Mercer K, Smith AK, Conneely K, Gapen M, et al. Trauma exposure and stress-related disorders in inner city primary care patients. Gen Hosp Psychiatry. 2009;31(6):505–14. https://doi.org/10.1016/j.genhosppsych.2009.05.003.
15. Greenberg PE, Kessler RC, Birnbaum HG, Leong SA, Lowe SW, Berglund PA, Corey-Lisle PK. The economic burden of depression in the United States: how did it change between 1990 and 2000? J Clin Psychiatry. 2003;64(12):1465–75.
16. Kuyken W, Warren FC, Taylor RS, Whalley B, Crane C, Bondolfi G, et al. Efficacy of mindfulness-based cognitive therapy in prevention of depressive relapse: an individual patient data meta-analysis from randomized trials. JAMA Psychiatry. 2016;73(6):565–74. https://doi.org/10.1001/jamapsychiatry.2016.0076.
17. Doerfler LA, Pbert L, DeCosimo D. Symptoms of posttraumatic stress disorder following myocardial infarction and coronary artery bypass surgery. Gen Hosp Psychiatry. 1994;16(3):193–9.
18. Carney RM, Freedland KE, Sheline YI, Weiss ES. Depression and coronary heart disease: a review for cardiologists. Clin Cardiol. 1997;20(3):196–200.
19. Borowicz L Jr, Royall R, Grega M, Selnes O, Lyketsos C, McKhann G. Depression and cardiac morbidity 5 years after coronary artery bypass surgery. Psychosomatics. 2002;43(6):464–71. https://doi.org/10.1176/appi.psy.43.6.464.
20. Connerney I, Shapiro PA, McLaughlin JS, Bagiella E, Sloan RP. Relation between depression after coronary artery bypass surgery and 12-month outcome: a prospective study. Lancet. 2001;358(9295):1766–71. https://doi.org/10.1016/S0140-6736(01)06803-9.
21. Cserep Z, Balog P, Szekely J, Treszl A, Kopp MS, Thayer JF, Szekely A. Psychosocial factors and major adverse cardiac and cerebrovascular events after cardiac surgery. Interact Cardiovasc Thorac Surg. 2010;11(5):567–72. https://doi.org/10.1510/icvts.2010.244582.
22. Edmondson D, Richardson S, Falzon L, Davidson KW, Mills MA, Neria Y. Posttraumatic stress disorder prevalence and risk of recurrence in acute coronary syndrome patients: a meta-analytic review. PLoS One. 2012;7:e38915.
23. Edmondson D, Shaffer JA, Denton EG, Shimbo D, Clemow L. Posttraumatic stress and myocardial infarction risk perceptions in hospitalized acute coronary syndrome patients. Front Psychol. 2012;3:144. https://doi.org/10.3389/fpsyg.2012.00144.
24. Berry E. Post-traumatic stress disorder after subarachnoid haemorrhage. Br J Clin Psychol. 1998;37(Pt 3):365–7.
25. Schelling G, Roozendaal B, Krauseneck T, Schmoelz M, De Quervain D, Briegel J. Efficacy of hydrocortisone in preventing posttraumatic stress disorder following critical illness and major surgery. Ann N Y Acad Sci. 2006;1071:46–53. https://doi.org/10.1196/annals.1364.005.

26. Schelling G, Stoll C, Haller M, Briegel J, Manert W, Hummel T, et al. Health-related quality of life and posttraumatic stress disorder in survivors of the acute respiratory distress syndrome. Crit Care Med. 1998;26(4):651–9.
27. Sembi S, Tarrier N, O'Neill P, Burns A, Faragher B. Does post-traumatic stress disorder occur after stroke: a preliminary study. Int J Geriatr Psychiatry. 1998;13(5):315–22. https://doi.org/10.1002/(SICI)1099-1166(199805)13:5<315::AID-GPS766>3.0.CO;2-P.
28. Dew MA, DiMartini AF, Switzer GE, Kormos RL, Schulberg HC, Roth LH, Griffith BP. Patterns and predictors of risk for depressive and anxiety-related disorders during the first three years after heart transplantation. Psychosomatics. 2000;41(2):191–2.
29. Stoll C, Schelling G, Goetz AE, Kilger E, Bayer A, Kapfhammer HP, et al. Health-related quality of life and post-traumatic stress disorder in patients after cardiac surgery and intensive care treatment. J Thorac Cardiovasc Surg. 2000;120(3):505–12.
30. Stukas AA Jr, Dew MA, Switzer GE, DiMartini A, Kormos RL, Griffith BP. PTSD in heart transplant recipients and their primary family caregivers. Psychosomatics. 1999;40(3):212–21.
31. Liberzon I, Abelson JL, Amdur RL, King AP, Cardneau JD, Henke P, Graham LM. Increased psychiatric morbidity after abdominal aortic surgery: risk factors for stress-related disorders. J Vasc Surg. 2006;43(5):929–34.
32. King AP, Abelson JA, Gholami B, Upchurch G, Henke P, Graham L, Liberzon I. Pre-surgical psychological and neuroendocrine predictors of psychiatric morbidity following major vascular surgery: a prospective longitudinal study. Psychosom Med. 2015;77(9):993–1005. https://doi.org/10.1097/PSY.0000000000000235.
33. Briere J, Jordan CE. Childhood maltreatment, intervening variables, and adult psychological difficulties in women: an overview. Trauma Violence Abuse. 2009;10(4):375–88. https://doi.org/10.1177/1524838009339757. Review. PubMed PMID: 19776086.
34. Kaplow JB, Dodge KA, Amaya-Jackson L, Saxe GN. Pathways to PTSD, part II: sexually abused children. Am J Psychiatry. 2005;162(7):1305–10. PubMed PMID: 15994713; PubMed Central PMCID: PMC2754170.
35. Briere J, Elliott DM. Prevalence and psychological sequelae of self-reported childhood physical and sexual abuse in a general population sample of men and women. Child Abuse Negl. 2003;27(10):1205–22. PubMed PMID: 14602100.
36. Zlotnick C, Johnson J, Kohn R, Vicente B, Rioseco P, Saldivia S. Childhood trauma, trauma in adulthood, and psychiatric diagnoses: results from a community sample. Compr Psychiatry. 2008;49(2):163–9. https://doi.org/10.1016/j.comppsych.2007.08.007. PubMed PMID: 18243889; PubMed Central PMCID: PMC2648973.
37. Kendler KS, Gardner CO, Prescott CA. Toward a comprehensive developmental model for major depression in women. Am J Psychiatry. 2002;159(7):1133–45. PubMed PMID: 12091191.
38. Kendler KS, Bulik CM, Silberg J, Hettema JM, Myers J, Prescott CA. Childhood sexual abuse and adult psychiatric and substance use disorders in women: an epidemiological and cotwin control analysis. Arch Gen Psychiatry. 2000;57(10):953–9. PubMed PMID: 11015813.
39. Xie P, Kranzler HR, Poling J, Stein MB, Anton RF, Brady K, Weiss RD, Farrer L, Gelernter J. Interactive effect of stressful life events and the serotonin transporter 5-HTTLPR genotype on posttraumatic stress disorder diagnosis in 2 independent populations. Arch Gen Psychiatry. 2009;66(11):1201–9. https://doi.org/10.1001/archgenpsychiatry.2009.153. PubMed PMID: 19884608; PubMed Central PMCID: PMC2867334.
40. Breslau N. Trauma and mental health in US inner-city populations. Gen Hosp Psychiatry. 2009;31(6):501–2. https://doi.org/10.1016/j.genhosppsych.2009.07.001. Erratum in: Gen Hosp Psychiatry. 2010;32(1):117. PubMed PMID: 19892206.
41. Binder EB, Bradley RG, Liu W, Epstein MP, Deveau TC, Mercer KB, Tang Y, Gillespie CF, Heim CM, Nemeroff CB, Schwartz AC, Cubells JF, Ressler KJ. Association of FKBP5 polymorphisms and childhood abuse with risk of posttraumatic stress disorder symptoms in adults. JAMA. 2008;299(11):1291–305. https://doi.org/10.1001/jama.299.11.1291. PubMed PMID: 18349090; PubMed Central PMCID: PMC2441757.

42. Felitti V, Anda R, Nordenberg D, Williamson DF, et al. Relationship of childhood abuse and household dysfunction to many of the leading causes of death in adults: the Adverse Childhood Experience (ACE) study. Am J Prev Med. 1998;14:245–58.
43. Anda RF, Brown DW, Dube SR, et al. Adverse childhood experiences and chronic obstructive pulmonary disease in adults. Am J Prev Med. 2010;34:396–403.
44. Dong M, Giles WH, Felitti VJ, et al. Insights into causal pathways for ischemic heart disease: Adverse Childhood Experiences Study. Circulation. 2004;110:1761–6.
45. Dube S, Fairweather D, Pearson W, et al. Cumulative childhood stress and autoimmune diseases in adults. Psychosom Med. 2009;71:243–50.
46. Dong M, Dube SR, Felitti VJ, Giles WH, Anda RF. Adverse childhood experiences and self-reported liver disease: new insights into a causal pathway. Arch Intern Med. 2003;163:1949–56.
47. Boscarino JA. A prospective study of PTSD and early-age heart disease mortality among Vietnam veterans: implications for surveillance and prevention. Psychosom Med. 2008;70:668–76.
48. Edmondson D, Cohen BE. Posttraumatic stress disorder and cardiovascular disease. Prog Cardiovasc Dis. 2013;55:548–56.
49. Lohr JB, Palmer BW, Eidt CA, Aailaboyina S, Mausbach BT, Wolkowitz OM, Thorp SR, Jeste DV. Is post-traumatic stress disorder associated with premature senescence? A review of the literature. Am J Geriatr Psychiatr. 2015;23:709–25.
50. Boscarino JA. Posttraumatic stress disorder and physical illness: results from clinical and epidemiologic studies. Ann N Y Acad Sci. 2004;1032:141–53. PubMed PMID: 15677401.
51. Roy SS, Foraker RE, Girton RA, Mansfield AJ. Posttraumatic stress disorder and incident heart failure among a community-based sample of US veterans. Am J Public Health. 2015;105:757–63.
52. Beristianos MH, Yaffe K, Cohen B, Byers AL. PTSD and risk of incident cardiovascular disease in aging veterans. Am J Geriatr Psychiatry. 2016;24(3):192–200. https://doi.org/10.1016/j.jagp.2014.12.003. PubMed PMID: 25555625.
53. Scherrer JF, Chrusciel T, Zeringue A, Garfield LD, Hauptman PJ, Lustman PJ, Freedland KE, Carney RM, Bucholz KK, Owen R. Anxiety disorders increase risk for incident myocardial infarction in depressed and nondepressed Veterans Administration patients. Am Heart J. 2010;159:772–9.
54. Gradus JL, Farkas DK, Svensson E, Ehrenstein V, Lash TL, Milstein A, Adler N, Sørensen HT. Associations between stress disorders and cardiovascular disease events in the Danish population. BMJ Open. 2015;5(12):e009334. https://doi.org/10.1136/bmjopen-2015-009334. PubMed PMID: 26667014; PubMed Central PMCID: PMC4679888.
55. Chen M-H, Pan T-L, Li C-T, Lin W-C, Chen Y-S, Lee Y-C, Tsai S-J, Hsu J-W, Huang K-L, Tsai C-F. Risk of stroke among patients with post-traumatic stress disorder: nationwide longitudinal study. Br J Psychiatry. 2015;206:302–7.
56. Boyko EJ, Jacobson IG, Smith B, Ryan MAK, Hooper TI, Amoroso PJ, Gackstetter GD, Barrett-Connor E, Smith TC, Millennium Cohort Study Team. Risk of diabetes in U.S. military service members in relation to combat deployment and mental health. Diabetes Care. 2010;33:1771–7.
57. Roberts AL, Agnew-Blais JC, Spiegelman D, Kubzansky LD, Mason SM, Galea S, Hu FB, Rich-Edwards JW, Koenen KC. Posttraumatic stress disorder and incidence of type 2 diabetes mellitus in a sample of women: a 22-year longitudinal study. JAMA Psychiatry. 2015;72:203–10.
58. Allison TG, Williams DE, Miller TD, Patten CA, Bailey KR, Squires RW, Gau GT. Medical and economic costs of psychologic distress in patients with coronary artery disease. Mayo Clin Proc. 1995;70(8):734–42.
59. Trask PC, Schwartz SM, Deaner SL, Paterson AG, Johnson T, Rubenfire M, Pomerleau OF. Behavioral medicine: the challenge of integrating psychological and behavioral approaches into primary care. Eff Clin Pract. 2002;5(2):75–83.

60. Druss BG, Rohrbaugh RM, Rosenheck RA. Depressive symptoms and health costs in older medical patients. Am J Psychiatry. 1999;156(3):477–9.
61. Unutzer J, Schoenbaum M, Katon WJ, Fan MY, Pincus HA, Hogan D, Taylor J. Healthcare costs associated with depression in medically Ill fee-for-service medicare participants. J Am Geriatr Soc. 2009;57(3):506–10. https://doi.org/10.1111/j.1532-5415.2008.02134.xJGS2134.
62. Etkin A, Wager TD. Functional neuroimaging of anxiety: a meta-analysis of emotional processing in PTSD, social anxiety disorder, and specific phobia. Am J Psychiatry. 2007;164(10):1476–88. https://doi.org/10.1176/appi.ajp.2007.07030504.
63. O'Doherty DCM, Chitty KM, Saddiqui S, Bennett MR, Lagopoulos J. A systematic review and meta-analysis of magnetic resonance imaging measurement of structural volumes in posttraumatic stress disorder. Psychiatry Res. 2015;232(1):1–33. https://doi.org/10.1016/j.pscychresns.2015.01.002.
64. Stark EA, Parsons CE, Van Hartevelt TJ, Charquero-Ballester M, McManners H, Ehlers A, et al. Post-traumatic stress influences the brain even in the absence of symptoms: a systematic, quantitative meta-analysis of neuroimaging studies. Neurosci Biobehav Rev. 2015;56:207–21. https://doi.org/10.1016/j.neubiorev.2015.07.007.
65. Kovács KJ. CRH: the link between hormonal-, metabolic- and behavioral responses to stress. J Chem Neuroanat. 2013;54:25–33. https://doi.org/10.1016/j.jchemneu.2013.05.003. Review. PubMed PMID: 23774011.
66. Kalin NH, Shelton SE, Davidson RJ. Cerebrospinal fluid corticotropin-releasing hormone levels are elevated in monkeys with patterns of brain activity associated with fearful temperament. Biol Psychiatry. 2000;47(7):579–85. PubMed PMID: 10745049.
67. Baker DG, West SA, Nicholson WE, Ekhator NN, Kasckow JW, Hill KK, Bruce AB, Orth DN, Geracioti TD Jr. Serial CSF corticotropin-releasing hormone levels and adrenocortical activity in combat veterans with posttraumatic stress disorder. Am J Psychiatry. 1999;156(4):585–8. Erratum in: Am J Psychiatry 1999;156(6):986. PubMed PMID: 10200738.
68. Bremner JD, Randall P, Vermetten E, Staib L, Bronen RA, Mazure C, et al. Magnetic resonance imaging-based measurement of hippocampal volume in posttraumatic stress disorder related to childhood physical and sexual abuse—a preliminary report. Biol Psychiatry. 1997;41(1):23–32.
69. Maren S, Phan KL, Liberzon I. The contextual brain: implications for fear conditioning, extinction and psychopathology. Nat Rev Neurosci. 2013;14(6):417–28. https://doi.org/10.1038/nrn3492. Review. PubMed PMID: 23635870; PubMed Central PMCID: PMC5072129.
70. Rauch SL, Whalen PJ, Shin LM, McInerney SC, Macklin ML, Lasko NB, et al. Exaggerated amygdala response to masked facial stimuli in posttraumatic stress disorder: a functional MRI study. Biol Psychiatry. 2000;47(9):769–76.
71. Liberzon I, Martis B. Neuroimaging studies of emotional responses in PTSD. Ann N Y Acad Sci. 2006;1071:87–109. https://doi.org/10.1196/annals.1364.009.
72. Quirk GJ, Russo GK, Barron JL, Lebron K. The role of ventromedial prefrontal cortex in the recovery of extinguished fear. J Neurosci. 2000;20(16):6225–31. PubMed PMID: 10934272.
73. Ochsner KN, Bunge SA, Gross JJ, Gabrieli JD. Rethinking feelings: an FMRI study of the cognitive regulation of emotion. J Cogn Neurosci. 2002;14(8):1215–29. PubMed PMID: 12495527.
74. Milad MR, Pitman RK, Ellis CB, Gold AL, Shin LM, Lasko NB, Zeidan MA, Handwerger K, Orr SP, Rauch SL. Neurobiological basis of failure to recall extinction memory in posttraumatic stress disorder. Biol Psychiatry. 2009;66:1075–82.
75. LeDoux JE, Cicchetti P, Xagoraris A, Romanski LM. The lateral amygdaloid nucleus: sensory interface of the amygdala in fear conditioning. J Neurosci. 1990;10(4):1062–9.
76. Campeau S, Davis M. Involvement of subcortical and cortical afferents to the lateral nucleus of the amygdala in fear conditioning measured with fear-potentiated startle in rats trained concurrently with auditory and visual conditioned stimuli. J Neurosci. 1995;15(3 Pt 2):2312–27. PubMed PMID: 7891169.
77. Quirk GJ. Extinction: new excitement for an old phenomenon. Biol Psychiatry. 2006;60(4):317–8. PubMed PMID: 16919520.

78. Milad MR, Wright CI, Orr SP, Pitman RK, Quirk GJ, Rauch SL. Recall of fear extinction in humans activates the ventromedial prefrontal cortex and hippocampus in concert. Biol Psychiatry. 2007;62:446–54.
79. Garfinkel SN, Abelson JL, King AP, Sripada RK, Wang X, Gaines LM, Liberzon I. Impaired contextual modulation of memories in PTSD: an fMRI and psychophysiological study of extinction retention and fear renewal. J Neurosci. 2014;34(40):13435–43. https://doi.org/10.1523/JNEUROSCI.4287-13.2014. PubMed PMID: 25274821; PubMed Central PMCID: PMC4262698.
80. De Bellis MD, Keshavan MS, Shifflett H, Iyengar S, Beers SR, Hall J, Moritz G. Brain structures in pediatric maltreatment-related posttraumatic stress disorder: a sociodemographically matched study. Biol Psychiatry. 2002;52(11):1066–78.
81. Hedges DW, Thatcher GW, Bennett PJ, Sood S, Paulson D, Creem-Regehr S, Brown BL, Allen S, Johnson J, Froelich B, Bigler ED. Brain integrity and cerebral atrophy in Vietnam combat veterans with and without posttraumatic stress disorder. Neurocase. 2007;13(5):402–10. https://doi.org/10.1080/13554790701851551. PubMed PMID: 18781439.
82. St Jacques PL, Botzung A, Miles A, Rubin DC. Functional neuroimaging of emotionally intense autobiographical memories in post-traumatic stress disorder. J Psychiatr Res. 2011;45(5):630–7. https://doi.org/10.1016/j.jpsychires.2010.10.011. PubMed PMID: 21109253; PubMed Central PMCID: PMC3081954.
83. Bryant RA, Kemp AH, Felmingham KL, Liddell B, Olivieri G, Peduto A, Gordon E, Williams LM. Enhanced amygdala and medial prefrontal activation during nonconscious processing of fear in posttraumatic stress disorder: an fMRI study. Hum Brain Mapp. 2008;29(5):517–23. PubMed PMID: 17525984.
84. Shin LM, Wright CI, Cannistraro PA, Wedig MM, McMullin K, Martis B, et al. A functional magnetic resonance imaging study of amygdala and medial prefrontal cortex responses to overtly presented fearful faces in posttraumatic stress disorder. Arch Gen Psychiatry. 2005;62(3):273–81. https://doi.org/10.1001/archpsyc.62.3.273.
85. Williams JB, Alexander KP, Morin JF, Langlois Y, Noiseux N, Perrault LP, et al. Preoperative anxiety as a predictor of mortality and major morbidity in patients aged >70 years undergoing cardiac surgery. Am J Cardiol. 2013;111(1):137–42. https://doi.org/10.1016/j.amjcard.2012.08.060.
86. Liberzon I, Abelson JL, Flagel SB, Raz J, Young EA. Neuroendocrine and psychophysiologic responses in PTSD: a symptom provocation study. Neuropsychopharmacology. 1999;21(1):40–50.
87. Pissiota A, Frans O, Fernandez M, von Knorring L, Fischer H, Fredrikson M. Neurofunctional correlates of posttraumatic stress disorder: a PET symptom provocation study. Eur Arch Psychiatry Clin Neurosci. 2002;252(2):68–75. PubMed PMID: 12111339.
88. Vermetten E, Schmahl C, Southwick SM, Bremner JD. Positron tomographic emission study of olfactory induced emotional recall in veterans with and without combat-related posttraumatic stress disorder. Psychopharmacol Bull. 2007;40(1):8–30. PubMed PMID: 17285093; PubMed Central PMCID: PMC3236699.
89. Driessen M, Beblo T, Mertens M, Piefke M, Rullkoetter N, Silva-Saavedra A, Reddemann L, Rau H, Markowitsch HJ, Wulff H, Lange W, Woermann FG. Posttraumatic stress disorder and fMRI activation patterns of traumatic memory in patients with borderline personality disorder. Biol Psychiatry. 2004;55(6):603–11. PubMed PMID: 15013829.
90. Morey RA, Dolcos F, Petty CM, Cooper DA, Hayes JP, LaBar KS, McCarthy G. The role of trauma-related distractors on neural systems for working memory and emotion processing in posttraumatic stress disorder. J Psychiatr Res. 2009;43(8):809–17. https://doi.org/10.1016/j.jpsychires.2008.10.014. PubMed PMID: 19091328; PubMed Central PMCID: PMC2684984.
91. Shin LM, McNally RJ, Kosslyn SM, Thompson WL, Rauch SL, Alpert NM, et al. A positron emission tomographic study of symptom provocation in PTSD. Ann N Y Acad Sci. 1997;821:521–3.

92. Bremner JD, Narayan M, Staib LH, Southwick SM, McGlashan T, Charney DS. Neural correlates of memories of childhood sexual abuse in women with and without posttraumatic stress disorder. Am J Psychiatry. 1999;156(11):1787–95.
93. Britton JC, Phan KL, Taylor SF, Fig LM, Liberzon I. Corticolimbic blood flow in posttraumatic stress disorder during script-driven imagery. Biol Psychiatry. 2005;57(8):832–40.
94. Lanius RA, Bluhm RL, Coupland NJ, Hegadoren KM, Rowe B, Theberge J, et al. Default mode network connectivity as a predictor of post-traumatic stress disorder symptom severity in acutely traumatized subjects. Acta Psychiatr Scand. 2010;121(1):33–40. https://doi.org/10.1111/j.1600-0447.2009.01391.x.
95. Phan KL, Britton JC, Taylor SF, Fig LM, Liberzon I. Corticolimbic blood flow during nontraumatic emotional processing in posttraumatic stress disorder. Arch Gen Psychiatry. 2006;63(2):184–92. PubMed PMID: 16461862.
96. Bremner JD, Vermetten E, Schmahl C, Vaccarino V, Vythilingam M, Afzal N, Grillon C, Charney DS. Positron emission tomographic imaging of neural correlates of a fear acquisition and extinction paradigm in women with childhood sexual-abuse-related post-traumatic stress disorder. Psychol Med. 2005;35(6):791–806. PubMed PMID: 15997600; PubMed Central PMCID: PMC3233760.
97. Alexopoulos GS, Hoptman MJ, Kanellopoulos D, Murphy CF, Lim KO, Gunning FM. Functional connectivity in the cognitive control network and the default mode network in late-life depression. J Affect Disord. 2012;139(1):56–65. https://doi.org/10.1016/j.jad.2011.12.002.
98. Anticevic A, Cole MW, Murray JD, Corlett PR, Wang XJ, Krystal JH. The role of default network deactivation in cognition and disease. Trends Cogn Sci. 2012;16(12):584–92. https://doi.org/10.1016/j.tics.2012.10.008.
99. Cole MW, Repovs G, Anticevic A. The frontoparietal control system: a central role in mental health. Neuroscientist. 2014;20(6):652–64. https://doi.org/10.1177/1073858414525995.
100. Hamilton JP, Chen MC, Gotlib IH. Neural systems approaches to understanding major depressive disorder: an intrinsic functional organization perspective. Neurobiol Dis. 2013;52:4–11. https://doi.org/10.1016/j.nbd.2012.01.015.
101. Fox MD, Snyder AZ, Vincent JL, Corbetta M, Van Essen DC, Raichle ME. The human brain is intrinsically organized into dynamic, anticorrelated functional networks. Proc Natl Acad Sci U S A. 2005;102(27):9673–8. https://doi.org/10.1073/pnas.0504136102.
102. Yeo BT, Krienen FM, Sepulcre J, Sabuncu MR, Lashkari D, Hollinshead M, et al. The organization of the human cerebral cortex estimated by intrinsic functional connectivity. J Neurophysiol. 2011;106(3):1125–65. https://doi.org/10.1152/jn.00338.2011.
103. Herringa RJ, Birn RM, Ruttle PL, Burghy CA, Stodola DE, Davidson RJ, Essex MJ. Childhood maltreatment is associated with altered fear circuitry and increased internalizing symptoms by late adolescence. Proc Natl Acad Sci U S A. 2013;110(47):19119–24. https://doi.org/10.1073/pnas.1310766110.
104. Rabinak CA, Angstadt M, Welsh RC, Kenndy AE, Lyubkin M, Martis B, Phan KL. Altered amygdala resting-state functional connectivity in post-traumatic stress disorder. Front Psychiatry. 2011;2:62. https://doi.org/10.3389/fpsyt.2011.00062.
105. Sripada RK, King AP, Garfinkel SN, Wang X, Sripada CS, Welsh RC, Liberzon I. Altered resting-state amygdala functional connectivity in men with posttraumatic stress disorder. J Psychiatry Neurosci. 2012;37(4):241–9. https://doi.org/10.1503/jpn.110069.
106. Sripada RK, King AP, Welsh RC, Garfinkel SN, Wang X, Sripada CS, Liberzon I. Neural dysregulation in posttraumatic stress disorder: evidence for disrupted equilibrium between salience and default mode brain networks. Psychosom Med. 2012;74(9):904–11. https://doi.org/10.1097/PSY.0b013e318273bf33.
107. Rabellino D, Tursich M, Frewen PA, Daniels JK, Densmore M, Theberge J, Lanius RA. Intrinsic connectivity networks in post-traumatic stress disorder during sub- and supraliminal processing of threat-related stimuli. Acta Psychiatr Scand. 2015;132(5):365–78. https://doi.org/10.1111/acps.12418.

108. Berridge CW, Waterhouse BD. The locus coeruleus-noradrenergic system: modulation of behavioral state and state-dependent cognitive processes. Brain Res Rev. 2003;42:33–84.
109. Sara SJ. The locus coeruleus and noradrenergic modulation of cognition. Nat Rev Neurosci. 2009;10:211–23.
110. van der Kolk B, Greenberg M, Boyd H, Krystal J. Inescapable shock, neurotransmitters, and addiction to trauma: toward a psychobiology of post traumatic stress. Biol Psychiatry. 1985;20:314–25.
111. Grant SJ, Huang YH, Redmond DE Jr. Behavior of monkeys during opiate withdrawal and locus coeruleus stimulation. Pharmacol Biochem Behav. 1988;30:13–9.
112. George SA, Knox D, Curtis AL, Aldridge JW, Valentino RJ, Liberzon I. Altered locus coeruleus-norepinephrine function following single prolonged stress. Eur J Neurosci. 2013;37:901–9.
113. Geracioti TD Jr, Baker DG, Ekhator NN, West SA, Hill KK, Bruce AB, Schmidt D, Rounds-Kugler B, Yehuda R, Keck PE Jr, Kasckow JW. CSF norepinephrine concentrations in post-traumatic stress disorder. Am J Psychiatry. 2001;158(8):1227–30. PubMed PMID: 11481155.
114. Geracioti TD Jr, Baker DG, Kasckow JW, Strawn JR, Jeffrey Mulchahey J, Dashevsky BA, Horn PS, Ekhator NN. Effects of trauma-related audiovisual stimulation on cerebrospinal fluid norepinephrine and corticotropin-releasing hormone concentrations in post-traumatic stress disorder. Psychoneuroendocrinology. 2008;33(4):416–24. https://doi.org/10.1016/j.psyneuen.2007.12.012. PubMed PMID: 18295412.
115. Southwick SM, Krystal JH, Bremner JD, Morgan CA III, Nicolaou AL, Nagy LM, et al. Noradrenergic and serotonergic function in posttraumatic stress disorder. Arch Gen Psychiatry. 1997;54(8):749–58.
116. Raskind MA, Peskind ER. Prazosin for post-traumatic stress disorder. N Engl J Med. 2018;378(17):1649–50. https://doi.org/10.1056/NEJMc1803171. PubMed PMID: 29694817.
117. Pietrzak RH, Gallezot JD, Ding YS, Henry S, Potenza MN, Southwick SM, et al. Association of posttraumatic stress disorder with reduced in vivo norepinephrine transporter availability in the locus coeruleus. JAMA Psychiatry. 2013;70:1199–205.
118. Naegeli C, Zeffiro T, Piccirelli M, Jaillard A, Weilenmann A, Hassanpour K, Schick M, Rufer M, Orr SP, Mueller-Pfeiffer C. Locus Coeruleus activity mediates hyperresponsiveness in posttraumatic stress disorder. Biol Psychiatry. 2018;83(3):254–62. https://doi.org/10.1016/j.biopsych.2017.08.021. PubMed PMID: 29100627.
119. Eichenbaum H. Hippocampus: cognitive processes and neural representations that underlie declarative memory. Neuron. 2004;44(1):109–20. https://doi.org/10.1016/j.neuron.2004.08.028.
120. Mizuno K, Giese KP. Hippocampus-dependent memory formation: do memory type-specific mechanisms exist? J Pharmacol Sci. 2005;98(3):191–7. https://doi.org/10.1254/jphs.CRJ05005X.
121. Jacobson L, Sapolsky R. The role of the hippocampus in feedback regulation of the hypothalamic-pituitary-adrenocortical axis. Endocr Rev. 1991;12(2):118–34.
122. Lathe R. Hormones and the hippocampus. J Endocrinol. 2001;169(2):205–31.
123. Richter-Levin G. The amygdala, the hippocampus, and emotional modulation of memory. Neuroscientist. 2004;10(1):31–9. https://doi.org/10.1177/1073858403259955.
124. Vertes RP. Interactions among the medial prefrontal cortex, hippocampus and midline thalamus in emotional and cognitive processing in the rat. Neuroscience. 2006;142(1):1–20. https://doi.org/10.1016/j.neuroscience.2006.06.027.
125. de Kloet ER, Karst H, Joels M. Corticosteroid hormones in the central stress response: quick-and-slow. Front Neuroendocrinol. 2008;29(2):268–72.
126. Sapolsky RM. Glucocorticoids and hippocampal atrophy in neuropsychiatric disorders. Arch Gen Psychiatry. 2000;57(10):925–35.
127. Starkman MN. Neuropsychiatric findings in Cushing syndrome and exogenous glucocorticoid administration. Endocrinol Metab Clin North Am. 2013;42(3):477–88. https://doi.org/10.1016/j.ecl.2013.05.010. Review. PubMed PMID: 24011881.
128. Karl A, Schaefer M, Malta LS, Dorfel D, Rohleder N, Werner A. A meta-analysis of structural brain abnormalities in PTSD. Neurosci Biobehav Rev. 2006;30:1004–31.

129. Kitayama N, Vaccarino V, Kutner M, Weiss P, Bremner JD. Magnetic resonance imaging (MRI) measurement of hippocampal volume in posttraumatic stress disorder: a meta-analysis. J Affect Disord. 2005;88:79–86.
130. Smith ME. Bilateral hippocampal volume reduction in adults with post-traumatic stress disorder: a meta-analysis of structural MRI studies. Hippocampus. 2005;15:798–807.
131. Logue MW, van Rooij SJH, Dennis EL, Davis SL, Hayes JP, Stevens JS, Densmore M, Haswell CC, Ipser J, Koch SBJ, Korgaonkar M, Lebois LAM, Peverill M, Baker JT, Boedhoe PSW, Frijling JL, Gruber SA, Harpaz-Rotem I, Jahanshad N, Koopowitz S, Levy I, Nawijn L, O'Connor L, Olff M, Salat DH, Sheridan MA, Spielberg JM, van Zuiden M, Winternitz SR, Wolff JD, Wolf EJ, Wang X, Wrocklage K, Abdallah CG, Bryant RA, Geuze E, Jovanovic T, Kaufman ML, King AP, Krystal JH, Lagopoulos J, Bennett M, Lanius R, Liberzon I, McGlinchey RE, McLaughlin KA, Milberg WP, Miller MW, Ressler KJ, Veltman DJ, Stein DJ, Thomaes K, Thompson PM, Morey RA. Smaller hippocampal volume in posttraumatic stress disorder: a multisite ENIGMA-PGC study: subcortical volumetry results from Posttraumatic Stress Disorder Consortia. Biol Psychiatry. 2018;83(3):244–53. https://doi.org/10.1016/j.biopsych.2017.09.006. PubMed PMID: 29217296.
132. Lindauer RJ, Vlieger EJ, Jalink M, Olff M, Carlier IV, Majoie CB, et al. Smaller hippocampal volume in Dutch police officers with posttraumatic stress disorder. Biol Psychiatry. 2004;56(5):356–63. https://doi.org/10.1016/j.biopsych.2004.05.021.
133. Lanius RA, Williamson PC, Densmore M, Boksman K, Gupta MA, Neufeld RW, Gati JS, Menon RS. Neural correlates of traumatic memories in posttraumatic stress disorder: a functional MRI investigation. Am J Psychiatry. 2001;158(11):1920–2. PubMed PMID: 11691703.
134. Shin LM, Orr SP, Carson MA, Rauch SL, Macklin ML, Lasko NB, Peters PM, Metzger LJ, Dougherty DD, Cannistraro PA, Alpert NM, Fischman AJ, Pitman RK. Regional cerebral blood flow in the amygdala and medial prefrontal cortex during traumatic imagery in male and female Vietnam veterans with PTSD. Arch Gen Psychiatry. 2004;61(2):168–76. PubMed PMID: 14757593.
135. Hou C, Liu J, Wang K, Li L, Liang M, He Z, Liu Y, Zhang Y, Li W, Jiang T. Brain responses to symptom provocation and trauma-related short-term memory recall in coal mining accident survivors with acute severe PTSD. Brain Res. 2007;1144:165–74. PubMed PMID: 17331476.
136. Yang P, Wu MT, Hsu CC, Ker JH. Evidence of early neurobiological alternations in adolescents with posttraumatic stress disorder: a functional MRI study. Neurosci Lett. 2004;370(1):13–8. PubMed PMID: 15489009.
137. Kim SJ, Lyoo IK, Lee YS, Kim J, Sim ME, Bae SJ, Kim HJ, Lee JY, Jeong DU. Decreased cerebral blood flow of thalamus in PTSD patients as a strategy to reduce re-experience symptoms. Acta Psychiatr Scand. 2007;116(2):145–53. PubMed PMID: 17650277.
138. Bryant RA, Felmingham KL, Kemp AH, Barton M, Peduto AS, Rennie C, Gordon E, Williams LM. Neural networks of information processing in posttraumatic stress disorder: a functional magnetic resonance imaging study. Biol Psychiatry. 2005;58(2):111–8. PubMed PMID: 16038681.
139. Semple WE, Goyer PF, McCormick R, Donovan B, Muzic RF Jr, Rugle L, McCutcheon K, Lewis C, Liebling D, Kowaliw S, Vapenik K, Semple MA, Flener CR, Schulz SC. Higher brain blood flow at amygdala and lower frontal cortex blood flow in PTSD patients with comorbid cocaine and alcohol abuse compared with normals. Psychiatry. 2000;63(1):65–74. PubMed PMID: 10855761.
140. Shin LM, Whalen PJ, Pitman RK, Bush G, Macklin ML, Lasko NB, Orr SP, McInerney SC, Rauch SL. An fMRI study of anterior cingulate function in posttraumatic stress disorder. Biol Psychiatry. 2001;50(12):932–42. PubMed PMID: 11750889.
141. Felmingham K, Kemp A, Williams L, Das P, Hughes G, Peduto A, Bryant R. Changes in anterior cingulate and amygdala after cognitive behavior therapy of posttraumatic stress disorder. Psychol Sci. 2007;18(2):127–9. PubMed PMID: 17425531.
142. King AP, Block SR, Sripada RK, Rauch SA, Porter KE, Favorite TK, Giardino N, Liberzon I. A pilot study of mindfulness-based exposure therapy in OEF/OIF combat veterans with PTSD: altered medial frontal cortex and amygdala responses in social-emotional processing.

Front Psychiatry. 2016;7:154. eCollection 2016. PubMed PMID: 27703434; PubMed Central PMCID: PMC5028840.
143. Lansing K, Amen DG, Hanks C, Rudy L. High-resolution brain SPECT imaging and eye movement desensitization and reprocessing in police officers with PTSD. J Neuropsychiatry Clin Neurosci. 2005;17(4):526–32. PubMed PMID: 16387993.
144. Seedat S, Warwick J, van Heerden B, Hugo C, Zungu-Dirwayi N, Van Kradenburg J, Stein DJ. Single photon emission computed tomography in posttraumatic stress disorder before and after treatment with a selective serotonin reuptake inhibitor. J Affect Disord. 2004;80(1):45–53. PubMed PMID: 15094257.
145. Bluhm R, Williamson P, Lanius R, Theberge J, Densmore M, Bartha R, et al. Resting state default-mode network connectivity in early depression using a seed region-of-interest analysis: decreased connectivity with caudate nucleus. Psychiatry Clin Neurosci. 2009;63(6):754–61. https://doi.org/10.1111/j.1440-1819.2009.02030.x.
146. Birn RM, Patriat R, Phillips ML, Germain A, Herringa RJ. Childhood maltreatment and combat posttraumatic stress differentially predict fear-related fronto-subcortical connectivity. Depress Anxiety. 2014;31(10):880–92. https://doi.org/10.1002/da.22291.
147. Miller DR, Hayes SM, Hayes JP, Spielberg JM, Lafleche G, Verfaellie M. Default mode network subsystems are differentially disrupted in posttraumatic stress disorder. Biol Psychiatry Cogn Neurosci Neuroimaging. 2017;2(4):363–71.
148. Krystal JH, Neumeister A. Noradrenergic and serotonergic mechanisms in the neurobiology of posttraumatic stress disorder and resilience. Brain Res. 2009;1293:13–23.
149. O'Donnell T, Hegadoren KM, Coupland NC. Noradrenergic mechanisms in the pathophysiology of post-traumatic stress disorder. Neuropsychobiology. 2004;50(4):273–83.
150. Hendrickson RC, Raskind MA. Noradrenergic dysregulation in the pathophysiology of PTSD. Exp Neurol. 2016;284(Pt B):181–95. https://doi.org/10.1016/j.expneurol.2016.05.014. Review. PubMed PMID: 27222130.
151. Jones E. Historical approaches to post-combat disorders. Philos Trans R Soc Lond B Biol Sci. 2006;361(1468):533–42. PubMed PMID: 16687259; PubMed Central PMCID: PMC1569621.
152. Orr SP, Metzger LJ, Pitman RK. Psychophysiology of post-traumatic stress disorder. Psychiatr Clin North Am. 2002;25(2):271–93.
153. Pitman RK, Orr SP. Psychophysiologic testing for post-traumatic stress disorder: forensic psychiatric application. Bull Am Acad Psychiatry Law. 1993;21(1):37–52.
154. Pitman RK, Orr SP, Steketee GS. Psychophysiological investigations of posttraumatic stress disorder imagery. Psychopharmacol Bull. 1989;25(3):426–31.
155. Pitman RK, Orr SP, Forgue DF, de Jong JB, Claiborn JM. Psychophysiologic assessment of posttraumatic stress disorder imagery in Vietnam combat veterans. Arch Gen Psychiatry. 1987;44(11):970–5.
156. Pitman RK, Orr SP, Shalev AY, Metzger LJ, Mellman TA. Psychophysiological alterations in post-traumatic stress disorder. Semin Clin Neuropsychiatry. 1999;4(4):234–41. https://doi.org/10.153/SCNP00400234.
157. Shalev AY, Orr SP, Pitman RK. Psychophysiologic response during script-driven imagery as an outcome measure in posttraumatic stress disorder. J Clin Psychiatry. 1992;53(9):324–6.
158. Hughes JW, Feldman ME, Beckham JC. Posttraumatic stress disorder is associated with attenuated baroreceptor sensitivity among female, but not male, smokers. Biol Psychol. 2006;71(3):296–302. PubMed PMID: 16011871.
159. Woodward SH, Kaloupek DG, Streeter CC, Kimble MO, Reiss AL, Eliez S, et al. Hippocampal volume, PTSD, and alcoholism in combat veterans. Am J Psychiatry. 2006;163(4):674–81. https://doi.org/10.1176/appi.ajp.163.4.674.
160. Minassian A, Geyer MA, Baker DG, Nievergelt CM, O'Connor DT, Risbrough VB, Team MRS. Heart rate variability characteristics in a large group of active-duty marines and relationship to posttraumatic stress. Psychosom Med. 2014;76(4):292–301. https://doi.org/10.1097/PSY.0000000000000056. PubMed PMID: 24804881; PubMed Central PMCID: PMC4062545.

161. Keary TA, Hughes JW, Palmieri PA. Women with posttraumatic stress disorder have larger decreases in heart rate variability during stress tasks. Int J Psychophysiol. 2009;73(3):257–64. https://doi.org/10.1016/j.ijpsycho.2009.04.003. PubMed PMID: 19374925.
162. Joshi S, Li Y, Kalwani RM, Gold JI. Relationships between pupil diameter and neuronal activity in the locus coeruleus, colliculi, and cingulate cortex. Neuron. 2016;89(1):221–34. https://doi.org/10.1016/j.neuron.2015.11.028. PubMed PMID: 26711118; PubMed Central PMCID: PMC4707070.
163. Cascardi M, Armstrong D, Chung L, Paré D. Pupil response to threat in trauma-exposed individuals with or without PTSD. J Trauma Stress. 2015;28(4):370–4. https://doi.org/10.1002/jts.22022. PubMed PMID: 26215078; PubMed Central PMCID: PMC4743760.
164. Kimble MO, Fleming K, Bandy C, Kim J, Zambetti A. Eye tracking and visual attention to threating stimuli in veterans of the Iraq war. J Anxiety Disord. 2010;24(3):293–9. https://doi.org/10.1016/j.janxdis.2009.12.006. PubMed PMID: 20138463; PubMed Central PMCID: PMC2838961.
165. De Bellis MD, Baum AS, Birmaher B, Ryan ND. Urinary catecholamine excretion in childhood overanxious and posttraumatic stress disorders. Ann N Y Acad Sci. 1997;821:451–5.
166. Wingenfeld K, Whooley MA, Neylan TC, Otte C, Cohen BE. Effect of current and lifetime posttraumatic stress disorder on 24-h urinary catecholamines and cortisol: results from the Mind Your Heart Study. Psychoneuroendocrinology. 2015;52:83–91. https://doi.org/10.1016/j.psyneuen.2014.10.023. PubMed PMID: 25459895; PubMed Central PMCID: PMC4297502.
167. Young EA, Breslau N. Saliva cortisol in posttraumatic stress disorder: a community epidemiologic study. Biol Psychiatry. 2004;56(3):205–9. PubMed PMID: 15271590.
168. Nicholson EL, Bryant RA, Felmingham KL. Interaction of noradrenaline and cortisol predicts negative intrusive memories in posttraumatic stress disorder. Neurobiol Learn Mem. 2014;112:204–11. https://doi.org/10.1016/j.nlm.2013.11.018. PubMed PMID: 24296460.
169. Keeshin BR, Strawn JR, Out D, Granger DA, Putnam FW. Elevated salivary alpha amylase in adolescent sexual abuse survivors with posttraumatic stress disorder symptoms. J Child Adolesc Psychopharmacol. 2015;25(4):344–50. https://doi.org/10.1089/cap.2014.0034. PubMed PMID: 25803321; PubMed Central PMCID: PMC4955591.
170. Shalev AY, Sahar T, Freedman S, Peri T, Glick N, Brandes D, Orr SP, Pitman RK. A prospective study of heart rate response following trauma and the subsequent development of posttraumatic stress disorder. Arch Gen Psychiatry. 1998;55(6):553–9. PubMed PMID: 9633675.
171. Pitman RK, Sanders KM, Zusman RM, Healy AR, Cheema F, Lasko NB, Cahill L, Orr SP. Pilot study of secondary prevention of posttraumatic stress disorder with propranolol. Biol Psychiatry. 2002;51(2):189–92. PubMed PMID: 11822998.
172. Donovan E. Propranolol use in the prevention and treatment of posttraumatic stress disorder in military veterans: forgetting therapy revisited. Perspect Biol Med. 2009;53(1):61–74.
173. McGhee LL, Maani CV, Garza TH, Desocio PA, Gaylord KM, Black IH. The effect of propranolol on posttraumatic stress disorder in burned service members. J Burn Care Res. 2009;30(1):92–7. https://doi.org/10.1097/BCR.0b013e3181921f51.
174. Nugent NR, Christopher NC, Crow JP, Browne L, Ostrowski S, Delahanty DL. The efficacy of early propranolol administration at reducing PTSD symptoms in pediatric injury patients: a pilot study. J Trauma Stress. 2010;23(2):282–7. https://doi.org/10.1002/jts.20517.
175. Sharp S, Thomas C, Rosenberg L, Rosenberg M, Meyer W III. Propranolol does not reduce risk for acute stress disorder in pediatric burn trauma. J Trauma. 2010;68(1):193–7. https://doi.org/10.1097/TA.0b013e3181a8b326.
176. de Kloet ER, Sibug RM, Helmerhorst FM, Schmidt MV. Stress, genes and the mechanism of programming the brain for later life. Neurosci Biobehav Rev. 2005;29(2):271–81. Erratum in: Neurosci Biobehav Rev. 2006;30(4):576. Schmidt, Mathias [corrected to Schmidt, Mathias V]. PubMed PMID: 15811498.
177. Meaney MJ, Szyf M, Seckl JR. Epigenetic mechanisms of perinatal programming of hypothalamic-pituitary-adrenal function and health. Trends Mol Med. 2007;13(7):269–77.

178. Viau V, Sharma S, Plotsky PM, Meaney MJ. Increased plasma ACTH responses to stress in nonhandled compared with handled rats require basal levels of corticosterone and are associated with increased levels of ACTH secretagogues in the median eminence. J Neurosci. 1993;13(3):1097–105.
179. Weaver IC, Diorio J, Seckl JR, Szyf M, Meaney MJ. Early environmental regulation of hippocampal glucocorticoid receptor gene expression: characterization of intracellular mediators and potential genomic target sites. Ann N Y Acad Sci. 2004;1024:182–212. https://doi.org/10.1196/annals.1321.099.
180. Anda RF, Brown DW, Felitti VJ, Bremner JD, Dube SR, Giles WH. Adverse childhood experiences and prescribed psychotropic medications in adults. Am J Prev Med. 2007;32(5):389–94.
181. Chapman DP, Whitfield CL, Felitti VJ, Dube SR, Edwards VJ, Anda RF. Adverse childhood experiences and the risk of depressive disorders in adulthood. J Affect Disord. 2004;82(2):217–25.
182. Huot RL, Thrivikraman KV, Meaney MJ, Plotsky PM. Development of adult ethanol preference and anxiety as a consequence of neonatal maternal separation in Long Evans rats and reversal with antidepressant treatment. Psychopharmacology. 2001;158(4):366–73. https://doi.org/10.1007/s002130100701.
183. Meaney MJ, Szyf M. Maternal care as a model for experience-dependent chromatin plasticity? Trends Neurosci. 2005;28(9):456–63.
184. Sanchez MM, Ladd CO, Plotsky PM. Early adverse experience as a developmental risk factor for later psychopathology: evidence from rodent and primate models. Dev Psychopathol. 2001;13(3):419–49.
185. Ladd CO, Thrivikraman KV, Huot RL, Plotsky PM. Differential neuroendocrine responses to chronic variable stress in adult Long Evans rats exposed to handling-maternal separation as neonates. Psychoneuroendocrinology. 2005;30(6):520–33. PubMed PMID: 15808921.
186. Liberzon I, Krstov M, Young EA. Stress-restress: effects on ACTH and fast feedback. Psychoneuroendocrinology. 1997;22(6):443–53.
187. Liberzon I, López JF, Flagel SB, Vázquez DM, Young EA. Differential regulation of hippocampal glucocorticoid receptors mRNA and fast feedback: relevance to post-traumatic stress disorder. J Neuroendocrinol. 1999;11(1):11–7. PubMed PMID: 9918224.
188. Ladd CO, Huot RL, Thrivikraman KV, Nemeroff CB, Plotsky PM. Long-term adaptations in glucocorticoid receptor and mineralocorticoid receptor mRNA and negative feedback on the hypothalamo-pituitary-adrenal axis following neonatal maternal separation. Biol Psychiatry. 2004;55(4):367–75. https://doi.org/10.1016/j.biopsych.2003.10.007.
189. Liu D, Diorio J, Tannenbaum B, Caldji C, Francis D, Freedman A, et al. Maternal care, hippocampal glucocorticoid receptors, and hypothalamic-pituitary-adrenal responses to stress. Science. 1997;277(5332):1659–62.
190. Morris MC, Compas BE, Garber J. Relations among posttraumatic stress disorder, comorbid major depression, and HPA function: a systematic review and meta-analysis. Clin Psychol Rev. 2012;32(4):301–15. https://doi.org/10.1016/j.cpr.2012.02.002.
191. Pfohl B, Sherman B, Schlechte J, Stone R. Pituitary-adrenal axis rhythm disturbances in psychiatric depression. Arch Gen Psychiatry. 1985;42(9):897–903.
192. Yehuda R. Neuroendocrine aspects of PTSD. Handb Exp Pharmacol. 2005;(169):371–403.
193. Young EA, Haskett RF, Murphy-Weinberg V, Watson SJ, Akil H. Loss of glucocorticoid fast feedback in depression. Arch Gen Psychiatry. 1991;48(8):693–9.
194. Heim C, Newport DJ, Heit S, Graham YP, Wilcox M, Bonsall R, et al. Pituitary-adrenal and autonomic responses to stress in women after sexual and physical abuse in childhood. JAMA. 2000;284(5):592–7.
195. Tyrka AR, Price LH, Gelernter J, Schepker C, Anderson GM, Carpenter LL. Interaction of childhood maltreatment with the corticotropin-releasing hormone receptor gene: effects on hypothalamic-pituitary-adrenal axis reactivity. Biol Psychiatry. 2009;66(7):681–5. https://doi.org/10.1016/j.biopsych.2009.05.012.
196. Bremner JD, Vythilingam M, Vermetten E, Adil J, Khan S, Nazeer A, Afzal N, McGlashan T, Elzinga B, Anderson GM, Heninger G, Southwick SM, Charney DS. Cortisol response to a

cognitive stress challenge in posttraumatic stress disorder (PTSD) related to childhood abuse. Psychoneuroendocrinology. 2003;28(6):733–50. PubMed PMID: 12812861.
197. Elzinga BM, Schmahl CG, Vermetten E, van Dyck R, Bremner JD. Higher cortisol levels following exposure to traumatic reminders in abuse-related PTSD. Neuropsychopharmacology. 2003;28(9):1656–65.
198. Baker DG, Ekhator NN, Kasckow JW, Dashevsky B, Horn PS, Bednarik L, Geracioti TD Jr. Higher levels of basal serial CSF cortisol in combat veterans with posttraumatic stress disorder. Am J Psychiatry. 2005;162(5):992–4. PubMed PMID: 15863803.
199. Rasmusson AM, Lipschitz DS, Wang S, Hu S, Vojvoda D, Bremner JD, Southwick SM, Charney DS. Increased pituitary and adrenal reactivity in premenopausal women with posttraumatic stress disorder. Biol Psychiatry. 2001;50(12):965–77. Erratum in: Biol Psychiatry 2002;52(7):771. PubMed PMID: 11750893.
200. Kellner M, Yassouridis A, Hübner R, Baker DG, Wiedemann K. Endocrine and cardiovascular responses to corticotropin-releasing hormone in patients with posttraumatic stress disorder: a role for atrial natriuretic peptide? Neuropsychobiology. 2003;47(2):102–8. PubMed PMID: 12707494.
201. Yehuda R, Kahana B, Binder-Brynes K, Southwick SM, Mason JW, Giller EL. Low urinary cortisol excretion in Holocaust survivors with posttraumatic stress disorder. Am J Psychiatry. 1995;152(7):982–6. PubMed PMID: 7793468.
202. Maes M, Lin A, Bonaccorso S, van Hunsel F, Van Gastel A, Delmeire L, Biondi M, Bosmans E, Kenis G, Scharpé S. Increased 24-hour urinary cortisol excretion in patients with posttraumatic stress disorder and patients with major depression, but not in patients with fibromyalgia. Acta Psychiatr Scand. 1998;98(4):328–35. PubMed PMID: 9821456.
203. Pitman RK, Orr SP. Twenty-four hour urinary cortisol and catecholamine excretion in combat-related posttraumatic stress disorder. Biol Psychiatry. 1990;27(2):245–7. PubMed PMID: 2294983.
204. Young EA, Breslau N. Cortisol and catecholamines in posttraumatic stress disorder: an epidemiologic community study. Arch Gen Psychiatry. 2004;61(4):394–401. PubMed PMID: 15066898.
205. Luecken LJ, Dausch B, Gulla V, Hong R, Compas BE. Alterations in morning cortisol associated with PTSD in women with breast cancer. J Psychosom Res. 2004;56(1):13–5. PubMed PMID: 14987959.
206. Wessa M, Rohleder N, Kirschbaum C, Flor H. Altered cortisol awakening response in posttraumatic stress disorder. Psychoneuroendocrinology. 2006;31(2):209–15. PubMed PMID: 16154709.
207. Neylan TC, Brunet A, Pole N, Best SR, Metzler TJ, Yehuda R, Marmar CR. PTSD symptoms predict waking salivary cortisol levels in police officers. Psychoneuroendocrinology. 2005;30(4):373–81. PubMed PMID: 15694117.
208. Heinrichs M, Wagner D, Schoch W, Soravia LM, Hellhammer DH, Ehlert U. Predicting posttraumatic stress symptoms from pretraumatic risk factors: a 2-year prospective follow-up study in firefighters. Am J Psychiatry. 2005;162(12):2276–86. PubMed PMID: 16330591.
209. Goenjian AK, Yehuda R, Pynoos RS, Steinberg AM, Tashjian M, Yang RK, Najarian LM, Fairbanks LA. Basal cortisol, dexamethasone suppression of cortisol, and MHPG in adolescents after the 1988 earthquake in Armenia. Am J Psychiatry. 1996;153(7):929–34. PubMed PMID: 8659616.
210. Yehuda R, Southwick SM, Krystal JH, Bremner D, Charney DS, Mason JW. Enhanced suppression of cortisol following dexamethasone administration in posttraumatic stress disorder. Am J Psychiatry. 1993;150(1):83–6. PubMed PMID: 8417586.
211. Newport DJ, Heim C, Bonsall R, Miller AH, Nemeroff CB. Pituitary-adrenal responses to standard and low-dose dexamethasone suppression tests in adult survivors of child abuse. Biol Psychiatry. 2004;55(1):10–20. PubMed PMID: 14706420.
212. Yehuda R, Golier JA, Halligan SL, Meaney M, Bierer LM. The ACTH response to dexamethasone in PTSD. Am J Psychiatry. 2004;161(8):1397–403. PubMed PMID: 15285965.

213. Bersani FS, Wolkowitz OM, Lindqvist D, Yehuda R, Flory J, Bierer LM, Makotine I, Abu-Amara D, Coy M, Reus VI, Epel ES, Marmar C, Mellon SH. Global arginine bioavailability, a marker of nitric oxide synthetic capacity, is decreased in PTSD and correlated with symptom severity and markers of inflammation. Brain Behav Immun. 2016;52:153–60. https://doi.org/10.1016/j.bbi.2015.10.015. PubMed PMID: 26515034.
214. Bruenig D, Mehta D, Morris CP, Harvey W, Lawford B, Young RM, Voisey J. Genetic and serum biomarker evidence for a relationship between TNFα and PTSD in Vietnam war combat veterans. Compr Psychiatry. 2017;74:125–33. https://doi.org/10.1016/j.comppsych.2017.01.015. PubMed PMID: 28160694.
215. Devoto C, Arcurio L, Fetta J, Ley M, Rodney T, Kanefsky R, Gill J. Inflammation relates to chronic behavioral and neurological symptoms in military personnel with traumatic brain injuries. Cell Transplant. 2017;26(7):1169–77. https://doi.org/10.1177/0963689717714098. PubMed PMID: 28933225; PubMed Central PMCID: PMC5657728.
216. Vidović A, Vilibić M, Sabioncello A, Gotovac K, Rabatić S, Folnegović-Šmalc V, Dekaris D. Changes in immune and endocrine systems in posttraumatic stress disorder - prospective study. Acta Neuropsychiatr. 2009;21(Suppl 2):46–50. https://doi.org/10.1017/S0924270800032725. PubMed PMID: 25384870.
217. Lindqvist D, Dhabhar FS, Mellon SH, Yehuda R, Grenon SM, Flory JD, Bierer LM, Abu-Amara D, Coy M, Makotkine I, Reus VI, Bersani FS, Marmar CR, Wolkowitz OM. Increased pro-inflammatory milieu in combat related PTSD - A new cohort replication study. Brain Behav Immun. 2017;59:260–4. https://doi.org/10.1016/j.bbi.2016.09.012. PubMed PMID: 27638184.
218. Himmerich H, Wolf JE, Zimmermann P, Bühler AH, Holdt LM, Teupser D, Kirkby KC, Willmund GD, Wesemann U. Serum concentrations of tumor necrosis factor-α and its soluble receptors in soldiers with and without combat-related posttraumatic stress disorder: influence of Age and Body Mass Index. Chin Med J (Engl). 2016;129(6):751–2. https://doi.org/10.4103/0366-6999.178039. PubMed PMID: 26960383; PubMed Central PMCID: PMC4804426.
219. Jergović M, Bendelja K, Savić Mlakar A, Vojvoda V, Aberle N, Jovanovic T, Rabatić S, Sabioncello A, Vidović A. Circulating levels of hormones, lipids, and immune mediators in post-traumatic stress disorder - a 3-month follow-up study. Front Psychiatry. 2015;6:49. https://doi.org/10.3389/fpsyt.2015.00049. eCollection 2015. PubMed PMID: 25926799; PubMed Central PMCID: PMC4396135.
220. Wang X, Xie H, Cotton AS, Duval ER, Tamburrino MB, Brickman KR, Elhai JD, Ho SS, McLean SA, Ferguson EJ, Liberzon I. Preliminary study of acute changes in emotion processing in trauma survivors with PTSD symptoms. PLoS One. 2016;11(7):e0159065. https://doi.org/10.1371/journal.pone.0159065. eCollection 2016. PubMed PMID: 27415431; PubMed Central PMCID: PMC4944986.
221. Zhou X, Wu X, An Y, Fu F. Longitudinal relationships between posttraumatic stress symptoms and sleep problems in adolescent survivors following the Wenchuan earthquake in China. PLoS One. 2014;9(8):e104470. https://doi.org/10.1371/journal.pone.0104470. eCollection 2014. PubMed PMID: 25105288; PubMed Central PMCID: PMC4126730.
222. Hoge EA, Brandstetter K, Moshier S, Pollack MH, Wong KK, Simon NM. Broad spectrum of cytokine abnormalities in panic disorder and posttraumatic stress disorder. Depress Anxiety. 2009;26(5):447–55. https://doi.org/10.1002/da.20564. PubMed PMID: 19319993.
223. Oganesyan LP, Mkrtchyan GM, Sukiasyan SH, Boyajyan AS. Classic and alternative complement cascades in post-traumatic stress disorder. Bull Exp Biol Med. 2009;148(6):859–61. PubMed PMID: 21116491.
224. Gola H, Engler H, Sommershof A, Adenauer H, Kolassa S, Schedlowski M, Groettrup M, Elbert T, Kolassa IT. Posttraumatic stress disorder is associated with an enhanced spontaneous production of pro-inflammatory cytokines by peripheral blood mononuclear cells. BMC Psychiatry. 2013;13:40. https://doi.org/10.1186/1471-244X-13-40. PubMed PMID: 23360282; PubMed Central PMCID: PMC3574862.

225. Hammad SM, Truman JP, Al Gadban MM, Smith KJ, Twal WO, Hamner MB. Altered blood sphingolipidomics and elevated plasma inflammatory cytokines in combat veterans with post-traumatic stress disordER. Neurobiol Lipids. 2012;10:2. PubMed PMID: 24403911; PubMed Central PMCID: PMC3882130.
226. Passos IC, Vasconcelos-Moreno MP, Costa LG, Kunz M, Brietzke E, Quevedo J, Salum G, Magalhães PV, Kapczinski F, Kauer-Sant'Anna M. Inflammatory markers in post-traumatic stress disorder: a systematic review, meta-analysis, and meta-regression. Lancet Psychiatry. 2015;2(11):1002–12. https://doi.org/10.1016/S2215-0366(15)00309-0. Review. PubMed PMID: 26544749.
227. Tursich M, Neufeld RW, Frewen PA, Harricharan S, Kibler JL, Rhind SG, Lanius RA. Association of trauma exposure with proinflammatory activity: a transdiagnostic meta-analysis. Transl Psychiatry. 2014;4:e413. https://doi.org/10.1038/tp.2014.56.
228. de Kloet CS, Vermetten E, Bikker A, Meulman E, Geuze E, Kavelaars A, et al. Leukocyte glucocorticoid receptor expression and immunoregulation in veterans with and without post-traumatic stress disorder. Mol Psychiatry. 2007;12(5):443–53.
229. de Kloet CS, Vermetten E, Heijnen CJ, Geuze E, Lentjes EG, Westenberg HG. Enhanced cortisol suppression in response to dexamethasone administration in traumatized veterans with and without posttraumatic stress disorder. Psychoneuroendocrinology. 2007;32(3):215–26.
230. Rohleder N, Joksimovic L, Wolf JM, Kirschbaum C. Hypocortisolism and increased glucocorticoid sensitivity of pro-Inflammatory cytokine production in Bosnian war refugees with posttraumatic stress disorder. Biol Psychiatry. 2004;55(7):745–51. PubMed PMID: 15039004.
231. Zieker J, Zieker D, Jatzko A, Dietzsch J, Nieselt K, Schmitt A, Bertsch T, Fassbender K, Spanagel R, Northoff H, Gebicke-Haerter PJ. Differential gene expression in peripheral blood of patients suffering from post-traumatic stress disorder. Mol Psychiatry. 2007;12(2):116–8. PubMed PMID: 17252001.
232. Yehuda R, Bierer LM, Sarapas C, Makotkine I, Andrew R, Seckl JR. Cortisol metabolic predictors of response to psychotherapy for symptoms of PTSD in survivors of the World Trade Center attacks on September 11, 2001. Psychoneuroendocrinology. 2009;34(9):1304–13. https://doi.org/10.1016/j.psyneuen.2009.03.018. PubMed PMID: 19411143; PubMed Central PMCID: PMC2785023.
233. Sarapas C, Cai G, Bierer LM, Golier JA, Galea S, Ising M, Rein T, Schmeidler J, Müller-Myhsok B, Uhr M, Holsboer F, Buxbaum JD, Yehuda R. Genetic markers for PTSD risk and resilience among survivors of the World Trade Center attacks. Dis Markers. 2011;30(2–3):101–10. https://doi.org/10.3233/DMA-2011-0764. PubMed PMID: 21508514. PubMed Central PMCID: PMC3825240.
234. Mehta D, Gonik M, Klengel T, et al. Using polymorphisms in FKBP5 to define biologically distinct subtypes of posttraumatic stress disorder: evidence from endocrine and gene expression studies. Arch Gen Psychiatry. 2011;68(9):901–10.
235. Breen MS, Maihofer AX, Glatt SJ, Tylee DS, Chandler SD, Tsuang MT, Risbrough VB, Baker DG, O'Connor DT, Nievergelt CM, Woelk CH. Gene networks specific for innate immunity define post-traumatic stress disorder. Mol Psychiatry. 2015;20(12):1538–45. https://doi.org/10.1038/mp.2015.9. PubMed PMID: 25754082; PubMed Central PMCID: PMC4565790.

Implementing Psychiatric Rehabilitation in the Mental Health System Services: From Theory to Practice

11

Afzal Javed and Paola Carozza

Abstract

Psychiatric rehabilitation services incorporate principles of recovery and wellness, community support, person-centred care and active involvement of individuals and families in the behavioural health system and services. Based on the definition from the Psychiatric Rehabilitation Association (PRA, formerly USPRA), psychiatric rehabilitation:

> …promotes recovery, full community integration and improved quality of life for persons who have been diagnosed with any mental health condition that seriously impairs their ability to lead meaningful lives. Psychiatric rehabilitation services are collaborative, person-directed and individualized. These services are an essential element of the health care and human services spectrum, and should be evidence-based. They focus on helping individuals develop skills and access resources needed to increase their capacity to be successful and satisfied in the living, working, learning, and social environments of their choice.

Because psychiatric rehabilitation is intended to be a person-directed and recovery-oriented service, the overall intent of this chapter is to establish broad parameters within which a variety of successful approaches can flourish, with particular reference about how the Italian field of mental health is dealing with the need of implementing rehabilitative practices in mental health services.

A. Javed
Warwick Medical School, University of Warwick, Warwick, UK

P. Carozza (✉)
Mental Health Department and Addiction Services of Ferrara, Ferrara, Italy

Evidence–Based and Recovery-Oriented Psychosocial Treatments, University of Ferrara, Ferrara, Italy
e-mail: paola.carozza@uni.net

L. Grassi et al. (eds.), *Person Centered Approach to Recovery in Medicine*, Integrating Psychiatry and Primary Care, https://doi.org/10.1007/978-3-319-74736-1_11

People with complex and enduring mental health problems are at the heart of current priorities in service developments in health and social care services [1, 2]. Rehabilitation psychiatry has also assumed an importance in mental health services and has emerged as an important subspecialty of mental health that offers a positive response to the needs of long-term mental health problems. These services are generating a promising interest to revive hope and open routes to personal achievements while acknowledging and accounting for our patients' chronic and continuing disability and impairments in personal and psychosocial functioning [3].

Psychiatric rehabilitation is generally defined as the process that aim reducing the impact of disabling and handicapping conditions related to the psychiatric conditions [4]. The concept of rehabilitation generally focuses on enabling the disabled people to achieve social integration and adapt or acquire the skills and competencies that may be helpful for their day-to-day activities. The practice of rehabilitation is not any new addition to treatment services as even during the time of institutionalization; efforts were made to provide some basic skills for day-to-day functioning to the inmates of the long-stay hospitals. The nineteenth and twentieth century's reforms including moral treatment, advances in social and community psychiatry and up rise of human right movements provided further evidence in the outcome of major mental illnesses to approaches that advocated dignity and respect for the patients. The emergence of "recovery" movement furthermore strengthened these concepts and emphasized the critical importance of such collaboration in the therapy and clinical practices.

The term "recovery" within the context of mental health services seems to be very popular as there have been a number of developments all around the world that have brought pioneering and innovative recovery-related changes in the psychiatric services in many areas of health and social care [5, 6]. It is argued that any ideal rehabilitation service should now provide a continuous, comprehensive and collaborative approach that should be patient orientated and aimed at promoting a culture of healing and hope. The key principles thus encourage interventions to be linked to individual needs and to the personal goals of patients embracing the outcomes of meaningful achievements. The significance of social impacts and consequences of psychiatric illnesses like loss of employment, loss of status, loss of support, loss of friends and loss of self-respect all result in a series of sufferings. The current dimensions of care thus make rehabilitation more and more important, and as documented by the UK Department of Health in the National Service Framework (NSF) document, rehabilitation principles and practice come up as a clear lead for people with chronic mental health problems [7].

11.1 Psychiatric Rehabilitation: International Perspectives

The current evidence fully supports the notion that psychiatric rehabilitation offers a positive hope to the current scenario of psychiatric care and meets the needs of people with long-term, complex and impairing mental health problems. In response to this, mental health services are getting redesigned and refined in almost all settings of health and social care. It is true that mental health rehabilitation services are still limited and enjoy less priority in many countries including both developing and developed world, and these gaps are not limited to any one country or one culture. On a positive side, it is however reassuring that the extent and severity of these issues are in fact being acknowledged all around the globe, and despite the limited resources, the treatment of mentally ill is now assuming a paramount importance in almost all countries with introduction of current philosophy and visions of overcoming the impacts of institutionalization and provision of services in the new format of community care, social inclusion and embracing the concepts of recovery [8].

There is however a general lack of mutual collaboration and consensus for joint working in different countries and cultures. In practice, every rehabilitation service is different and may have its limitations depending on its scope and application. Historically many different models of psychosocial rehabilitation were practised using sheltered workshops, transient employment schemes, workplace incentives and occupational placements. The clubhouse model also came up as an important addition to these endeavours and highlighted the importance of different dimensions of rehabilitation for the mentally ill [9]. This model was started in the USA in the 1950s for setting support to its members in areas of community settlement and supporting for their preparation for future employment. The residents of clubhouse were called members, and they were expected to participate in all aspects of running of the clubhouse like its management, sharing responsibilities with staff, preparing meals, working in the office and doing other related work. Following a period of pre-vocational training, employment placements were arranged in a variety of jobs with mainstream employment [10]. This concept enjoyed a worldwide recognition, and many such facilities are now working in Europe, Asia and other parts of the world. In Europe, many of the clubhouses are involved with small business ventures and are run by and/or employ significant number of disabled persons. A similar facility that runs in Pakistan with the name of Fountain House has shown its noticeable effectiveness for psychiatric rehabilitation services in a developing country where resources are scanty and infrastructure for psychiatric services are very limited [11].

11.2 Challenges, Needs and Opportunities

Looking at the current developments in the field of general health care, one can generally be positive and optimistic with the care and management of patients, but mental health have been the forgotten need in many local health-care services. There has been a number of shortfalls in the system, and it is true that despite high prevalence and extent and severity of mental health problems, due recognition has not been given to the needs of the mentally ill. Although current epidemiological data continues backing the WHO and World Bank reports that strongly supports the findings that mental disorders are causing considerable sufferings and burden to a large population, mental health services unfortunately still shows big gaps.

Rehabilitation psychiatry, in particular, has faced a number of uncertainties and dilemmas as well. This is a forgotten speciality in many aspects, but it is reassuring that a number of current innovations are taking place in this area of care. Starting from the philosophy of moral treatment to the emerging concepts of recovery, rehabilitation psychiatry is coming up with a range of models for dealing with impairments and disabilities.

One of the key issues for contemporary health and social services is the promotion of social inclusion for our patients. Based on the principles of inclusion, there has been a way forward for promoting recovery and continuing care for chronic and enduring mental illnesses [12]. The centrality of users and carers' experiences is strengthening the new foundations of our current practices in different fields of psychiatric rehabilitation. The potential users of rehabilitation services are now chosen not only from different diagnostic perspective, but the consequent stigma and multiple indices of social exclusion are also important determinants for these services [13].

The other challenges for present-day health and social services are how to put the viewpoint of patients, users or consumers and families within the perspectives of their care. This obviously needs a change that would require a keen understanding of all stakeholders' role in mental health services. Some service users have little understanding with the recovery principles and do not believe they will ever recover. The reasons may be multiple varying from realism to pessimism or even the fear that they will never be able to take control for their lives. The carers have their own limitations that could be related to their unmet expectations and lack of resources to meet their demands. The professionals, who may be highly enthusiastic, do have some worries about the implications of service provisions. They may become sceptical about the resources required for remit of recovery as it could equate to raising false hope that could endanger unrealistic expectations in patients and families. There are also issues about professional's expertise to be aware of patients or users' perspectives, experiences and their training for listening to their patients. The notion of dialogue requires further acceptance for introducing the centrality of user and carer experiences in our therapeutic approaches. It is worth noting that the term "dialogue" that essentially means a listening to and a hearing of the viewpoints of two equal partners is reinforced by the patients and carers' groups [14].

These concepts are thus important for establishing a long-lasting and purposeful engagement with the users and carers. There is no doubt that in the developed countries, involvement of families and carers is becoming an integral component of treatment processes, but in low-income countries where families play an important role in the care of mentally ill, there is still a long way to get this accepted in a more formal way [15]. There is strong evidence that if patients and carers are involved in the treatment processes and if there is a joint decision, it will certainly make the prognosis of mental illnesses more favourable and promising. Looking at the core concept of recovery, this involvement becomes even more meaningful as the distribution of responsibilities in making any treatment plan effective does increase the value of the joint working.

There are also some differences and disagreements about the understanding of the principles of rehabilitation between different professional groups and individual members of the groups [16]. The differences may involve individual or collective processes for rehabilitation including assessment, diagnosis and treatment modalities. For example, some common dilemmas may revolve around whose views are more important for assessment of needs – the professionals, users, carers or the families. What are the meanings of diagnosis and what purpose diagnosis fulfil in therapeutic domains? Similarly is it best to name a disorder and if so how can this be used in alleviating the anxieties and apprehension of our patients and their families? Information sharing, breaking confidentiality and what to choose for selective information are some other challenges that can have ongoing implications. Furthermore treatment choices may differ from patient to patient or clinician to clinician. That also brings the disputed question of when compulsory treatment is justified and what is it justified forcing people to live in a particular setting not of their choice?

Another major challenge lies in training of the professionals in the field of psychiatric rehabilitation [17]. There are very few countries where comprehensive training programmes are offered to the mental health professionals in different areas of PSR [18]. With the changing needs, it is becoming imperative to emphasize the importance of training in the field of rehabilitation. There are some good examples that can be used as a starting point. The Royal College of Psychiatrists in the UK sets out a vision for training the recovery-oriented and user-focused approaches for rehabilitation services and has adapted a policy of getting carers and families involved in training programmes for psychiatrists [19]. This outlines the needs in the area of professional training along with efforts for capacity building and has helped in increasing knowledge, awareness and responsiveness of the trainee psychiatrists at their work place. The College has implemented a requirement for service users and carers to be involved in the higher training programmes for the trainee psychiatrists. This also challenges the paternalistic values of the medical curriculum and supports the notion of working with the patients and service users rather than working "on" them. The *Ten Essential Shared Capabilities* developed by the UK Department of Health, the National Institute for Mental Health in England and the Sainsbury Centre [19] also provide a recommended set of general skills for ensuring high-quality training in the field of rehabilitation and recovery. These include working in partnership, respecting diversity, practising ethically, challenging inequality, promoting recovery, identifying people's needs and strengths, providing service user-centred care, making a difference, promoting safety and positive risk taking and personal development and learning. These recommendations provide a framework that looks at the attitudes as well as a high degree of competence appropriate to the role of professionals engaged with rehabilitation and recovery services.

Despite the current inequalities and shortcomings in our mental health systems, it is worth mentioning some of the notable work done by a number of regional and international organizations. The World Psychiatric Association (WPA), a representative organization of psychiatrists, is very keen to raise the profile of this particular issue by flagging the importance of this aspect of care by developing partnership for better mental health in a global perspective. During the 2008 to 2011 triennium, the WPA appointed a task force on developing partnership for best practices in working with service users and carers. The task force provided a set of recommendations and directions for the member societies of WPA for implementation in their respective countries [20]. The World Association for Psychosocial Rehabilitation (WAPR www.wapr.info), another organization that works in the field of psychiatric rehabilitation, gives a lot of importance to patients, carers and family for their role in the treatment and rehabilitation programmes [21]. WAPR is promoting the concept of rehabilitation, recovery and empowerment of patients over the last many decades in a meaningful way and has got representatives of patients, carers and families on their executive board who take full responsibility in making decisions in formulating the policies of this international organization.

The Royal College of Psychiatrists (UK) has also given a significant importance to the work of patients and carers, and the College regularly approaches local carers and users groups for contributing to the policies of the College [22]. The Royal College of Psychiatrist in collaboration with the Prince's Royal Trust for carers also took a number of initiatives and proposed a triangle of care as an approach that has been developed by carers and the professionals to improve carer's engagement in treatment services. These guidelines outline key elements in achieving the partnership with examples of good practice and are also supported by work from many other organizations [23].

Mental health is indeed experiencing an exciting time. We have moved from asylums to community, and as most of our patients are living in the community, their needs for psychiatric rehabilitation and adjustment in the community require a paramount importance in planning service provision policies. It is strongly felt that rehabilitation psychiatry needs a conceptual change in theory as well as in practice and requires additional strengths of support from various stakeholders. This can be achieved by prioritizing and highlighting the needs for our patients and their carers and families and reviewing training curriculum for mental health professionals in the field of psychosocial rehabilitation. With the changing trends in mental health, it becomes imperative that all other organizations should also take a proactive role in promoting this initiative and help and assist in gaining further successes in the processes of rehabilitation and recovery.

Mental health should adapt policies based on social inclusion and participation of service users, professionals and carers with emphasis on attention to the rights of people with mental ill health, as well as to fairness, equality and justice. It is the need of the time that the future work should focus on examining the resilience of families looking at families' strengths and the protective factors. It is also desired that in-depth understanding of the long-term consequences of care giving and the support and training that are essential to families in various stages of patient's illness also needs to be formalized. There is equally a strong need that professionals should plan for interventions with a thorough assessment of family member's strengths, as well as their limitations. More specifically mental health professionals must have a reliable and valid understanding of what families have and do not have in terms of resources for coping and living with those who are mentally ill.

It is also expected that mental health professionals and policy makers will continue developing empathetic attitude towards the issues of capacity building and will advocate the needs to develop innovative teaching and training programmes for patients, families and carers [24]. While supporting the families and easing their burdens, it could be similarly effective to involve families as active members of the health-care teams by using experiences of users and families for training purposes and their involvement as employees, trainers and researchers for future work in this area [25]. We should also be familiar with the cultural factors that influence our learning and thus having an influence in shaping our attitudes towards service developments.

11.3 The Psychosocial Treatments EB: An Integral Part of the Care and Recovery Processes

The need to integrate psychosocial treatments EB with psychopharmacology in the treatment of mental illness is based on the evidence that etiopathogenesis of mental illness is related to psychological, biological and social factors and that mental illness impacts psychological, biological and social dimensions of human being [26, 27].

In the last decades, other two remarkable scientific acquisitions have given a significative contribution to growth of knowledges in the mental health field: the spread of the concept of recovery for which the improvements of mental health are not only related to the symptoms but also to the ability to take a perspective of life again, to perform valid social roles, to increase the ability to choose and to drive own life, to improve cognition, to cope with stressors and to recognize and manage intense feelings and emotions and the findings of neuroscience (in particular social neuroscience) that have strongly highlighted the influences of social and environmental factor both on human genome and functional behaviours [28].

It is evidence that more than 60% of people with mental illness don't receive all appropriate treatments which would require and that at least 70% of people with schizophrenia have already cognitive impairment concurrent or previous the onset, often resistant to the effects of drugs. Therefore, we believe that is urgent to adopt treatment strategies that are effective on the psychological and social consequences of mental illness, other than on those one biological [29].

The practice of psychiatric rehabilitation includes all psychosocial treatments EB in order to protect from vulnerability to stress-induced relapses. They are

Table 11.1 Main EBPs

• Boston University Choose-Get-Keep (BU CGK) approach
• Clubhouse approach
• Wellness Recovery Action Plan (WRAP)
• Motivational interviewing (MI)
• Illness management and recovery (IMR)
• Supported employment: individual placement and support (IPS)
• Family psychoeducation (FPE)
• Peer support
• Wellness coaching
• Cognitive enhancement therapy (CET)
• Social skills training
• Cognitive behaviour therapy (CBT)
• Integrated treatment for dual diagnosis
• Supported employment
• Assertive community treatment

articulated in programmes for skill development so that the patient can deal with stressors and life situations that require adaptation and more independence and in supported environment programmes (employment, housing and education supported).

Psychiatric rehabilitation services (PRS) are expected to use evidence-based and best practices that are effective in responding to the needs of individuals participating in the programme [30, 31]. Evidence-based and emerging best practices often utilized in PRS programmes are listed below [32, 33]. The provider may employ any or all of the evidence-based/emerging practices to meet an individual's preferences and needs (Table 11.1).

The Italian experience has allowed to conclude that every psychosocial treatments EB must have determined principles that are the core of psychosocial rehabilitation, already cited above.

11.4 Outcomes Measurement

Psychiatric rehabilitation programmes (PRP) have been noted to be of significant value to individuals living with serious mental health conditions. All PRP should design and document a process to gather and analyse outcomes of participation in treatment [34–36].

Outcomes documented in research studies of psychiatric rehabilitation services are listed in Table 11.2 [37].

It is recommended to collect and to share results with the individual from the progress measure every 3 months, to incorporate them into the rehabilitation planning process and to review IPR for 6 months, which may coincide with IRP updates. The progress measure can be used to empower individuals in service in their care and to improve communication between providers and individuals, around domains important to psychiatric rehabilitation service delivery [38, 39].

Table 11.2 Outcomes of psychiatric rehabilitation

1.	Increased community tenure
2.	Increased social connectedness
3.	Reduced psychiatric hospitalization
4.	Reduced involvement with criminal justice
5.	Decreased use of illicit drugs and/or decreased misuse of prescription drugs
6.	Improved member satisfaction with:
	(a) Behavioural health services received
	(b) Quality of life
7.	Increased active participation in treatment and service planning
8.	Improved adherence to agreed-upon services
9.	Active self-notation of progress
10.	Heightened self-esteem (self-report)
11.	Improved vocational functioning
12.	Improved educational status
13.	Improved stability of housing status
14.	Improved self-perception of overall wellness
15.	Improving the level of functioning as much as possible
16.	Encouraging the widest possible participation in main domain of life: work, family, friendship, leisure, housing, physical health, etc
17.	Encouraging the greatest possible participation of the patient in setting personal objectives and in planning own treatment
18.	Encouraging less dependence possible from professional services
19.	Learning skills and functional behaviours
20.	Improving cognitive function
21.	Improving social cognition
22.	Developing motivation to change
23.	Learning coping strategies
24.	Reconnecting emotions and events
25.	Understanding mental illness and changing distorted beliefs
26.	Reducing external and internal stigma
27.	Regaining the ability to choose and lead own life

11.5 To Transfer EB Principles in Practice: A Great Challenge

It's known in the field that introducing a scientific and methodological approach in daily clinical practice is very hard. Implementing EBPs requires a change in the usual organizational models and in the current policies, as well as in the staff training and supervision [40, 41]. Therefore, effective treatments are rarely available for the vast majority of people for whom they were thought, except for the new antipsychotic medication, quickly accepted and prescribed by psychiatrists, thanks to the efforts of the pharmaceutical market.

The purpose of putting into daily practice the principles of some of the most important EBPs implies to modify the cultural and organizational dimensions of most of mental health services systems, focused on symptoms stabilization rather than recovery [42] .

The indicators of this trend are listed in Table 11.3.

In fact, the implementation of psychiatric rehabilitation services requires (Table 11.4):

Table 11.3 Characteristics of a mental health services system not psychiatric rehabilitation and recovery oriented

1.	Many mental health professionals think that serious mental illnesses are almost associated with a poor prognosis
2.	The psychosocial practices have to gain a dignity of techniques, given that they have a marginal role if compared with biological treatments
3.	Increased awareness of the inadequacy of stabilization paradigm (intervention only in acute phase of mental illness, desired outcome: symptoms remission)
4.	The programmes lack of interventions aimed to provide the patients with abilities and support, so that they could get and maintain valid social roles in the community
5.	The personnel working in the mental health services is not always been equipped with effective tools to link own practice to client's goals, purposes and perspectives. Most of the activities are an end to theirselves
6.	Many persons with severe mental disorders are replaced in psychiatric residential facilities, often reproducing a disconnected and isolated way of living, being onerous for the citizenship, disempowering people and increasing internal stigma
7.	The practice is more oriented to efficiency than to efficacy. Lack of monitoring the quality and outcomes of treatments

Table 11.4 Implementing psychiatric rehabilitation services

1.	Coordination between different agencies
2.	Long period of time to acquire the skills to deliver treatments
3.	Skills to face the resistance and inertia of the practitioners to change the way they deliver services
4.	Commitment to teach staff new techniques and learn from this
5.	Clear mandate from the leadership and its commitment to provide resources and support
6.	Familiarizing practitioners with EBPs, fitting the workplace so that EBPs can be easily used by the staff
7.	Continuous on-site staff training and selection of patients to demonstrate the efficacy of new treatments
8.	Development of criteria for setting standards and measures of clinical quality that include the use of new practices
9.	Courage to eliminate inefficient practices often defended by many practitioners, families, politicians and other stakeholders

11.6 The Italian Perspective: Law 180/78—Main Principles

Approved in 1978, the Law 180, generally referred to as the "Basaglia Law", marks the "Italian Revolution" in the field of mental health, developing a radical process of change in services delivery: from guardianship to the beginning of the patient's de-institutionalization. Let us try to summarize the main points of this change. First, the law stated that citizens' mental health had to be promoted by means of three levels of intervention, all deeply interrelated: prevention, treatment and rehabilitation. Second, the law affirmed that the people with psychiatric disabilities had the right to receive effective treatments in the environment where they lived, trying both to reduce hospitalizations and desocialization and to maintain the connections with significative others. Third, the law introduced the concept of social inclusion as result of a range of interventions focused on helping the person with psychiatric disabilities to maintain or achieve valued roles in the community. At least, the law forbade further admissions in the mental hospital and established a wide net of services that should have met the main needs both of people with mental illness and their family members (crisis, enrichment, treatment, rehabilitation, relationships, etc.).

For a better understanding, it is appropriate to describe the current organization of mental health services in Italy, the Mental Health Department, that is the organization that collects the whole array of community-based psychiatric services. In the Italian health reform, the terms "department" means integrated organization of complementary services (operational units), each of them pursuing specific objectives, all concurring for a common goal.[1]

Anyway, a law isn't sufficient to change old practices. In fact, despite the existence of the Italian Law 180/78, there is a lot of evidence that most of services' systems are mainly oriented to "stabilize" the symptoms as unique outcome and to "replace" many clients in the psychiatric residential facilities, often reproducing a marginalized way of living instead of orienting towards recovery processes.

Currently, there is an increased awareness of the inadequacy of the stabilization paradigm (interventions only in acute phase of mental illness, desired outcome: symptoms remission) and of his consequence: many people with mental illness who are stabilized but disabled and isolated. In fact, the Italian mental health services system shows some weaknesses, among which the main are low clients' families involvement in their relatives' treatment plan and lack of support to patients' families; an increased number of clients placed into public and private psychiatric residential facilities with increased costs; a lack of monitoring of the quality, of the effectiveness and of outcomes of treatments; and most importantly, insufficiency of community-based professional competence of practitioners.

During the past years, we learned that the traditional treatments (medication and crisis interventions) have shown theirselves inadequate to meet the different needs of people with psychiatric disabilities and insufficient to increase role functioning in the real world. It follows that it's necessary to pay a greater attention to the tools and the methods with which to counteract the disabling effects of the mental illness on the individuals that suffer from it.

---

[1] • Community mental health centres. Model of care: community assertive treatment, the services are delivered in the environment of life of people with mental illness (outpatient services) with the mission of helping them to obtain and to maintain valid social roles. • Psychiatric ward (inpatient service), where people with emotional and behavioural disorganization are helped to regain acceptable level of psychosocial balance. • Psychiatric rehabilitation unit, compounded by residential facilities and centres of psychiatric rehabilitation, whose function is to develop effective programmes for people with severe mental illness that will strengthen their skills and capacities to live independently and meaningfully in the community as more as possible. • Apartments settled in urban area, to help people discharged from residential facilities to gain tenant role, according "supported housing" care model. • Neuropsychiatry children services, aimed to deliver treatments and cognitive rehabilitation to people with psychomotor deficit, language troubles and intellective disability under 18 years of age. • Community services for drug and alcohol abuse or dependence

11.7 Building a Rehabilitation and Recovery-Oriented Mental Health Department

As mentioned above, considerations prompt to promote a radical services system's change through a change of the paradigm: from biomedical paradigm to biopsychosocial paradigm, focused on a holistic approach. In other words, it means that people with psychiatric disabilities, before being defined as sick, cases or diagnosis are regarded as unique persons, each of them with three closely connected dimensions: biological, psychological and social.

In fact, the biopsychosocial model is powerful in counteracting the risk of fragmentation of interventions and, therefore, of the person.

In this approach, the whole array of services, each for own specific field of action, has the purpose to increase the personal and social functioning and subjective well-being of people with psychiatric disability, in order to be able to perform successfully a valid social role in the environment of choice (job, housing, education, meaningful activities in the community) with the least professional support.

The principles and values inspiring process of change are listed in Table 11.5 and the actions to promote the change in Table 11.6 [43].

Table 11.5 Principles and values

1.	Limiting disability's impact through psychosocial treatment and social supports
2.	Encouraging client's involvement in own treatment
3.	Strengthen successes; don't blame the person for his/her failures
4.	Building close relationship with the person with mental illness, who is allowed to risk, to mistake and to have the same aspirations all human beings have
5.	Focusing on strengths; don't amplify deficits

Table 11.6 Actions to promote change

1.	Increasing practitioners' knowledges, attitudes and skills about psychosocial evidence practices and concept of recovery
2.	Orienting daily practices to scientific evidence
3.	Spreading culture of outcomes' assessment
4.	Increasing the number of people discharged from the psychiatric residential facilities through supported housing and vocational programmes
5.	Helping to change the beliefs of many mental health professionals which think that serious mental illnesses have almost a poor prognosis and that the people with psychiatric disabilities cannot lead a meaningful life without the continuous support of psychiatric services
6.	Helping family members to recognize the outcomes of recovery, even those one minimal
7.	Implementing psychosocial programmes that counteract:
	(a) Desocialization (detachment between the individual and his environment)
	(b) Internal stigma (powerlessness, shame, worthlessness, inability to take over own life)
	(c) Giving up hope, purposes and every effort to change
8.	Training programmes' coordinators in order to learn leadership skills
9.	Strengthening partnership with families and with associations of families
10.	Encouraging the birth of associations of users and their participation in services' quality assessment
11.	Implementing person-centred programmes for specific targets of population

11.8 The Training of the Workforce: The "Core" of the Process of Change

In the process of change of the mental health services system, great importance must be attributed to the personnel training.There was an evident need to increase professional competence of the workers that stems from the lack of adequate tools to cope with psychiatric disability and to make the workers competent to help the disabled people to achieve personal goals and to develop processes of recovery [44].

As mentioned above, to adopt evidence-based practices and to measure the outcomes, it's necessary to supply the personnel with effective tools, through a continuous learning process (intensive training in the workplace and regular supervisions) [45].

The importance of recruiting skilled and motivated practitioners has also often been highlighted. It is well-known how the lack of appropriate knowledges and abilities and negative attitudes of the professionals to assist users in their processes of rehabilitation and recovery influences the consumers' outcomes, reduces personnel effectiveness and gives rise to repeated failures and intense emotional reactions that may put into some negative behaviours like:

- Avoiding relationship with user
- Using diagnostic labels to explain failures
- Considering dysfunctional behaviours an expression of seriousness of mental illness and of progressive deterioration
- Repeating every day the same intervention, even if clearly ineffective
- Taking up role of entertainer, baby-sitter, guardian or substitute of familiars
- Devaluing own professional role

The training should be organized in two levels: training for people working day to day with patients and training to develop new competences for the leadership.

The first level of training, intended to psychiatrists, psychologists, nurses, social workers and occupational therapists, should be aimed to the development of staff professional competence, with particular reference to the following abilities (Table 11.7) [46].

The other level of training, focused on leadership competences, should be the purpose to increase the leadership's abilities (orienting staff to change, motivating

Table 11.7 Staff professional competences

1.	Building a relationship of support and partnership with clients and their families
2.	Using motivational techniques
3.	Adopting care planning oriented to the patients' objectives
4.	Delivering group treatments of social skill training
5.	Supporting patients in the community through practising social roles
6.	Relating with social referees supporting user's social role (employers, teachers, neighbours, etc.)
7.	Listening, understanding, supporting, involving and orienting clients' families, helping them to cope with dysfunctional behaviours of relative

staff, helping them to overcome resistance to change, supporting and supervising staff, checking patients' care planning and assessing outcomes and promoting peer support and supervision) [47, 48].

The fourth action, carrying on a process of de-institutionalization from residential facilities, should increase the number of persons discharged from the public and private psychiatric residential facilities, through developing effective programmes in the public and private residential facilities, helping people with severe mental illness enhance their skills and choice, drawing up a rehabilitation treatment individual plan for each patient living in public and private residential facilities, highlighting personal objective and the desired outcome, using the supported housing and vocational programmes to promote discharge, planning a re-entry in their places of origin of patients placed in extra-provincial residential facilities, improving the quality of the long-term treatment for patients with serious disability and progressive deterioration (so-called patient without hope) and opening the MHDt to the community.

With respect to the last point, the mental health services system is not self-sufficient, but must develop and implement integration strategies with all the stakeholders, with the aim both to reduce the dependence of the service users on the mental health system and to acquire the appropriate resources (jobs, houses, leisure facilities, educational opportunities) that are essential for the social inclusion in the ordinary community environments.

The need of building a partnership between families and professionals has already been highlighted. It stems from the evidence that a high percentage of people with psychiatric disabilities lives in family (more than 60%) and that most of the patients dwelling independently or in the residential facilities has frequent contacts with the parents. Furthermore, the family both strongly influences the outcomes of treatments and plays a crucial role in the recovery of his relative. The experience has demonstrated that the most important attitudes of the mental health community practitioners towards families are to listen, understand, support, involve and orient clients' families, helping them to cope with dysfunctional behaviours of relative, to understand their meanings, to grasp the relative's progresses and to maintain hope also when there are steps backwards and relapses.

Great attention must be devoted to encouraging the birth and growth of associations of users and their participation in services' quality assessment [49].

11.9 Person-Centred Programmes: Overcoming Fragmentation Between the Different Component of MHDt and Between Mental Health Services and Other Health Services and Social Agencies

In the last decades, a number of people with mental illness that need integrated multidimensional interprofessional treatments increased dramatically. So there is even greater need of going beyond services that works each on their own (failure of parallel model as well as sequential model).

In this context, the "core" is person and his/her treatment plan and not services or professionists. Different competences are involved on the basis of the different

Table 11.8 Targets of population are suitable for person-centred programmes

1.	People with dual diagnosis (practitioners "lended" from community mental health centres, psychiatric rehabilitation unit, community services for drug and alcohol abuse or dependence, social services)
2.	People with severe personality disorders (practitioners "lended" by community-based mental health centres, psychiatric rehabilitation unit, community services for drug and alcohol abuse or dependence, social services)
3.	Early intervention for young people with psychiatric disorders and disadaptive behaviours (practitioners "lended" by community-based mental health centres, psychiatric rehabilitation unit, neuropsychiatry children services, community services for drug and alcohol abuse or dependence, social services, family clinic)
4.	People with autistic spectrum disorder
5.	People with mental illness in phase of remission that have basic social needs (housing, employment, subsidies, economic resources to access meaningful social activities) (practitioners "lended" by community-based mental health centres, psychiatric rehabilitation unit, social services)
6.	People with intellectual disability (practitioners "lended" by community-based mental health centres, neuropsychiatry children services, primary care)
7.	Elderly people with physical and mental illness (practitioners "lended" by community-based mental health centres, primary care, social services)

needs of people and not because practitioners belong to a specific unit or service. This model implies to build an interprofessional team (practitioners come from different unit and service) and to plan periodical meetings between all practitioners involved with the aim to review the treatment plan [43].

What targets of population are suitable for person-centred programmes? The categories of patients that can benefit from this approach are listed in Table 11.8.

In order to increase effectiveness of person-centred programmes, it is necessary to define a network manager for each programme, who joins together with the team at least weekly in order to review the treatments' plans and warrants that practitioner share information and all know the objective of interventions delivered by colleagues.

In this programme model, the whole team is trained according to the most recent acquisitions in the field and is responsible of expected outcomes.

11.10 Problems, Barriers and Contradictions from Process of System Change

Some issues could rise from process of system change (Table 11.9) [50].

11.10.1 Resistance to Change Own Practices

Usually, in the psychiatric field, the resistance to change is motivated by the following arguments:

- The scientific results may not always be used to meet the real and complex needs of patients as it is the "clinical wisdom" coming from his own experience.

Table 11.9 Issues related to system change process

1.	Resistance to change own practices
2.	Resistance to adopt a scientific method
3.	Resistance due to prejudices towards mental illness
4.	Obstacles due to the organizational model
5.	Barriers due to resources constraints

- Even if no one is satisfied with the quality of the services we currently have, it is difficult for the system to incorporate new approaches. Practitioners are aware that the change could be just "window dressing", especially when innovation is linked to leader unreliable or transient.
- The EBP cannot address the problems of the real world, being applied to patient samples other than those who usually turn to public services.

11.10.2 Resistance to Adopt a Scientific Method

- Fear that techniques, procedures and outcomes cause a sort of "methodological cast" which resets the human component, creativity and flexibility
- Belief that the possession of techniques delivers the same service for all, denying individual needs and characteristic
- Difficulties in transforming a job for certain aspects idealized, because it is essentially based on human components, to a measurable one
- Tendency to abstraction and generalization paying little attention to the objective data
- Paying little attention to identify and to evaluate the results

11.10.3 Resistance Due to Prejudices Towards Mental Illness

- The belief that people with serious psychiatric disabilities are not able to choose appropriate roles and environments and do not wish to change their situation for the better
- Pessimism about their ability to learn and grow
- The belief that the mental illness destroys the desires, goals, dreams and perspectives

11.10.4 Obstacles Due to Organizational Model

- The same clinician has the responsibility of specific functions (delivering EB treatment) as well as of generic functions (liaison with general practitioners and general hospital, forensic psychiatry, bureaucratic and administrative tasks, night or holiday shifts in psychiatric ward). So, there is a conflict between generalist model and EB practices model

- Most of practitioners struggle to shift from a role very dependent on doctors to a professional role with a high level of responsibility and autonomy.
- Many psychiatrists struggle to support and to orient the staff in the learning process and the implementation of new practices. They don't accept the increased responsibility and autonomy of non-medical personnel.
- Italian managers and practitioners aren't used to work in team, to share knowledges, to peer supervision, to life-long learning and to workplace continuous training
- Sometimes new way to approach the complexity breeds strong resistance to change, especially among those who have been used to intervene on symptoms only and not on the whole person.
- Excessive bureaucracy activities, disconnected from practice and wasteful of time and of energy that should, instead, be used to accelerate the process of change.
- Difficulty to follow all patients who need systematic, continuous and coordinated EB treatment. Therefore, a problem arises: On which target of patients we must invest more resources since they are limited and not subject to increase, at least at present?

11.10.5 Barriers Due to Resources Constraints

At the conference about clinical psychiatric practice in Italy, which was recently held in Florence, the Italian Society of Psychiatry presented the results of a regional-level survey on mental health departments.

The picture that comes out of the analysis of more than 30% of DSMs in 14 regions is alarming. In the last 10 years, reorganization, mergers and resources constraints have led to the reduction of 50% of human resources (doctors, nurses, psychologists, social health-care workers, social workers, educators) dedicated to the care of patients with psychiatric disorders. The ratio between practitioners and population has risen from 0.8 to 0.4 per 1500 inhabitants.

Conclusion

The experience, supplied with data from the literature, indicates that specific factors are critical to introduce the psychosocial EBPs in services system.

First, a leadership seriously committed to promote change. This means developing a new type of leadership, beginning from the thesis that many, if not most, of the basic differences between organizations are due to differences in the quality and effectiveness of the leadership.

Second, building consensus within the organization on the advantage and the opportunity to use EBP. Meeting with staff periodically to discuss the critical issues that emerge as the organization moves towards EBPs is an effective mean in order to increase consensus and motivation.

The usual way of working can be a set of behaviours difficult to change. Staff often returns to the old patterns and you need to remind them of the benefits of providing new practices both for themselves and for the people they serve.

Third, assessing carefully and constantly knowledges, skills, attitudes and level of training of personnel. Fourth, supporting staff to find the time to learn and implement new practices reviewing workloads, preventing the person finds himself in conflict between two equally binding mandates.

Remembering that new practices must be replaced to old did not represent an additional burden.

Fifth, defining on what targets of patients to invest the resources, if the implementation does not involve an increase of resources.

Lastly, paying attention to build consensus among all stakeholder interested in the mental health and sensitive to the need of new practices (regional and local health administrators, city officials, associations of families, social services, etc.).

References

1. World Health Organization. Global Burden of Disease Report, WHO. 2008. http://www.who.int/healthinfo/global_burden_disease/estimates_country/en/index.html.
2. Collins PY, Patel V, Joestl SS, et al. Grand challenges in global mental health. Nature. 2011;475(7354):27–30.
3. Anthony WA, Liberman RP. The practice of psychiatric rehabilitation: historical, conceptual & research base. Schizophr Bull. 1986;12:542–9.
4. Rosler W. Psychiatric rehabilitation today: an overview. World Psychiatry. 2006;5(3):151–7.
5. Davidson L, Lawless MS, Leary F. Concepts of recovery: competing or complementary. Curr Opin Psychiatry. 2006;19(suppl. 6):619–24.
6. Leamy M, Bird V, Le Boutillier C, et al. A conceptual framework for personal recovery in mental health: systematic review and narrative synthesis. Br J Psychiatry. 2011;199:445–52.
7. Department of Health. National Service Framework for mental health: modern standards & service models. London: Department of Health; 1996.
8. Wykes T, Holloway F. Community rehabilitation: past failures and future prospects. Int Rev Psychiatry. 2000;12:197–205.
9. Beard JH, Propst RN, Malamud TJ. The fountain house model of rehabilitation. Psychiatr Rehabil J. 1982;5:47–53.
10. Hänninen E, Javed A, Wahlb H. Community-based rehabilitation and the Clubhouse Model as means to recovery and mental health services reform. Rehabilitación basada en la comunidad y el modelo Clubhouse como medio de recuperación y reforma de los servicios de salud mental. Rev Neuropsiquiatria. 2013;76(1):3–12.
11. Javed MA, Chaudhry MR. Rehabilitation psychiatry-description of a pioneering facility in Pakistan. Int J Rehabil Res. 2000;23(4):331–2.
12. Royal College of Psychiatrists Social Inclusion Scoping Group. Mental Health and Social Inclusion: Making Psychiatry and Mental Health Services Fit for the 21st Century, Position Statement PS01/2009. London: Royal College of Psychiatrists; 2009.
13. Sartorius N. Stigma and mental health. Lancet. 2007;370(9590):810–1.
14. Amering M, Schmolke M. Recovery in mental health: reshaping scientific and clinical responsibilities. Chichester: Wiley-Blackwell; 2009.
15. Simpson EL, House AO. User and carer involvement in mental health services: from rhetoric to science. Br J Psychiatry. 2004;183(2):89–91. https://doi.org/10.1192/bjp.183.2.89.
16. Thornicroft G, Tansella M. Growing recognition of the importance of service user involvement in mental health service planning and evaluation. Epidemiol Psichiatr Soc. 2005;14(1):1–3.
17. Rudnick A, Eastwood D. Psychiatric rehabilitation education for physicians. Psychiatr Rehabil J. 2013;36(2):126–7.

18. Pelletier JF, Tourette-Turgis C. Recovery-oriented medical training: a narrative literature review for the University of Recovery as a new concept of co-learning between patients and (future) healthcare providers. J Commun Med Health Educ. 2016;6:495. https://doi.org/10.4172/2161-0711.1000495.
19. Hope R. The ten essential shred capabilities: a framework for the whole of the mental health workforce. London: Department of Health; 2004. www.dh.gov.uk/assetRoot/04/08/70/04087170pdf.
20. Wallcraft J, Amering M, Freidin J, Javed A, et al. Partnerships for better mental health worldwide: WPA recommendations on best practices in working with service users and family carers. World Psychiatry. 2011;10:229–36.
21. World Association for Psychosocial Rehabilitation website. www.wapr.infor.
22. Royal College of Psychiatrists. Rehabilitation & recovery now: council report CR 121. London: Royal College of Psychiatrists; 2004.
23. Royal College of Psychiatrists. Royal College of Psychiatrists Position statement—Mental Health and Social Inclusion. PS01/2009, June 2009. London: Royal College of Psychiatrists; 2009.
24. Crawford MJ, Rutter D, Manley C, et al. Systematic review of involving patients in the planning and development of health care. BMJ. 2002;325:1263–5.
25. Campbell J. In: Wallcraft J, Amering M, Schrank B, editors. Handbook of service user involvement in mental Health Research. Chichester: Wiley-Blackwell; 2009. p. 113.
26. Lehman AF, Steinwachs DM. Patterns of usual care for schizophrenia: initial results from the Schizophrenia Patient Outcome Research Team (PORT) Client Survey. Schizophrenia Bull. 1998a;24(1):11–20.
27. Kopelowicz A, Liberman RP, Wallace CJ. Psychiatric rehabilitation for schizophrenia. Int J Psychol Psychol Ther. 2003;3(2):283–98.
28. Fassino S, Abbate Daga G, Leombruni P. Manuale di psichiatria biopsicosociale. Torino: Centro Scientifico Editore; 2007.
29. Lehman AF, Steinwachs DM. Translating research into practice: The Schizophrenia Patient Outcome Research Team (PORT) treatment reccomendations. Schizophrenia Bull. 1998b;24(1):1–10.
30. Drake RE, Goldman H, Leff HS, Lehman AF, Dixon L, Mueser K. Implementing evidence-based practices in routine mental health service settings. Psychiatr Serv. 2001;52(2):179–82.
31. Falloon IR, Held T, Roncone R, Coverdale JH, Laidlaw TM. Optimal treatment strategies to enhance recovery from schizophrenia. Aust N Z J Psychiatry. 1998;32(1):43–9.
32. Meuser KT, Torrey WC, Lynde L, Singer P, Drake RE. Implementing evidence-based practices for people with severe mental illness. Behav Modif J. 2008;27(3):387–411.
33. Substance Abuse and Mental Health Services Administration (SAMHSA). Evidence best practices toolkits. Washington, DC: Washington Press; 2008.
34. Gingerich S, Meuser K. Illness management and recovery. Princetown: Substance Abuse and Mental Health Services Administration (SAMHSA), Centre for Mental Health Services (CMHS), and tThe Robert Wood Johnson Foundation; 2006.
35. Ruggeri M, Dall'Agnola RB. Come valutare l'esito nei Dipartimenti di Salute Mentale. Roma: Il Pensiero Scientifico; 2000.
36. World Health Organization (2001), International classification of functioning, disability and health, Geneve.
37. Wing JK, Curtis RH, Beevor AS. HoNOS: Health of the Nation Outcome Scales: report on research and development. London: Royal College of Psychiatrists; 1996.
38. McDonald-Wilson K, Henry A, Wilkniss S, Nicholson J. Assessment in psychiatric rehabilitation for planning interventions and tracking outcomes. Washington, DC: USPRA, Assessment Institute; 2007.
39. Lasalvia A, Ruggeri M, Mazzi MA, Dall'Agnola RB. The perception of needs of care in staff and patients in community-based mental health services. The South-Verona outcome project 3. Acta Psychiatr Scand. 2000;102:366–75.

40. Iowa Practice Improvement Collaborative Project, Iowa Consortium for Substance Abuse Research and Evaluation at the University of Iowa. Evidence-Based Practices: an Implementation Guide for Community-Based Substance Abuse Treatment Agencies; 2003.
41. Fixsen DL, Naoom SF, Blase KA, Friedman RM, Wallace F. Implementation research: a synthesis of the literature. Tampa, FL: University of South Florida, Louis de la Parte Florida Mental Health Institute, The National Implementation Research Network; 2005.
42. Essock SM, Goldman HH, Van Tosh L, Anthony WA, Appell CR, Bond GR, Dixon LB, Dunakin LK, Ganju V, Gorman PG, Ralph RO, Rapp CA, Teague GB, Drake RE. Evidence-based practices: setting the context and responding to concerns. Psychiatr Clin N Am. 2003;26:919–38.
43. Carozza P. Dalla centralità dei servizi alla centralità della persona. L'esperienza di cambiemnto di un Dipartimento di salute mentale. Milano: Franco Angeli Editore; 2014.
44. Nordt C, Rössler W, Lauber C. Attitudes of mental health professionals toward people with schizophrenia and major depression. Schizoprehnia Bullettin. 2006;32(4):709–14.
45. Joint Commission on Accreditation of Healthcare Organizations. Meeting the competency challenge in behavioral health: the resource tool for behavioral health care human resource professionals who must meet the rigorous requirements of JCAHO. Washington, DC: C & R Publications; 2000.
46. Joint Commission on Accreditation of Healthcare Organizations. Hospital accreditation standards. Oakbrooke Terrace: Joint Commission Resource; 2002.
47. Coursey RD, Curtis L, Marsh DT, Campbell J, Harding C, Spaniol L, et al. Competencies for direct service staff members who work with adults with severe mental illnesses in outpatient public mental health/managed care systems. Psychiatr Rehabil J. 2000a;23(4):378–92.
48. Hoge MA, Tondora J, Marrelli AF. The fundamentals of workforce competency: implications for behavioral health. Admin Pol Ment Health. 2005;32:509–31.
49. Marrelli AF, Tondora J, Hoge MA. Strategies for developing competency models. Admin Pol Ment Health. 2005;32:540–61.
50. Carozza P. La psichiatria di comunità tra scienza e soggettività. Linee di pratica Clinica nei Servizi di Salute Mentale. Milano: Franco Angeli Editore; 2010.

Rehabilitation-Oriented Treatment and Care in Psychosomatic Medicine Under a Lifespan Perspective

12

Michael Linden

Abstract

Many illnesses and especially mental disorders take a long-term course. In these cases, the diagnosis and treatment must adopt a long-term or lifespan perspective. Lifespan research examines the development of individuals from conception to death, recognizing biological, psychological and social factors alike. There is a need for the classification and assessment of courses, the description of determinants of course and the identification of critical developmental phases. In respect to treatment, questions are when to intervene, how, how long and how to evaluate treatment outcome. As treatment of chronic disorders is multidimensional and applied by different therapists and helpers parallel or successively, treatment coordination and case management over time are of great importance, which gives primary care physicians a special role. Finally, patients with chronic disorders are often disabled because of capacity limitations. Treatment must therefore not only focus on symptoms/functions but even more on capacity limitations and impairment of participation. Additionally there is a need for forensic evaluation in providing social support or early retirement. The care for patients with chronic disorders can be described as medical rehabilitation, which is a medical specialty of its own right. As there is a lack of related research, most medical guidelines, which mostly focus on episode treatment, are not valid in medical rehabilitation, which is why experimental and rule-based knowledge is of prime importance.

For publication in: Grassi L, Riba L, Wise T. Psychosomatic medicine: a guide for integrating recovery-oriented care and treatment. New York: Springer.

M. Linden
Research Group Psychosomatic Rehabilitation, Charité University Medicine Berlin, Berlin, Germany
e-mail: michael.linden@charite.de

L. Grassi et al. (eds.), *Person Centered Approach to Recovery in Medicine*, Integrating Psychiatry and Primary Care, https://doi.org/10.1007/978-3-319-74736-1_12

12.1 Chronicity in Mental and Psychosomatic Disorders

A greater part of mental disorders takes a chronic course. This is by definition the case for dementia, schizophrenia, substance abuse, generalized anxiety disorder or personality disorders but also true in a relevant proportion for anxiety disorders, somatoform disorders or depression. Chronic diseases in general and chronic mental and psychosomatic disorders in particular represent a substantial part of burden of disease in modern societies [1]. They regularly impair coping with demands of daily life and cause restrictions in participation. They must therefore be considered as "disabilities" [2]. Even mild symptoms, like in dysthymia or social phobia, can lead to significant negative consequences in the long run [3]. A bio-psycho-social perspective is needed, as given in the International Classification of Functioning, Disability and Health (ICF) of the World Health Organization [4]. Therefore, it is not sufficient to deal with such disorders cross-sectionally. A long-term, course or rather lifespan perspective is needed in diagnosis and treatment.

12.2 Lifespan Perspective

Lifespan research is a transdisciplinary scientific approach, dealing with the development of organisms from conception to death, their maturing, ageing and the factors which influence this process [5–7]. This includes changes in personality, social roles or need for social support across life. Of interest are genetic factors, early adversities during pregnancy, biological ageing processes and the living and social environment [8–10]. The lifespan perspective is well acknowledged in medicine, as many of the widespread diseases are long-term illnesses [11–14]. In this perspective, the present status of an illness is of less interest than the earlier course and the developmental options in the future. This needs concepts for the classification of illness courses and developmental stages, knowledge on factors which can modify illness courses and long-term treatment concept under a bio-psycho-social perspective.

12.3 Classification of Illness Courses and Developmental Stages

Chronic diseases can take very different courses which have different clinical meanings and consequences. Therefore a classification of courses is needed. An overview is given in Table 12.1. First, there are asymptomatic premorbid states or risk constellations like obesity, or lack of physical fitness, or an anxious personality. Secondly, there are asymptomatic states, which nevertheless are seen as an illness like osteoporosis, increased blood sugar or compensated generalized anxiety disorder.

Next there are recurrent diseases with full or partial remission between illness phases like depression or migraine. The frequency of episodes can be high or low

Table 12.1 Course of diseases over the lifespan

Course	Form
Asymptomatic	• Risk factor, but no illness • Risk factor and illness
Episodic-recurrent	• High or low frequency • Accelerating, stable or decelerating frequency • Changing or identical symptomatology
Persistent	• Stable • Fluctuating • Exacerbating • Deteriorating • Improving
Progressive	• Linear development • Comorbid development

and can be stable across time, decreasing or increasing. Also, the symptomatology can be the same or differ from episode to episode.

Furthermore, there are disorders with symptom persistence. Symptomatology can be stable over a long time, but it also can be fluctuating in intensity, exacerbating, improving or deteriorating. There are progressive courses where one disease merges into another, like an anxious personality leading to phobia. There can also be the development of comorbidity, like an anxious personality resulting on alcohol dependency.

In summary, it is not enough to describe the present syndrome and apply diagnostic algorithms according to ICD [15]. The previous and future courses are at least as important. A problem is that there is a lack of concepts on the systematization, classification, and assessment of course [16].

12.4 Determinants and Critical Phases of Illness Course

Knowledge on determinants of the illness course is needed to guide treatment. There are single factors, which can lead to a disorder, like an accident resulting in PTSD. In most cases, there is a "risk accumulation", which means that several risk factors are present and interact, like genetic disposition, environmental influences, health-damaging behaviour, negative effects of treatment, subjective coping with illness or social resources [17, 18]. Risk constellations can vary considerably from person to person even with the same disorder.

Knowledge about risk factors often is coming from epidemiological studies, providing correlational data, but not necessarily information on causal relationships and treatment options. Depression may be correlated with cardiological illnesses but is not a causal factor, and antidepressant treatment is not changing their course [19].

Furthermore, risk factors can have very different effects depending on the point of time. There are "critical periods" across the lifespan, in which risk factors may be especially detrimental. This starts with "early adversities" during pregnancy, which can lead to metabolic disorders or stress-related disorders in later life, or physical and emotional maltreatment in early childhood, which can result in lifelong problems. Critical developmental or vulnerability phases can be biologically or socially determined, like osteoporosis and hip fracture in old age or parenthood in adolescents [8–10, 20].

There are also critical phases in the course of illness, which can make treatment necessary [21, 22]. These include changes in the course of the disease, like the transition of regular alcohol consumption to alcohol abuse or even dependency. Biographical critical events such as divorce may be relevant in the course of a depressive illness or diabetes, be it because of the associated stress or changes in the living condition. Sickness absence from work is also a critical event in the course of an illness as it indicates problems either in the illness status or the environment and as it can develop into long-term incapacity to work.

12.5 Medical Rehabilitation Treatment

As stated before, long-term treatment requires a holistic approach to patients, which is another expression of the well-known bio-psycho-social model in medicine and especially psychosomatic medicine [23, 24]. It can also be called "medical rehabilitation", which has been defined as the medical specialty for the treatment of chronic illness and disability [25]. While acute medicine is focusing on the treatment of illness episodes, rehabilitation medicine is dealing with the course of illness across years. It has the task "to prevent, treat, improve, stabilize, and compensate chronic diseases and associated limitations in capacity and participation", as is stated, for example, in the German social security statute book (§ 26 SGB IX). To achieve this target, all possible interventions are used like medication, psychotherapy, capacity training, patient education, counselling of relatives, referral to specialists, inpatient treatment, or occupational training and procurement of domestic help or early retirement. Medical rehabilitation is more complex and demanding than acute medical care. As a substantial part of diseases takes a chronic course, medical rehabilitation is not a marginal but central part in health care [26]. It is a special type of medical service of all physicians who provide long-term care, like general practitioners or specialists working in outpatient facilities. Furthermore, it is a task for specialized rehabilitation hospital and institutions [25]. Finally also self-help groups, counselling centres or sheltered living and working facilities are of importance [16, 27].

Treatment management in medical rehabilitation is characterized by some peculiarities like when to intervene, how to intervene, how to assess treatment effects, how long to intervene and how to coordinate different therapists over time and at a given point in time.

When to intervene: In acute episodes, treatment starts when there is an acute deterioration in health, like a depressive episode. In long-term illness like dysthymia, there is no such starting point. In most treatment guidelines, precise prescriptions are given on what to do in episode treatment but almost no recommendations on when to do what in long-term illness.

Indications to start treatment could be changes in the illness status but also long times without any positive development. It could be the occurrence of risk factors. Changes in the environment can pose new demands on the patient and therefore require therapeutic help.

How to intervene: When the indication is given, the question remains how to intervene. First of all, treatment for episodes is often not helpful or even contraindicated in chronic disorders. An opioid medication may be justified to alleviate acute back pain, but it is contraindicated after a quarter of a year in chronic back pain. Similarly, psychotherapy for acute adjustment disorder is different from adjustment problems over years. Furthermore, treatment for chronic disorders must be multidimensional, i.e. focusing on the disorder and treatment process but also on illness behaviour or on capacity limitations and restrictions in participation. Often many options are conceivable, but not everything can be made at the same time, which requires a decision on what is most effective but also what is feasible at this particular moment in the illness development. Finally, the patient has an important word to say. While in acute medicine the physician is the primary player, in chronic illness, preferences of the patient play a crucial role, and because of this, shared decision-making, in spite of known difficulties, is indispensable [28].

A general problem in the treatment of long-term illness is the lack of scientific evidence. Most studies on treatment effects come from short-term trials. Similar studies on long-term treatment are more complicated and costly and in most cases not available. Any treatment decision is therefore largely based on medical experience rather than scientific evidence [29].

How long to intervene: In acute illness episodes, there is most of the time a defined end to treatment, mostly with remission of symptoms, or after a defined period of ensuing treatment to prevent early recurrence. In chronic illness, the decision to stop or prolong treatment is more complex. If there are persistent symptoms in spite of ongoing treatment, as it often is the case, one could either argue that a prolongation of treatment is needed as the patient is still ill or that it should be ended, as it does not reach its goal. Similarly, if there is symptomatic remission, one could think that treatment is no longer needed but also that treatment worked and therefore should be continued. A linkage between treatment and illness developments is often impossible, as these can be spontaneous changes of time or results of other intervening variables. Again preferences of patients play a major role. Some want to play it safe and prefer long-term over intermittent treatment, while others want to get rid of any therapy as soon as possible.

Coordination of multidimensional treatment: As already discussed, rehabilitation medicine is interdisciplinary and multidimensional. There are comorbidities which require interventions by different experts. Help is needed with social problems, be it at work or at home. Patients also tend to have their own ways and contact professionals and non-professionals according to their idiosyncratic illness interpretations and hopes. There are preventive, curative and compensatory needs. Patients need help not only by primary care physicians but also specialists of all kind. There are furthermore physicians and non-physician specialists, self-help groups, the internet and family members and friends. They all have different options to help, they are all important, and they should all work in the same direction. Coordination is necessary, as uncoordinated actions can cause harm to the patient. Therefore, an important problem is how to coordinate different players at a given time, but also across time, and who can do this. General practitioners are in this respect of great importance as they take care of patients over years, which make them primary case managers [30].

Evidence-based guidelines: As already stated earlier, there is a lack of scientific studies on many of the aforementioned diagnostic and therapeutic problems. Medical guidelines are in their majority dealing with acute episode treatment. They are based on reviews of controlled studies, which are preferably coming from short-term interventions. As far as long-term courses are mentioned, they give mostly only expert advice. Chronic disorders are characterized by the fact that every case is different, even when the same illness is diagnosed. "Over a long-term effective therapy … little is known" and "from a systematic review of randomized controlled trials … no safe and generalized conclusions" to longer-term therapy effects can be concluded [31]. Many guidelines may therefore not only lack validity in respect to the treatment of chronic disorders but could even result in negative effects, as has been demonstrated in pharmacotherapy [32, 33].

Rational treatment in chronic disorders must therefore refer to procedural and experiential knowledge. This is rather rule than content based. Instead of recommending a certain treatment, the question is, what has been done so far and what has worked and what not [21]? When the question is whether treatment should be prolonged or ended, the question is, what is the preference of the patient? If treatment does not show sufficient results, why not first increase or intensify the ongoing treatment before trying another one? This is in line with modern concepts of personalized and individualized medicine [34, 35].

12.6 Forensic Assessment and Social Support

Most chronic disorders are associated with impairment and restrictions in participation in family life, at work or in leisure activities [36]. Only chronic illnesses can cause long-term inability to work and early retirement. It is therefore an important part of care to assess disability and to give these patients social support as needed. This includes the assessment and, if possible, improvement of limitations of capacities and of context demands. It also must make judgements on the foreseen course and prognosis.

Capacities: These are not the symptoms which decide about disability but the resulting inability to perform activities according to life requirements. Activity has been defined in the ICF [4] as "the execution of a task or action by an individual". Capacity is the ability to execute activities. "Participation" is described as the "involvement in a life situation". It is present when the person can execute all activities that are needed in her or his life situation, with or without given assistance.

There are some established instruments which can be used to quantify capacity limitations. Well-known examples are the ADL und IADL scales (instrumental activities of daily living) which are used in the evaluation of need of basic care, like eating or washing oneself [37, 38]. The GAS, GAF, PSP and SOFAS are instruments which ask for global ratings on the ability to execute complex psychological tasks [39–42]. Published by WHO is the *WHODAS 2.0* (World Health Organization Disability Assessment Schedule II) [43], which covers a broad spectrum of activity limitations and participation restrictions in respect to "comprehension and communication", "mobility", "caring for themselves", "handling other people", "activities in daily life" or "participation in social life". In reference to the ICF, "ICF Core Sets" [44] have been developed, which list activities which are of special relevance for certain disorders.

An instrument which has been specifically designed to asses capacity limitations in reference to specified environments is the Mini-ICF-APP (Mini instrument in reference to the ICF for the assessment of the component Activities and Participation in persons with Psychological Problems) [45, 46]. It describes capacities according to the ICF component activities/participation which are typically impaired by mental problems and specifies the context which is needed for "qualifying" the degree of impairment. It can be used by clinicians and researchers alike. The capacity dimensions include (1) adjustment to rules and routines, (2) planning and structuring of tasks, (3) flexibility, (4) applying knowledge, (5) decision-making, (6) proactivity, (7) endurance, (8) assertiveness, (8) interaction with other persons, (10) integration in groups, (11) building dyadic relations, (12) self-care and (13) mobility. Anchor definitions and interview questions are provided. Seven references for qualifying each dimension are recommended: (a) the present workplace to make a judgement on sickness absence; (b) the profession to evaluate the ability to fulfil job requirements in general; (c) the general labour market (like a job in a hotel corresponding to the individual constitution and education), which allows a judgement whether a person can sustain himself; (d) a restaurant to asses a need for care; (e) a therapeutic setting, like activities in occupational therapy in hospitals; and also (f) the premorbid status of this particular patient to evaluate the course of treatment.

Context: The meaning and qualifying of capacities is dependent on context requirements. If a person runs 100 m in 15.5 s, then this may be very good for a 60-year-old person but very bad for an Olympian. Similarly, the grading of capacities in writing and calculating in school is depending on the class level, or a given degree of social competency will be graded differently if someone is a sales person or a bricklayer. Disability is context dependent. Persons are not disabled as such, but everybody is disabled to different degrees in different contexts. Everybody has capacity limitations if the demands are high enough. Crucial are the capacity-context-interaction and the person-environment fit [47, 48].

Treatment of person environment fit: The capacity-context-interaction model has direct implications for the treatment of chronic illnesses and disability. Symptoms/functions, capacities, and the environment alike provide targets for interventions. Functions/symptoms can be improved by psychotherapy or pharmacotherapy. There are specific trainings to enhance capacities, like assertiveness training or even the direct training of professional skills [49, 50].

Next, changes in the environment can be made to improve participation. If capacity limitations do not allow to execute a certain activity, still the environment can be changed in a way so that the activity is no longer needed, or support can be installed so that demands can again be fulfilled. To focus on the environment when dealing with chronically ill and disabled persons is in compliance with the United Nations' "Convention on the Rights of Persons with Disabilities" [51], which recommends that living conditions are provided in a way so that disabled persons can participate and be included in community life, independent of individual capacity limitations.

Prognosis: Disability is per se a chronic state of affairs. Transitional impairment is of no great relevance. When it comes to treatment decisions or forensic assessments, knowledge or assumptions on the prospective course are of crucial importance. The earlier course can help to predict the future course. The type and present state of illness also can help to make predictions. Of importance is whether appropriate treatments have been applied, as chronicity must be understood as treatment resistance [52]. Only if it has been shown that treatment cannot lead to remission, chronicity can be assumed.

12.7 Conclusion

A lifespan orientation is needed to meet the challenges of chronic disorders. It implies a bio-psycho-social perspective. As many mental disorders take a long-term course, it is plausible that this concept is best recognized in psychosomatic medicine [23–25]. Recovery in chronic disorders cannot mean "restitution ad integrum" but helping to compensate symptoms and impaired functions, to train capacities and provide supportive living conditions. The motto of the day is to help rather than to cure. This rehabilitation perspective opens a broad range of treatment options and can give great relief to patients.

Nevertheless, this approach needs more scientific attention, as there is a lack of empirical data in many respects, like the classification, assessment and treatment of courses, of determinants of course, of selection and steering of treatment and time points of intervention, the coordination of therapists and measures of social support.

References

1. Linden M, Linden U, Schwantes U. Disability and functional burden of disease because of mental in comparison to somatic disorders in general practice patients. Eur Psychiatry. 2015;30:789–92.
2. Linden M. Krankheit und Behinderung. Das ICF-Modell. Nervenarzt. 2015;86:29–35.
3. Grant BF, Hasin DS, Stinson FS, Dawson DA, Ruan WJ, Goldstein RB, Smith SM, Saha TD, Huang B. Prevalence, correlates, co-morbidity, and comparative disability of DSM-IV generalized anxiety disorder in the USA: results from the National Epidemiologic Survey on Alcohol and Related Conditions. Psychol Med. 2005;35:1747–59.
4. World Health Organization (WHO). International Classification of Functioning, Disability and Health: ICF. Geneva: World Health Organization; 2001.

5. Cheng S, Mao L. Physical activity continuum throughout the lifespan: is exercise medicine or what? J Sport Health Sci. 2016;5:127–8.
6. Baltes PB, Reuter-Lorenz P, Rosler F, editors. Life-span development and the brain. Cambridge: Cambridge University Press; 2006.
7. Rudolph CW. Lifespan developmental perspectives on working: a literature review of motivational theories. Work Aging Retirement. 2016;2:130–58.
8. Entringer S, Buss C, Wadhwa PD. Prenatal stress and developmental programming of human health and disease risk: concepts and integration of empirical findings. Curr Opin Endocr Diabetes Obes. 2010;17:507–16.
9. Plagemann A, Harder T, Rodekamp E. Prävention der kindlichen Adipositas während der Schwangerschaft. Monatsschr Kinderheilkd. 2010;158:542–52.
10. Chaney A, Carballedo A, Amico F, et al. Effect of childhood maltreatment on brain structure in adult patients with major depressive disorder and healthy participants. J Psychiat Neurosci. 2014;39:50–9.
11. Hubbard-Turner T, Wikstrom EA, Guderian S, Turner MJ. An acute lateral ankle sprain significantly decreases physical activity across the lifespan. J Sports Sci Med. 2015;14:556–61.
12. Mezuk B, Heh V, Prom-Wormley E, Kendler KS, Pedersen NL. Association between major depression and type 2 diabetes in midlife: findings from the screening across the lifespan twin study. Psychosom Med. 2015;77:559–66.
13. Crowley SJ. Sleep behavior across the lifespan: how a model can expand our current understanding. Sleep Med Rev. 2015;28:1–4.
14. Lynch J, Smith GD. A life course approach to chronic disease epidemiology. Annu Rev Public Health. 2005;26:1–35.
15. World Health Organization (WHO). The ICD-10 Classification of mental and behavioural disorder. Geneva: World Health Organization; 1992.
16. Bernert S, Linden M. Die Klassifikation von Verläufen chronischer Erkrankungen unter einer Lebensspannenperspektive als Grundlage der medizinischen rehabilitation. Präv Rehabil. 2011;23:87–103.
17. Michishita R, Matsuda T, Kawakami S, Kiyonaga A, Tanaka H, Morito N, Higaki Y. The accumulation of healthy lifestyle behaviors prevents the incidence of chronic kidney disease (CKD) in middle-aged and older males. Environ Health Prev Med. 2016;21:129–37.
18. Sheridan S, Pignone M, Mulrow C. Framingham-based tools to calculate the global risk of coronary heart disease. J Gen Intern Med. 2003;18:1039–52.
19. Lichtman JH, Bigger JT, Blumenthal JA, Frasur-Smith N, Kaufmann PG, Lespérance F, Mark DB, Sheps DS, Taylor CB, Froelicher ES. AHA science advisory. Depression and coronary heart disease. Prog Cardiovasc Nurs. 2008;24:19–26.
20. Speerin R, Slater H, Li L, et al. Moving from evidence to practice: models of care for the prevention and management of musculoskeletal conditions. Best Pract Res Clin Rheumatol. 2014;28:479–515.
21. Linden M. Critical incidents und sozialmedizinische Weichenstellungen in der stationären psychosomatischen rehabilitation. Präv Rehabil. 2013;25:62–70.
22. Nicholas MK, Linton SJ, Watson PJ, Main CJ. Early identification and management of psychological risk factors ("yellow flags") in patients with low back pain: a reappraisal. Phys Ther. 2011;91:1–17.
23. Engel GL. The need for a new medical model: a challenge for biomedicine. Science. 1977;196:129–36.
24. Fava GA, Ruini C, Tomba E, Wise TN. The biopsychosocial factor. Psychother Psychosom. 2012;81:1–4.
25. Linden M. Psychosomatic inpatient rehabilitation. The German model. Psychother Psychosom. 2014;83:205–12.
26. Sachverständigenrat zur Begutachtung der Entwicklung im Gesundheitswesen im BMG. Bedarfsgerechte Versorgung—Perspektiven für ländliche Regionen und ausgewählte Leistungsbereiche Gutachten; 2014.

27. Noess O, Hernes FH, Blane D. Life course influences on mortality at older ages: evidence from the Oslo Mortality Study. Soc Sci Med. 2016;62:329–36.
28. Herlitz A, Munthe C, Törner M, Forsander G. The counseling, self-care, adherence approach to person-centered care and shared decision making: moral psychology, executive autonomy, and ethics in multi-dimensional care decisions. J Health Commun. 2016;31:964–73.
29. World Health Organization (WHO). Adherence to long-term therapies. Evidence for action. Geneva: World Health Organization; 2003.
30. Linden M. Chronische psychische Erkrankungen in der Hausarztpraxis. Hausarzt. 2016;53:56–7.
31. Arbeitsgemeinschaft Adipositas im Kinder Jugendalter. S3-Leitlinie zur Therapie der Adipositas im Kindes- und Jugendalter. 2009. http://www.aga.adipositas-gesellschaft.de/index.php?id=9.
32. Linden M, Müller WE. Rehabilitations-Psychopharmakotherapie. Arzneimittelbehandlung chronifizierender und chronifizierter psychischer syndrome. Köln: Deutscher Ärzteverlag; 2005.
33. Linden M, Westram A. Results of controlled clinical trials comparing guidelined exposed and "guideline naive" physicians in the treatment of depression, hypertension, and diabetes: what can be learned? Curr Psychiatr Rev. 2011;7:43–9.
34. Hamburg MA, Collins FS. The path to personalized medicine. New England J Med. 2010;363:301–4.
35. Mezzich J, Snaedal J, van Weel C, Heath I. Toward person-centered medicine: from disease to patient to person. Mt Sinai J Med. 2010;77:304–6.
36. Livneh H. Quality of life and coping with chronic illness and disability. Rehabil Counsel Bull. 2015;59:67–83.
37. Katz S, Moskowitz RW, Jackson BA. Studies of illness in the aged. The Index of ADL: a standardized measure of biological and psychosocial function. J Am Med Assoc. 1963;185:914–9.
38. Mahoney FJ, Barthel DW. Functional evaluation: the Barthel index. Md State Med J. 1965;14:61–5.
39. Endicott J, Spitzer RL, Fleiss JL, Cohen J. The sickness rating scale: a procedure for measuring overall severity of psychiatric disturbance. Arch Gen Psychiatry. 1976;33:766–71.
40. American Psychiatric Association. Diagnostic criteria from DSM-IV. Washington, DC: American Psychiatric Association; 1994.
41. Nasrallah H, Morosini PL, Gagnon DD. Reliability, validity and ability to detect change of the personal and social performance scale in patients with stable schizophrenia. Psychiatry Res. 2008;161:213–24.
42. Morisini PL, Magliano L, Brambilla L, Ugolini S, Pioli R. Development, reliability and acceptability of a new version of the DSM-IV social and occupational functioning assessment scale (SOFAS) to assess routine social functioning. Acta Psychiatr Scand. 2000;1001:323–9.
43. World Health Organization. WHODAS II—Disability Assessment Schedule Training Manual: a guide to administration. Geneva: World Health Organization; 2004.
44. Cieza A, Ewert T, Üstün TB, Chatterji S, Kostanjsek N, Stucki G. Development of ICF core sets for patients with chronic conditions. J Rehabil Med. 2004;44:9–11.
45. Linden M, Baron S, Muschalla B, Molodynski A. Mini-ICF-APP social functioning scale. Oxford: Hogrefe; 2014a.
46. Linden M, Baron S, Muschalla B, Ostholt-Corsten M. Fähigkeitsbeeinträchtigungen bei psychischen Erkrankungen. Diagnostik, Therapie, und sozialmedizinische Beurteilung in Anlehnung an das mini-ICF-APP. Bern: Huber; 2014b.
47. Ky Y. Affective influences in person-environment fit theory: exploring the role of affect as both cause and outcome of P-E fit. J Appl Psychol. 2009;94:1210–26.
48. Hesketh B, Griffin B. Person-environment-fit. Encyclopedia of adulthood and ageing. New York, NY: Wiley; 2015. p. 1–5.
49. Smith MJ, Boteler Humm L, Fleming MF, Jordan N, Wright MA, Ginger EJ, Wright K, Olsen D, Bell MD. Virtual reality job interview training for veterans with posttraumatic stress disorder. J Vocat Rehabil. 2015;42:271–9.

50. Mesa F, Le TA, Beidel DC. Social skill-based treatment for social anxiety disorder in adolescents. In: Ranta K, La Greca AM, Garcia-Lopez LJ, Marttunen M, editors. Social anxiety and phobia in adolescents. New York: Springer; 2015.
51. United Nations. Convention on the rights of persons with disabilities. New York, NY: UN; 2006.
52. Thase ME, Rush AJ. When at first you don't succeed: sequential strategies for antidepressant nonresponders. J Clin Psychiatry. 1997;58:23–9.

A Psychosomatic Approach of Anorexia Nervosa

13

Thibaut Lebailly, Stéphane Saint-André, Stephane Laplace, Anne-Sophie Lancien-Dereine, Adeline Gourbil, and Michel Botbol

Abstract

Based on the literature review and on experiences with clinical cases, this paper presents a psychosomatic approach of anorexia nervosa. Psychosomatic is defined here as the entanglement of a double formation of symptoms: somatic symptoms on the one hand and psychological symptoms on the other. Are considered psychosomatic, psychological functioning favoring a somatic symptom or impacting its evolution. Coming within this scope, the psychosomatic school of Paris (Marty in particular) described operational thinking as a form of thinking frequently associated with psychosomatic disorders corresponding to this global definition. This paper shows that this form of thought can be seen as a failure of integration of the imaginary and affective life. By several aspects, operational thinking overlaps with alexithymia as described by Sifneos and the Boston School. The consequence of operational thinking functioning is a personality, often rigid, leaving little space to fantasies and to psychic elaboration. This functioning induces a body unbalance due to the arousal that cannot be elaborated otherwise, particularly during adolescence. The main aim of this paper is to consider if the approach proposed by the psychosomatic schools can have a clinical interest in the understanding and the cares of adolescent patients with anorexia nervosa.

T. Lebailly · S. Saint-André · A. S. Lancien-Dereine · A. Gourbil
Child and Adolescent Psychiatry Department of the Brest University Hospital, University of Western Brittany, Brest, France

S. Laplace
Psychologist, Child and Adolescent Psychiatry Department of the Brest University Hospital, University of Western Brittany, Brest, France

M. Botbol (✉)
Child and Adolescent Psychiatry Department of the Brest University Hospital, University of Western Brittany, Brest, France

Service Universitaire de Psychiatrie Infanto-Juvénile, Hôpital de Bohars, Bohars, France

L. Grassi et al. (eds.), *Person Centered Approach to Recovery in Medicine*, Integrating Psychiatry and Primary Care, https://doi.org/10.1007/978-3-319-74736-1_13

13.1 Introduction

Anorexia nervosa (AN) is an eating disorder (ED) defined by the DSM 5 according to three diagnostic criteria [1]:

- A. Restriction of energy intake relative to requirements, leading to a significantly low body weight in the context of age, sex, developmental trajectory, and physical health. Significantly low weight is defined as a weight that is less than minimally normal or, for children and adolescents, less than that minimally expected.
- B. Intense fear of gaining weight or of becoming fat or persistent behavior that interferes with weight gain, even though at a significantly low weight.
- C. Disturbance in the way in which one's body weight or shape is experienced, undue influence of body weight or shape on self-evaluation, or persistent lack of recognition of the seriousness of the current low body weight.

In this paper, Psychosomatic is defined as the entanglement of a double formation of symptoms: somatic symptoms on one hand and psychological symptoms on the other. Are considered psychosomatic, psychological functionning seen as determinants of a somatic symptom or of its evolution. The *operational thinking,* described by the psychosomatic school of Paris [2] comes within the scope of this global definition [3]. As we shall see in this paper, this school defines this form of thought as a failure of integration of the imaginary and affective life. By several aspects, it includes alexithymia as described by Sifneos and the Boston School [4]. The consequence of this functioning is a personality, often rigid, leaving little space to phantasmatic life and to psychic elaboration, resulting in a body unbalance due to the excitements that cannot be elaborated otherwise. In this paper, we will try to consider if the approach proposed by the psychosomatic schools can have a clinical interest in the understanding and in the care of patients with anorexia nervosa.

Starting with a brief literature review on anorexia nervosa and on the point of view of the Paris School of Psychosomatic, this paper will present a clinical vignette of an adolescent with AN followed by the team of our child psychiatry ED unit in Western Brittany (France).

13.2 Psychosomatic Approach of the School of Paris: Operational Thinking

Psychosomatic disorders are somatic affections in which the psychic part seems to be preponderant, if not determinant. Our objective, here, is to consider to what extent the psychosomatic approach proposed by the School of Psychosomatic of Paris may have an interest in cases of adolescent AN. Indeed, our experience has led us to question this particular relationship, on cases of patients whose mental functioning is caught in major difficulties determining the part played by the body in their disorder.

For that purpose, we have first to define precisely what psychosomatic disorders are and especially what they are not. Therefore, we must differentiate them from somatoform disorders, which are psychic manifestations taking the form of an organic attack but where no somatic lesion can be found. Psychosomatic disorders present a somatic lesion whose origin is not necessarily psychic but whose durability is considered to be related to the patient's psychic functioning [5].

Several disorders cannot therefore be considered psychosomatic [6]:

- First, the secondary psychological reactions to somatic diseases, which are more likely to be maladaptive
- Then the aggravations of somatic diseases due to psychological difficulties
- Finally, conversional hysterical functional disorders, even if the limit with psychosomatic disorders is not always clear

For Alexander [7], however, only the voluntary and sensory neuromuscular systems can be affected by hysterical conversions. According to him, nevertheless, the vegetative system and the organism as a whole can be impacted "by the emotional tensions likely to spread in all parts of the body, through the cortico-thalamic pathways and the autonomous fibers." For him, a chronic or excessive stimulation or inhibition, by this emotional tension, of the functioning of the organs can give rise to what he calls an "organ neurosis." This "functional disorder" does not therefore have a symbolic meaning, as hysterical conversions might have, but these organ neuroses could pave the way for a psychosomatic disorder [8].

In the 1960s, Marty and his successors at the Psychosomatic School of Paris developed the notion of "operational thinking", which they extended in the 1980s to the notion of "operational life." It is a psycho-behavioral way of thinking and functioning, centered on logic and pragmatics, the current and the factual, and where the speech does not imply any elaboration or association. It can be said that the patient is very close to the materiality of facts and objects, without any space for fantasies or representations. The operational thinking is essentially concerned with things and avoids systematically what is related to affects and emotions. According to Marty, this lack of imaginative life in the patient's functioning favors somatic disturbances, by a mechanism similar to the one developed by Freud in relation with anxiety and traumatic neuroses: the insufficiency of the protective-shield system provided by mental representations results in the inefficiency of the psychic apparatus to protect the self against the psychosensory arousal. Consequently, the lack of symbolization leads to a shift of all or part of the conflicts and tensions, on the body or on the body functions.

Besides the cases related to a structural deficiency, the same mechanism could also result from a psychotraumatic life event. In both cases, it would be the too strong intensity of the arousal that overwhelms the mentalization capacities of the psychic apparatus and the person's ability to adapt his behavior accordingly, thus prompting him to export these tensions on the somatic apparatus.

Several characteristics of the operational functioning can be clinically identified. Firstly, a certain monotony of the discourse, as if it was detached. The symptoms are described in an impersonal manner giving an impression of "echolalia" or "echo speech." The patient puts the physician in a position of omniscience, as if he knew the whole story without having to be told of, causing blurring and confusion [9].

For Corcos [10], the affect is not absent, it is neutralized in an alexithymic functioning. He notes here an abrasion of the auto-representative processes. To fill the void left by the neutralization of affects, the subject sticks to an ideological and technical ambient discourse, in a movement of identification, giving the impression of a discourse that is not his own.

13.3 Psychosomatic in Childhood

The Psychosomatic School of Paris has also been interested in early "mother-child"[1] interactions, from a psychosomatic perspective. One could say indeed that there is nothing more "psychosomatic" than an infant [5]: the body has a major role in the interactions with the entourage, the interactions basing on the various physiological functions (nutrition, sphincter elimination, tonus, etc.), and the communication of the behavioral elements to the persons of his entourage; these persons, who are mainly the caregivers, will have to mentalize these elements, using the "mother's anticipatory illusions" that is to say the capacity of the caregivers to anticipate the infant's psychic development. The mentalization is of paramount importance here because, through it, the caregivers endorse, on behalf of the infant, the protective-shield functions the baby is not yet able to perform [11].

In line with this point of view, Spitz classifies psychosomatic disorders according to two major types of "maternal" attitudes [12]: *psychotoxic* disorders responding to qualitatively inappropriate mother-child relationships and disorders caused by *impairment* responding to quantitatively insufficient mother-child relationships, the latter being associated with anaclitic depression and marasmus.

It seems important therefore to evaluate not only the impact of the "maternal" attitude on the child but also the modification of this attitude according to the symptoms of the child. Indeed, the "mother" and more generally the caregivers are particularly sensitive to the psychosomatic manifestations of the baby, leading them to adopt new behaviors in front of the infant's somatic expressions. Infant's psychosomatic disorders are, therefore, eminently relational because they provoke reactions in the infant entourage, they often worry: it can involve the digestive (colic, vomiting, and merycism) or respiratory (asthma, spasms of the sob) or dermatological (eczema, alopecia aureate) spheres. Thus, the aggressiveness underlying the

[1] The notion of "mother" involves, in this context, much more than the sole person of the mother; the concept of "mother-environment" has been proposed by Winnicott to define all of the infant's caring environment, generally, but not always, represented by the biological mother or the main caregiver but involving also other caregivers who are not differentiated from her. In this paper, the term "mother" refers to this Winnicottian concept.

mother-child relationship is often completely forgotten when the psychosomatic symptoms appear. It is not rare in those cases to observe that this aggressive aspect is displaced on the mother-doctor relationship, the mother becoming a mother-therapist as described by Winnicott [13]. She would then no longer be *good enough* but, responding either too early or too late to her child's needs and subsequently encroaching upon her child's space, would "nurse" him without giving him any possibility of experimenting new situations and new affects. The infant is therefore exposed to the development of a "false-self" in which the child neglects his inner needs and wishes to become as adapted as possible to what he feels his caregiver expects from him. Consequently, he reduces his capacity of containing his projections, illusions, and fantasies in his transitional space. This brings us back to Marty's operative thinking.

Brazelton points out that psychosomatic disorders are not only psychological for the children, because the fear they trigger in their parents involves them concretely [14]. He notes that many children with asthma tend to attract the attention of their parents, or to express their fears, using this symptom as a way to communicate with them. Parents allow themselves to be drawn into this situation because of their own anxiety [15]. If they cannot control these symptoms, their feelings of guilt, anger, and anxiety cause tension in the family and with their child. He proposes a preventive model to avoid the structuration of this psychosomatic relationship. This model is about reassuring the child by allowing him to find solutions giving him the impression of being able to take control of his symptoms. The aim is to avoid that the child would be left with the freezing anxiogenic feelings related to the organic disorder and to allow him to elaborate and symbolize his fear or his pain. When this can be reached, the child can avoid the operational regression of the thinking, limiting the psychosomatic reaction to a more congruent portion.

13.4 Anorexia and Adolescence

The evolution of the cares of AN results from the evolution of the understanding of this disorder. Indeed, AN has been known, since at least the seventeenth century, when it was described by R. Morton who labeled them "nervous phthisis" whose origin would be due to an alteration of the vital impulse. However, it was with the descriptions of Gull and Lasègue that the first standardized cares were formalized. Gull spoke of "anorexia apepsia" and then of "anorexia nervosa" when Lasègue made a connection with hysteria under the term "hysterical anorexia" in his description of 1873 [16]. Lasègue emphasized the importance of family relationships in the disease: "the family has only two methods that are both exhausting: praying or threatening (…) the greater the concern, the lower the appetite. (…) Excessive insistence calls for an excess of resistance" and further "the environment in which the patient lives has an influence that it would be unfortunate to omit or be unaware of." It is now agreed that anorexia is not so much a hysterical pathology as a pathology of the links, which has led, especially in France, to an evolution of the therapeutic proposals, based on separation of the anorectic patient from his family and familial environment. In this model, separation is no longer an aversive treatment; it aims at quiescing the family's interactions and links that are difficult to bear by the adolescent because of the "adolescence paradox" [17]; this paradox is triggered by the separation induced by the sexualization of the links due to puberty and to the social injunction toward autonomy related to his becoming adult. While the adolescent needs the most to be helped or soothed by the persons of his environment, to overcome the anxiogenic effects of this imposed separation and of the body changes due to puberty, he also needs to show to himself and to others how independent and autonomous he is, particularly in his family relations. As stated by P Jeammet [17], "what he needs the most is what threatens him the most, because he needs it." This psychopathological understanding dates back to the Göttingen Symposium of 1965, when experts reached a consensual position on the psychopathology of anorexia nervosa, around two central notions: first, the conflict is at the level of the body (mainly at the level of sexually invested food functions), and second, anorexia expresses a disability to assume the genital role and the bodily transformations related to puberty. The symptom is not only the outcome of the instinctual conflict but also the result of a defect in the organization of the self. We shift from a model close to hysteria to that of a severe pathology of the self with the failure of the process of separation-individuation.

Typical anorexia nervosa affects most often young girls at the beginning of their puberty, classically after their first menstruation. Puberty and access to genital sexuality appear as sources of disturbance of the adolescent's psychic balance [18]. The question of the image of the body is central at this age; the silhouette changes both for the teenager and for her entourage. The body is then upset both in its function as spatial landmark (altering sensorially the relation to the world and the environment) and in its function as a symbolic representative of the self. The body is thus at the forefront for the modifications of the adolescent's self and for her identity quest.

This is associated with another important intrapsychic movement, related to the loss of the influence of the significant figures of childhood and to the change in the relational modes with them. This movement has been compared to a work of mourning because it destroys "the infantile megalomaniac ideal" in which the child projects his feeling of being able to realize everything on his parents.

This psychic task, to achieve the detachment from their parental authority and their infantile objects, leads the adolescent to live moments of depression that are ultimately inherent to their developmental process [10].

AN is a particularly efficient solution to refuse this task and avoid this depression. Through the effect of denutrition, it freezes the sexualization of the body, and through this it avoids actively the sexualization of the links and, consequently, the need to separate from her infantile objects. At the same time, the concerns AN causes to the parents increase their psychological and physical proximity to their child; like Donkey Skin, the young anorexic girls are protected by their body against the sexual lust their puberty changes trigger in others. It is the rationale behind the quiescing interest of the separation contract mentioned earlier.

13.5 Anorexia and Alexithymia

Adolescence is then a troubled period in which the quest for identity and autonomy threatens the narcissistic bases of the adolescent and, consequently, exposes him to a risk of depression. To fight against this risk, the adolescent uses various defense mechanisms and among them not only the common ones (as repression, or displacement), leading to a classical neurotic functioning, but also mechanisms, like intellectualization, asceticism, and splitting, which are rather favoring a psychosomatic functioning.

According to A. Freud, intellectualization is a defensive mechanism of the ego aiming at controlling the impulses at the level of thoughts [19]. It is frequently associated with asceticism she sees as a defense mechanism of the ego at better controlling the drives at the level of the body. Anorexia nervosa can be considered as an extreme form of these defense mechanisms. Intellectualization also allows the adolescent to rationalize his emotions and his sexual drives, contributing to the splitting between body and mind and to the operational functioning of the self. Alexithymia is an extreme form of this splitting, giving it its characteristic features: a difficulty in identifying and verbalizing emotions, in differentiating emotions and associated bodily sensations, and in getting in touch with their fantasmatic life. A thinking oriented toward the concrete aspects of existence at the expenses of their affective aspects is the result of this functioning, i.e., the common features defining Sifneos's alexithymia.

13.6 Anorexia and Operative Thinking

Unlike alexithymia, the concept of operative thinking comes from the psychoanalytic field. It presents four main aspects, which cover more or less the concept of alexithymia:

- Difficulties in communicating feelings to others.
- Inability to identify one's feelings and to distinguish them from bodily sensations.
- Poverty of imaginary life.
- Thought turned outward (concrete thinking) and not inwardly.

Marty suggests that these subjects have neither affects nor fantasies. This would be due to the lack of caregivers' interpretations both at the quantitative level, leading to a low "stock" of representations and interpretations, and at the qualitative level, leading to poverty in the range of available affects. Once this structured deficit appears, it seems to be not much reversible, early interactions having a major role in the subsequent development of psychosomatic disorders. This also applies to the complex of "dead mother" introduced by Green [20], in which, because of her pervasive depressive feelings and thoughts, the "mother" cannot invest her infant, impacting the child's development and his adult affective and emotional functioning. Compared with alexithymia, operative thinking has an additional dimension: the inability to mentalize the conflicts with a risk of discharging the excess of excitement and anxiety in the somatic and behavioral spheres. We could therefore consider operative thinking as a risky mode of alexithymic functioning. Anorexic dietary behaviors are an example of such functioning.

Thus, the "alexithymic operativity" that can be observed in anorexic patients is not much modifiable, explaining the chronicity of the disorder and the persistence of an operative psychic functioning. In a review of several works focusing on this question, Joergen-Grabe et al. [21] describe some major obstacles determining cold contact, avoiding pattern of attachment, great impairment in object investment, to which we have to add insensitivity to emotional indicators generating additional obstacles to an introspective work [22]; all these characteristics make difficult for these patients, the construction of a therapeutic alliance, in spite of their, often severe, psychological distress.

Corcos ultimately assumes that there is a maternal "failure" in the mothers of anorexic patients, particularly in the investment of their child's autonomous, living, and erotic body. He thinks that this failure would not favor, in these patients, a good integration of their feminine and would participate in the advent of a sadomasochistic organization that fixed their infantile objects. Thus, in AN, two puberty-driven metamorphoses would be neutralized: the becoming woman and the becoming mother [10]. The adolescent's body, still largely undifferentiated from her mother's one, undergoes passively the pubertal modifications, reactivating the problematic of separation-individuation. AN could therefore be described as *a silent revolt in a passive resistance*. In this perspective, to separate the patient from his family would also have the effect of giving her the illusion that it is possible to become a woman, a process metaphorized by weight gain and body forms.

13.7 Clinical Vignette

Our therapeutic system in Western Brittany is centered on ambulatory cares. These cares are provided by a small team involving a child psychiatrist and a nurse, both members of the child psychiatric team, and a pediatrician belonging to the pediatric team. This ambulatory team follows the majority of the eating disorder patients in an outpatient consultation unit. When hospitalization criteria are met in a patient, according to the French High Authority for Health's recommendations [23], she is first hospitalized in the pediatric inpatient unit, focusing on weight-regaining objectives to recover clinical safety. If, in spite of this pediatric hospitalization, these therapeutic objectives are not met, the patient shifts in the child and adolescent psychiatry inpatient unit, if the parents accept it; at that stage, a contract of separation is generally decided for 1–4 weeks to quiesce the family ties put at stake by the AN symptom. During this period of separation, the patient does not meet her parents who are regularly received in clinical interviews by the child psychiatrist in charge of the inpatient child and adolescent psychiatry unit. The contract states that after the period of separation, the patient will remain hospitalized until she reaches a threshold weight decided jointly with her, the therapeutic staff, and the family. The contract mentions also the threshold of the patient's weight that will allow her to return home on leave during the weekends. When she is discharged from the hospitalization, the patient returns home with an ambulatory follow-up. In some cases, the patient will not return home immediately after being discharge from the inpatient unit; an intermediary step will be proposed to her and her family, in a *therapeutic boarding school*, a facility, specific to France health system. This facility offers to adolescents and young adults with psychiatric disorders, a long-term program (from 6 months to 2 years) associating institutional psychiatric cares to ordinary high school or college studies in this therapeutic context [24].

"O is 14 years old when she is admitted in our child and adolescent psychiatry inpatient unit for AN. She is the second of a sibling of two; her older brother is 17 years old.

Her mother suffered from an episode of agoraphobia and eating disorders between 21 and 25 years old and was successfully treated with a psychotherapy.

The father's childhood has been strongly affected by his parents' chronic alcoholism and by related family violence. Both parents are now dead.

The family relates the beginning of O's eating disorders to the death of her maternal grandmother, 2 years ago, from an oncological relapse and after several hospitalizations for severe denutrition imposing enteral feeding. O was 12 years old at that time and begun progressively to reduce her intake of sweet and fat food, losing weight significantly; it was not the first time she was losing weight. When she was 11 years old, she had lost 3.5 kg after the breaking of a love relation with a boyfriend and of a friendship with her best girlfriend, both prompting in her a feeling of betrayal and a drastic drop in her self-esteem. She benefited from the counseling of her pediatrician and from some sessions with a psychologist; she recovered a normal weigh rapidly thereafter.

After the death of her grandmother, O became hyperactive with a sharp increase of her exercise time (dancing, body building). She shows signs of dysmorphophobia, a permanent control of her calorie intake. Her comments are intellectualized and do not express much affects. She is hospitalized in a pediatric unit when she is 13 years old. She is submitted to the installation of a nasogastric tube to receive a nocturnal enteral feeding, but she cannot stand it and removed it. However, she succeeds in stabilizing her weight with the help of dietary supplements. In spite of the pediatric follow-up and a new psychological counseling, this stabilization does not last long, and her weight loss starts again after a few weeks, conducting the pediatric team to address her to our specialized eating disorders ambulatory team.

In that setting, her follow-up imposes rapidly a new hospitalization in a pediatric ward due again to weight loss. O cannot stand being separated from her parents and runs away for the ward. Her parents decide not to bring her back to the hospital and to keep her at home.

O kept losing weight and a new hospitalization is necessary. To avoid the repetition of the previous experience, and taking into account the important rigidity of her psychological functioning, the hospitalization will, this time, take place in the child and adolescent psychiatric inpatient unit, with a *separation contract* between the parents and the medical staff; this contract set up a period of separation between her and her family for 4 weeks, followed by a period of hospitalization in which she will be able to see her parents regularly but will remain hospitalized until she reaches a weight threshold decided jointly; the contract set up also that she will resume her ambulatory treatment after being discharged from the hospital.

O expresses very rapidly how difficult it is for her to be separated from her family, but she cannot say much more about her feelings. For the staff members, it is difficult to develop a relation with her. O remains always in a mastering position, controlling her emotions, as shown by the rigidity and the ritualization of her thoughts. She always complies with the staff's requests as perfectly as she can, trying to avoid any criticism. She never says any negative comments about her parents.

During the regular family meetings with the medical staff, every 2 weeks, the staff observes that the family functioning is excessively closed in on itself, with a very high level of intra-familial co-dependency between its members. Few spaces are left for the others. The family is united around the idea that they need to struggle against the external world seen as threatening.

The mother explains that she has been sexually assaulted in the street by some unknown individual when she was a child; she was not able to disclose it to her parents at once and did it only many years later, some months after O's birth. She reports that she has had, at that time, periods of strong anxiety around this event. O was informed when she was 10 years old; the parents report that she was terrorized by this information during some months, fearing to go out of home; they also say that she felt guilty for not having got aware of her mother suffering.

The questions related to sexuality or puberty are difficult for O who expresses her disgust and her fear of becoming sexualized. Her parents explain spontaneously that when she was 9 years old, O became very intrusive with her father, a behavior they understand as "a late oedipal complex"; it reached such an intensity that the mother asked the father to be more "distant" from her.

In the inpatient unit, O's evolution is exclusively ponderal. She eats well, gains weight, and is less hyperactive.

At the end of the 4 weeks separation period, she sees her parents, as scheduled in the separation contract. She does not express much emotion in their first meeting, where staff members are present. However, rapidly thereafter, the parents show obvious difficulties to maintain the project they contracted 1 month ago and put an end to O's hospitalization. However, they ask for an ambulatory follow-up, we accept of course".

13.8 Discussion

We feel that this clinical case can illustrate how psychosomatic consideration can be helpful in cases of anorexia nervosa. The body is an object of hatred, possessed by a bad object, an internal persecutor confused with it [25]. The patient's ego is in a state of distress, exacerbating her underlying depression in front of the threat of an ever-growing sexualized body. O struggles, therefore, against the sensation of hunger. The splitting between the body and the mind induces extrapsychic and intracorporeal projection of the bad object. It illustrates the Jeammet's already mentioned quotation "what threatens her most is what she needs most" [26]. Here the symptoms appear clearly to be a way to master the relationship with the significant others, i.e. as much the parents as the professionals.

The operative thinking can be observed here, not because affects are absent but because they remain unrecognized, not worked through, not fantasized. Affects are seen only as a succession of concrete events with utilitarian and concrete representations.

Brusset [27] observes that beside this splitting, one can observe, in these patients, a narcissistic investment of the body claiming to avoid a libidinal investment of the others. The body becomes the support of a defensive megalomaniac idealization. This leads to a paradoxical position where there are at the same time an idealized body, object of desire, and a real body, object of denial.

Considering this case, we could say that it is "the mother-daughter" relationship which is psychosomatic. This relationship is expressed through the body of the other. As a consequence, **the** patient does not recognize her emotional states because they are not totally her own. The anorexic patient ceases to eat and thus to grow and to be able to emancipate herself, maintaining the relationship of dependence with her parents and a nourishing model of recursive loop [28, 29].

In these situations, the objective of the treatment is to bring the patient out of this functioning, transforming her symptom into a family symptom to build up and work through.

Conclusion

Finally, the psychosomatic approach of AN allows to consider it as a "transitional pathology," in which "alexithymic operativity" is a predominant feature. This understanding suggests a therapeutic perspective focusing on the treatment of the alexithymic or operative dimensions of these patients' disorder through therapeutic individual or group therapeutic mediations, enhancing creativity, mentalization, and pleasurable experiences. Separation may be at the beginning, a condition to allow these pleasurable and creative experiences.

References

1. American Psychiatric Association. DSM-5: diagnostic and statistical manual of mental disorders. Washington, DC: American Psychiatric Publishing; 2013.
2. Marty P. La psychosomatique de l'adulte. Paris: Presses universitaires de France; 2011. 126 p.
3. Marty P, de d M'UM. La « pensée opératoire ». Rev Fr Psychosom. 2016;6(2):197–208.
4. Sifneos PE. The prevalence of 'Alexithymic' characteristics in psychosomatic patients. Psychother Psychosom. 1973;22(2–6):255–62.
5. Marcelli D, Cohen D. Enfance et psychopathologie. Issy-les-Moulineaux: Elsevier Masson; 2012. 672 p.

6. Kreisler L, Fain M, Soulé M, Lebovici S. L'enfant et son corps : études sur la clinique psychosomatique du jeune âge. Paris: Presses universitaires de France; 1974. 516 p.
7. Alexander F, Baendek T. La Médecine psychosomatique, ses principes et ses applications. Paris: Payot; 1967. 256 p.
8. Jadoulle V. Les dérives de la pensée psychosomatique. L'évolution Psychiatr. 2003;68(2):261–70.
9. Roussillon RAD de la Publication, Brun A, Chabert C, Ciccone A, Ferrant A, Georgieff N, et al. Manuel de psychologie et de psychopathologie clinique générale. Issy-les-Moulineaux: Elsevier Masson; 2014.
10. Corcos M, Atger F, Jeammet P. Évolution des approches compréhensives des troubles des conduites alimentaires. Ann Méd-Psychol. 2003;161(8):621–9.
11. Aulagnier P. La violence de l'interprétation : du pictogramme à l'énoncé. Paris: Presses universitaires de France; 1991. 363 p.
12. Spitz RA. De la naissance à la parole : la première année de la vie. Paris: PUF; 1984. 306 p.
13. Winnicott DW. Jeu et réalité: l'espace potentiel. Paris: Gallimard; 2002. 276 p.
14. Brazelton TB. Points forts. I: les moments essentiels du développement de votre enfant. Librairie générale française: Paris; 2007. 607 p.
15. Garralda ME. Somatisation in children. J Child Psychol Psychiatry. 1996;37(1):13–33.
16. Lasègue C. De l'anorexie hystérique et Les exhibitionnistes. Paris: Théraplix; 1970. 35 p.
17. Jeammet P. Anorexie, boulimie: les paradoxes de l'Adolescence. Paris: Hachette littératures; 2011.
18. Anzieu D, Bowlby J, Chauvin R. L'attachement. Zazzo R, éditeur. Neuchâtel, Suisse, France; 1979. 250 p.
19. Freud A. Le moi et les mécanismes de défense. Paris: Presses universitaires de France; 1990. 166 p.
20. Green A. Narcissisme de vie, narcissisme de mort. Paris: Minuit; 2016. 384 p.
21. Grabe HJ, Frommer J, Ankerhold A, Ulrich C, Gröger R, Franke GH, et al. Alexithymia and outcome in psychotherapy. Psychother Psychosom. 2008;77(3):189–94.
22. de Tychey C. Alexithymie et pensée opératoire : Approche comparative clinique projective franco-américaine, Abstract, Resumen. Psychol Clin Proj. 2010;16:177–207.
23. Recommandations de bonne pratique. Anorexie mentale : prise en charge. Médecine Thérapeutique. 2012;17(4):334–61.
24. Botbol M, Mammar N, Barrère Y. Institutions soins etudes en psychiatrie de l'adolescent et du jeune adulte (Care and study institutions in adolescent and young adult psychiatry).
25. Selvini M. L'Anoressia mentale. Milano: Feltrinelli; 1963. xi+245.
26. Jeammet P. Réalité externe et réalité interne. Importance et spécificité de leur articulation à l'adolescence. Rev Fr Psychanal. 1980;44(3–4):481–522.
27. Brusset B, Widlöcher D. L'assiette et le miroir: l'anorexie mentale de l'enfant et de l'adolescent. Toulouse: Privat, impr; 1991. 274 p.
28. Minuchin S, Rosman BL, Baker L, Minuchin S. Psychosomatic families: anorexia nervosa in context. Cambridge, MA: Harvard University Press; 2009. 366 p.
29. Neuburger R. L'autre demande: psychanalyse et thérapie familiale. Paris: Payot & Rivages, DL; 2003. 195 p.

Part III

Integrated Intervention

The Role of Integrated Interventions in Psychosomatic Diseases

14

Massimo Biondi, Francesco Saverio Bersani, and Massimo Pasquini

Abstract

Based on the evidence that there can be no health without mental health, psychosomatic medicine recognizes the complexity of the interface between psychiatry, lifestyle and medicine. At the clinical level, psychosomatic medicine integrates interdisciplinary evaluation and management involving diverse specialties including psychiatry, psychology, neurology, internal medicine, allergology, dermatology, rheumatology and endocrinology. At the research level, the fields of psychoneuroimmunology and psychoneuroendocrinology integrate findings from neuroscience, experimental psychology, physiology, genetics, pharmacology and molecular biology to understand the mechanistic underpinnings of psychosomatics. A clinical approach based on personalized and scientifically based integrated interventions, consistent with the bio-psycho-social model of medicine, is the best way to actually promote clinically significant physical and mental health improvements.

14.1 Introduction

The fifth edition of the Diagnostic and Statistical Manual of Mental Disorders (DSM-5) formally recognizes the category of "somatic symptom and related disorders", which includes a range of conditions characterized by the tendency to experience or communicate psychological distress in the form of physical symptoms such

M. Biondi · F. S. Bersani · M. Pasquini (✉)
Department of Human Neurosciences, Sapienza University of Rome, Rome, Italy
e-mail: massimo.pasquini@uniroma1.it

L. Grassi et al. (eds.), *Person Centered Approach to Recovery in Medicine*, Integrating Psychiatry and Primary Care, https://doi.org/10.1007/978-3-319-74736-1_14

as somatic symptom disorder, illness anxiety disorder, conversion disorder (or functional neurological symptom disorder), psychological factors affecting other medical conditions, and factitious disorder [1, 2]. Taken together, these conditions represent the current psychiatric diagnostic characterization of the broader concept of "psychosomatic medicine", which is a rapidly evolving interdisciplinary medical field aimed at the exploration of the influence of social, psychological, neurological and behavioural factors on biological bodily processes (and vice versa) [3].

Based on the evidence that there can be no health without mental health, psychosomatic medicine recognizes the complexity of the interface between psychiatry, lifestyle and medicine [3–5]. At the clinical level, psychosomatic medicine integrates interdisciplinary evaluation and management involving diverse specialties including psychiatry, psychology, neurology, internal medicine, allergology, dermatology, rheumatology and endocrinology [3]. At the research level, the fields of psychoneuroimmunology and psychoneuroendocrinology integrate findings from neuroscience, experimental psychology, physiology, genetics, pharmacology and molecular biology to understand the mechanistic underpinnings of psychosomatics [3].

Over the last 20 years, the World Health Organization (WHO) has supported the bio-psycho-social model of health as the most reliable theoretical framework for the understanding of medical disorders [6]. The model implies (1) that health and disease result from intricate, variable, bidirectional interactions of biological factors (e.g. genetic, biochemical), psychological factors (e.g. mood, personality, behaviour), and social factors (e.g. cultural, familial, socioeconomic), and (2) that it is essential to manage the three types of factors together in order to achieve satisfactory clinical outcomes [6]. The bio-psycho-social model applies to virtually all disciplines of medicine, and it is of particular relevance for the psychosomatic conditions [6].

There are individuals in which psychological distress is expressed in the form of somatic symptoms or it worsens the clinical course/severity of a pre-existing medical condition, and there are subjects in which a medical condition induces a reactive psychiatric syndrome or it worsens the clinical course/severity of a pre-existing psychiatric condition. In all these cases, in which psychosomatic phenomena play a crucial role, an approach based on integrated interventions, consistent with the bio-psycho-social model of medicine, is the best way to promote clinically significant physical and mental health improvements.

14.2 Function-Oriented Rather than Diagnosis-Oriented Integrated Treatments in Somatizing Patients

There is no clear consensus on how to treat subjects with a DSM-defined diagnosis of a somatic symptom disorder. The categorical approach to define diagnoses used in the DSM-5, in fact, presents certain disadvantages which limit its actual usefulness in predicting treatment outcomes.

Given that all mental disorders are considered syndromes rather than diseases, the boundaries between normality and pathology are often close, and sometimes rather artificial [7]. Diagnoses of somatic and related disorders are often formulated based on the magnitude of subjective suffering or on quantitative rather than qualitative criteria [7, 8]. The great variability in the clinical presentation of somatic and related disorders and their "continuums" can be explained as a result of their multifactorial, non-deterministic and stochastic aetiologies and of the interactions between genetic, biological, environmental and psychosocial factors, disposition and resilience [7, 8]. Categorical models cannot accommodate and satisfactorily describe the inter-individual psychopathological continuous-quantitative or discrete-qualitative phenomena, and therefore a categorical diagnosis per se does not represent a safe ground to set up a psychopharmacological or psychotherapeutic intervention [7, 8].

Subjects with the same diagnosis of a somatic symptom disorder, for example, can be extremely different in terms of clinical features and of expression of psychopathological dimensions. Consistently with the model of a "dimensional psychopathology", the clinical intervention should be based on the individual symptom profile and the underlying neurobiology of each patient partially independently of the DSM-defined diagnosis.

The Rapid Dimensional Assessment Scale (RADAS) is one of the few instruments that can be used to rate the severity of a range of psychopathological dimensions and symptoms at the same time; while it lacks in terms of measurement of biological correlates of the explored conditions, the scale presents several strengths among short administration duration, low costs, and good prediction of clinical outcomes [9–15]. It is considered a reliable and valid dimensional tool in both research and clinical settings. The items are rated on a 5-point scale ranging from 0 to 4, with higher scores indicating greater severity. Scores of 1 indicate the presence of a condition intermediate between normality and psychopathology, while scores of 2 or more indicate the presence of symptoms of definite clinical relevance [9–15].

Through the use of the RADAS (or other similar instruments) it is possible to identify the prominent dimensions of psychological suffering, thus facilitating the decision-making process and the treatment choice. As discussed in a previous paper [8], Fig. 14.1 shows the RADAS profile of three subjects with the DSM-5 diagnoses of illness anxiety disorder and of conversion disorder (or functional neurological symptom disorder). While all the patients have similarly high levels of somatization, they differ markedly in terms of severity of other psychiatric symptoms such as sadness, apathy, reality distortion, obsessiveness or impulsivity; as each of these dimensions can be targeted differently through a range of possible interventions, it is the individual profile of psychopathology of each patient that should drive the choice of the intervention (both psychopharmacological and psychotherapeutic) rather than the condition of being a "somatizer" per se. The same approach [8] can be used for the psychiatric or psychological treatment of patients having medical disorders with known psychosomatic underpinnings such as fibromyalgia and inflammatory bowel disease (IBD), as shown in Fig. 14.2.

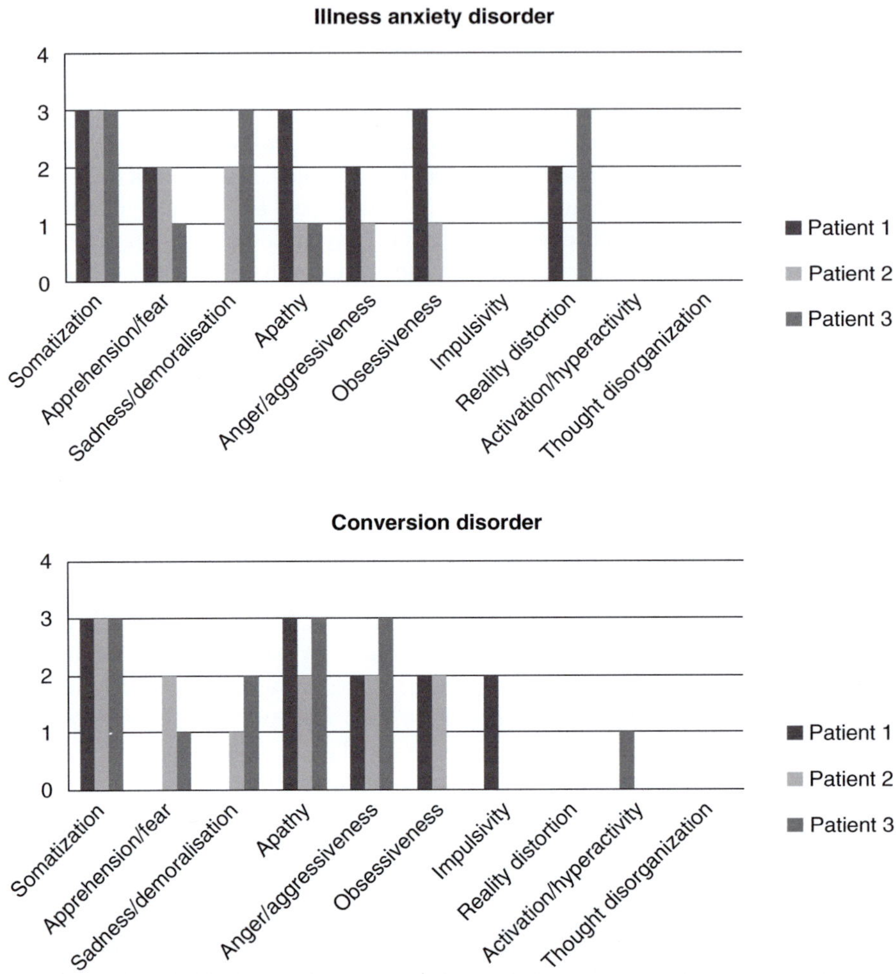

Fig. 14.1 Different dimensional psychopathological profiles of three patients affected by illness anxiety disorder (top) and conversion disorder (bottom). Adapted from [8]

In terms of psychopharmacology, for example, among the patients affected by an illness anxiety disorder (Fig. 14.1), patient 1 could be treated with an antidepressant of the class of selective serotonin reuptake inhibitors (SSRIs) to target apprehension, apathy and obsessiveness plus a mood stabilizer or a D2 blocker for the treatment of anger and reality distortion, patient 2 could be treated with a SSRI to target sadness and apprehension, and patient 3 could be concomitantly treated with an SSRI and a D2 blocker as sadness and reality distortion are the most prominent clinical manifestations [8]; among the patients affected by conversion disorder (Fig. 14.1), patient 1 could be treated with a mood stabilizer (e.g. valproic acid) plus a benzodiazepine because of concomitant presence of symptoms of anger and impulsivity, patient 2 could be treated with an antidepressant with strong serotonergic properties

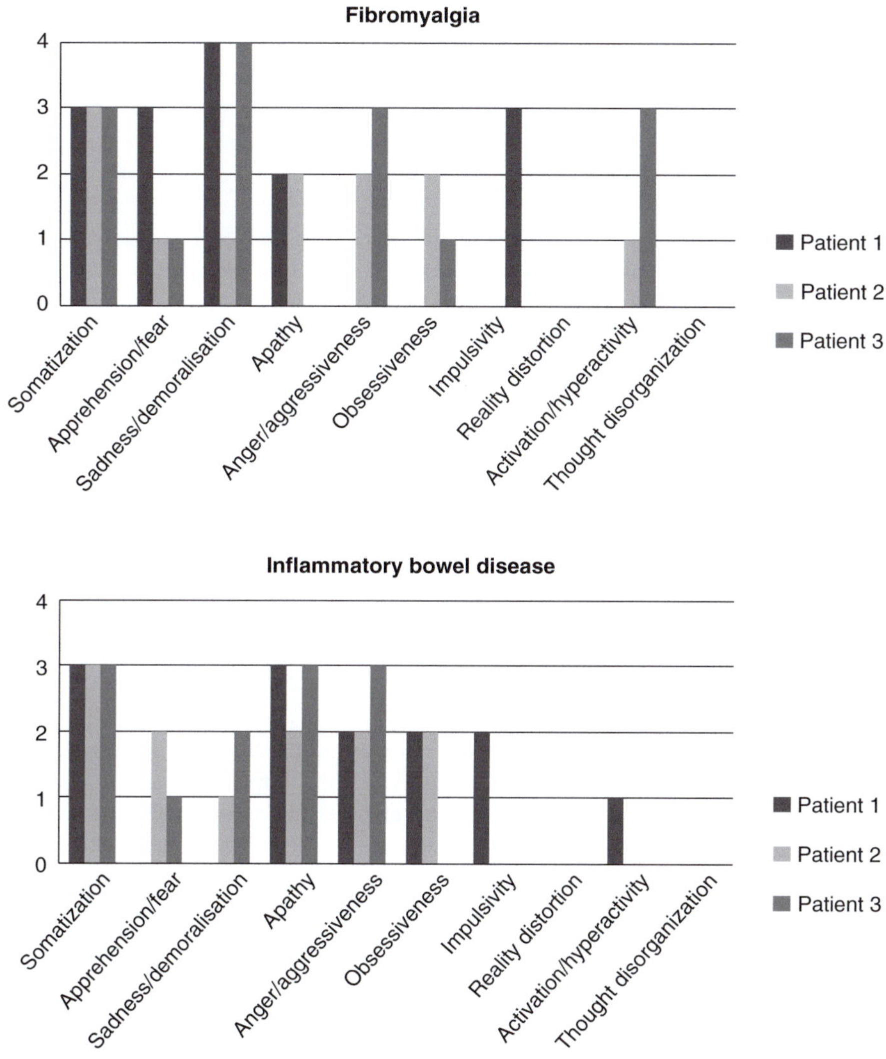

Fig. 14.2 Different dimensional psychopathological profiles of three patients affected by fibromyalgia (top) and inflammatory bowel disease (bottom). Adapted from [8]

(e.g. SSRI or a tricyclic antidepressants) due to the moderate severity of symptoms of apprehension, apathy and obsessiveness, and patient 3 could be treated with a serotonin-norepinephrine reuptake inhibitor (SNRI) or SSRI plus a mood stabilizer (e.g. valproic acid or gabapentin) to target sadness, apathy, activation and anger [8]; among the patients affected by fibromyalgia (Fig. 14.2), patient 1 could be treated with a SNRI medication, a SSRI medication or mirtazapine for the predominance of sadness and apprehension plus amisulpride to target apathy, patient 2 could be treated with a SSRI to target sadness, apprehension, apathy and obsessiveness, plus a mood stabilizer for the presence of mildly severe symptoms of anger and hyperactivity, and patient 3 could be treated with the combination of an SSRI plus a mood stabilizer (for the presence of anger and activation in addition to sadness and low levels of apprehension and obsessiveness) [8]; among the patients affected by IBD (Fig. 14.2), patient 1 could be initially treated with a mood stabilizer because of the presence of moderately severe symptoms of anger, impulsivity and activation, and then a SSRI could be added for obsessiveness and apathy, patient 2 could be treated with an antidepressant with prominent serotonergic properties (e.g. of SSRI or tricyclic class) due to the presence of apprehension, apathy and obsessiveness, plus a mood stabilizer (e.g. valproate, lamotrigine or gabapentin) to target symptoms of anger, and patient 3 could be treated with the combination of an SSRI plus a mood stabilizer for the presence of anger in addition to sadness and apathy [8].

These examples of psychopharmacological therapy are given to show how subjects with similar psychosomatic conditions can differ markedly in the severity of other underlying psychiatric or psychological aspects, and therefore the choice of the intervention (taking into consideration the heterogeneity of the effects of psychiatric medications) should be driven by the individual profile of psychopathological needs.

14.3 Psychotherapy for Psychosomatic Conditions: Clinical Effectiveness and Psychobiological Underpinnings

The major pathways linking psychological distress to the function of somatic cells throughout the body include the hyperactivity of the sympathetic nervous system, the alteration of hypothalamic–pituitary–adrenal (HPA) axis functioning and the adoption of certain stress-related behaviours (e.g. use of tobacco, alcohol or other substances) [16]. These three pathways are therefore among the major mediators of psychosomatic disturbances and can be targeted or modulated for therapeutic purposes through a range of non-pharmacological interventions.

Accumulating evidence suggests that impaired neuroendocrine physiology at the HPA level in subjects with depressive and anxiety disorders can be affected and restored by psychotherapy [16–18]. A mechanism through which psychotherapy may affect psychobiological responses to stress includes the modulation of cognitive appraisal. Cognitive appraisal, the subjective interpretation of the stressor, has been shown to be crucial in starting the cascade of psychobiological responses to stress: a failure to regulate the biological stress response following a stressful or traumatic episode may result in a cascade of psychobiological alterations that lead to psychiatric symptoms of anxiety and depression associated with increased rates of medical comorbidity (e.g. subjects exposed to chronic psychological stress present decreased immunity measures, high rates of cardiovascular and metabolic disturbances, upregulated inflammatory response, increased oxidative damage and early mortality) [19–22].

Lazarus and Folkman's transactional theory of stress of 1984 proposed that mental appraisals in response to a stressful situation (including the diagnosis of a medical condition such as cancer) were related to health outcomes [23]. Appraisal is a process whereby individuals decide whether stressful situations are threats to their well-being or not (primary appraisals), and determine whether they have the resources to deal with the stressor if it is viewed as a threat (secondary appraisals) [23, 24]. As reported by Bigatti et al. [24], according to Lazarus and Folkman's model primary appraisals are typically categorized as one of four subtypes, based on their effect on well-being: "benign appraisals are made when individuals believe the situation poses no threat to their well-being; harm/loss appraisals are made if an individual believes the stressor has already caused him/her damage; threat appraisals are similar to harm/loss appraisals, except that they are focused on the possibility of future damage; challenge appraisals are made when individuals see the stressful situation as an opportunity for growth or development".

Appraisals may determine the degree and type of biological stress responses, and "threatening" rather than "challenging" stress appraisals may be a psychological mechanism linking psychological stress to health disturbances [19–21]. Subsequently, as summarized in Fig. 14.3, in subjects affected by psychosomatic conditions the modulation of cognitive stress appraisal through psychotherapy can induce a more physiological hormonal HPA response finally resulting in clinical improvements and better health outcomes.

An additional mechanism through which psychotherapy may affect psychobiological responses to stress includes the modulation of resilience and coping styles. It is known that being primary caregivers of a chronically ill person can represent a relevant source of chronic psychological stress that may negatively affect physical and mental health [25]. However, despite the large body of literature on health risks associated with caregiving, preliminary evidence showed that certain resilient attitudes including problem-solving skills, personal mastery, low subjective perception of stress, positive religious coping and positive self-efficacy may contribute to protect caregivers from stress-related psychobiological disturbances [19, 26, 27].

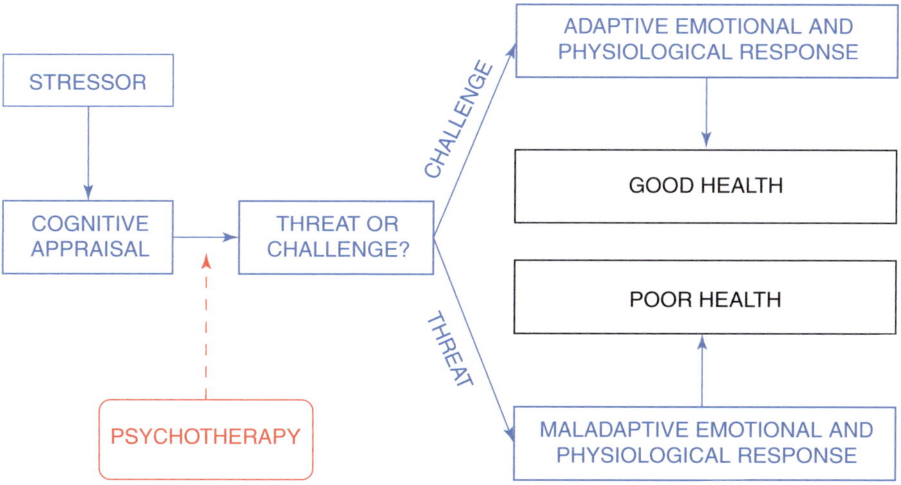

Fig. 14.3 Schematic representation of how psychotherapy can influence health outcomes through the modulation of cognitive appraisals according to Lazarus and Folkman's model

Effective defensive coping may buffer the HPA acute stress response and may protect individuals from being overwhelmed [19, 26, 27]. Therefore it is possible that the condition of caregiving (i.e. chronically high levels of psychological stress) does not represent a deterministic "sentence of unhealthy life" per se, but rather the poor health outcomes of caregivers may at least partially depend on how caregivers respond to the stressors; this aspect can be effectively modulated through psychological approaches.

In relation to medical conditions for which there is a known psychosomatic influence on disease course, accumulating evidence suggests a role of psychotherapy as a treatment to be integrated with other medical and pharmacological interventions.

McCombie et al. in 2013 performed an extended review on the role of psychotherapy in the treatment and clinical management of IBDs [28]. IBDs (Crohn's disease, ulcerative colitis, indeterminate colitis) are chronic relapsing–remitting inflammatory conditions of the intestines, presenting with symptoms of bloody stools, diarrhoea, fatigue, abdominal pain, anaemia, loss of appetite, weight loss and fever [28]. The aetiology of these conditions is unclear, although it is considered to be related to a complex interplay between genetic, environmental and immunological factors [28–30].

Several studies have reported the profound impact of IBDs on the psychological well-being of patients; despite this recognized association, psychiatric comorbidities are often underdiagnosed and undertreated (for a review, see [28]). As pointed out by McCombie et al., psychological characteristics such as neurotic personality, stress or coping styles can influence psychological or disease-related outcomes, while behaviours such as medication adherence or smoking cessation are critical in preventing disease episodes [28]. Therefore, psychotherapies targeting stress management, improving coping strategies and reducing detrimental behaviours may ameliorate psychological well-being and disease course of IBD patients [28].

In the meta-analysis of McCombie et al., which included 18 studies and 924 subjects, the authors found mixed evidence on whether psychotherapy improves anxiety, depression, and quality of life and disease progression, but found psychotherapy to show promise in reducing pain, fatigue, relapse rate and hospitalization, and in improving medication adherence [28].

Preliminary evidence suggesting a role of psychotherapy as a valid treatment option to be integrated with medical interventions have also been found in relation to other psychosomatic conditions such as migraine [31], fibromyalgia [32], tinnitus [33, 34] and certain chronic dermatitis [35]. Interestingly, some form of psychological intervention is nowadays often successfully used also in a range of diseases in which the psychosomatic nature is less evident. For example, the psychoeducational approaches (originally used for subjects with chronic psychiatric conditions, especially bipolar disorder [36]) focused on lifestyle habits are increasingly used in combination with standard treatments in subjects with cardiovascular and metabolic disturbances [37, 38].

Of interest in the field of psychotherapy for medical conditions, specific forms of psychological interventions have been conceptualized in order to specifically address the existential needs of individuals with cancer in advanced phases, such as the supportive-expressive group psychotherapy, the meaning-centred psychotherapy and the dignity therapy (DT). The DT is a recent and specific form of therapy developed by Chochinov and colleagues [39]. As reviewed by Costantini et al., DT addresses the existential needs of patients in palliative care; it is focused on the fundamental theme of dignity as the cornerstone of humanization in medicine [40]. DT is initiated via specific questions such as "Tell me a little of your personal history, the things you remember best; which do you think are most important?" "What would you like your family to know about you; are there things that you would like to be remembered for?" [40]. The individual sessions (which can take place at the bedside of hospitalized patients) are structured in order to highlight aspects of life that have been meaningful for the person, and, in the last session, the therapist, after having transcribed and re-edited them, reads the "manuscript" to the patient [40]. As Costantini et al. point out, *"the aim of the intervention is to draw up a document that represents the "legacy" of the person, something that is meaningful and will survive, thus helping to restore a sense of meaning, value, and dignity"* [40]. A study comparing DT with standard palliative care and client-centred care showed that DT had a significant effect in improving quality of life, increasing sense of dignity and helping the families [40].

14.4 The Molecular Mediators of Cellular Ageing as a Possible New Target of Integrated Intervention in Psychosomatic Medicine

Blackburn and colleagues defined telomeres as tandem repeats of hexameric sequence units (TTAGGG) that, together with protective proteins, cap chromosomal ends and support chromosomal stability and genomic integrity [41–43]. When somatic cells divide, telomeres may not be fully replicated due to the "end replication problem"; subsequently, telomeres tend to shorten over time [41–44]. Blackburn et al have showed that when telomeres shorten sufficiently, cells can become senescent and molecular mechanisms are activated that promote growth arrest, mitochondrial impairment, inflammation, apoptosis and genomic instability [41–43]; furthermore oxidation and inflammation appear to be additional strong telomere shortening stimuli [41–44]. Telomere length is determined also genetically, with heritability estimates ranging from 44 to 80% [45]. It has been observed that human telomere length (TL) (often assessed in leukocytes—LTL) tends to shorten with age unless counterbalanced by telomerase (i.e. the major telomere-lengthening enzyme) or by alternative mechanisms [41–44]. This, plus the fact that short LTL is related to somatic morbidity and premature mortality, suggests that LTL is a mechanistic indicator of "biological age" (as opposed to just "chronological age") and may represent a cumulative log of number of cell divisions and exposure to cytotoxic processes [44–47]. The possible significance of telomere shortening for human disease is highlighted by population studies that have linked shortened LTL to cardiovascular risk and to a number of adverse disease outcomes, including early mortality [48–50].

Telomerase is a reverse transcriptase enzyme that rebuilds telomere length, thereby delaying cell senescence and apoptosis; it exerts its protective action by adding DNA sequence repeats (TTAGGG) onto the 3′ telomeric ends [42, 44]. This regulated action of telomerase is a major mechanism responsible for lengthening and protecting telomeres, thereby maintaining cellular functioning [42, 44]. Blackburn et al have showed that telomerase has a functional RNA component (TERC), which serves as a template for telomeric DNA synthesis, and a catalytic protein component with reverse transcriptase activity (TERT), which adds the telomeric repeats [42]. In addition to its canonical effects on telomere maintenance, telomerase has a variety of TL-independent actions (e.g. induction of growth-promoting factors, induction of DNA methyltransferase I with subsequent epigenetic influences, improvement of mitochondrial function, decreases of reactive oxygen species, DNA repair enhancement) that support cellular survival and/or function [51, 52].

Mitochondria are ubiquitous organelles of eukaryotic systems considered the "power generators" of the cell, converting oxygen, energy substrates and other compounds into adenosine triphosphate [53, 54]. In addition to energy production, mitochondria also play crucial roles in other cellular processes including apoptotic and necrotic cell death, gene expression, and signal transduction [54, 55]. It has been shown that cells of different tissues contain multiple mitochondria, which contain multiple copies of their own genome, i.e. the mitochondrial DNA (mtDNA), encoding 37 genes essential to energy production [56–58]. Changes in the number of mtDNA molecules per cell (namely the mitochondrial DNA copy number—mtDNAcn) are tightly regulated and reflect variations in mitochondrial biogenesis (i.e. the formation of new mitochondria) [57–60]. Reduced mtDNAcn is associated with ageing [57, 61, 62] and somatic morbidity [63–71]. This has recently led to the idea that mtDNAcn is also a novel indicator of "biological age" reflecting variations in mitochondrial energetic function and biogenesis. Consistently with this idea, several molecular pathways mechanistically link mtDNAcn with the telomere-telomerase system. For example, critically shortened telomeres elicit sustained DNA damage responses, such as activation of tumour suppressor protein p53, with outcomes that include decreased expression of PGC-1a (the master regulator of mitochondrial biogenesis) and subsequent decrease of mitochondrial function and mtDNAcn [47, 58, 72]. Further, mtDNAcn has been found directly correlated with LTL in several recent reports [73–76].

TL, telomerase activity (TA) and mtDNAcn have recently been investigated in relation to psychiatric disorders and treatments [47, 58, 44]. An increasing number of studies suggest that several psychological conditions and psychiatric disorders are associated with short LTL, altered TA and reduced mtDNAcn [47, 58, 44]. Despite the underlying mechanisms and the causal direction of these associations are not totally clear yet, this evidence support the idea that, at the cellular level, the telomere-telomerase-mitochondria system is a novel and relevant locus of interest in the interface between psychiatry and medicine, as it may represent a common molecular mediator of both physical and psychiatric disturbances.

Consistently with this several studies have recently been performed on the relationship of psychopharmacology and psychotherapy with the molecular markers of

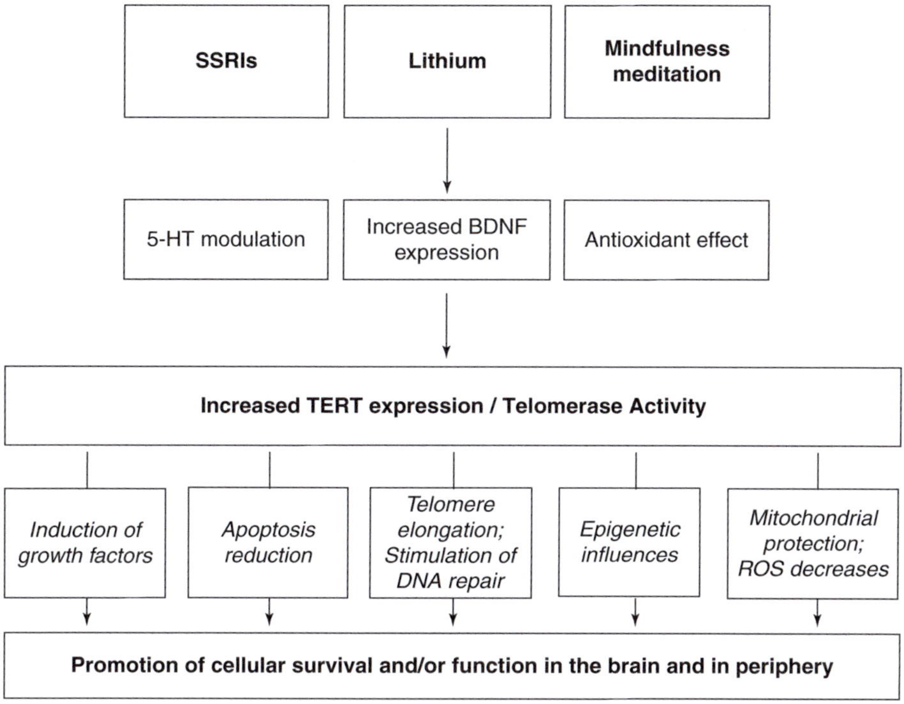

Fig. 14.4 Schematic representation of possible pathways linking psychopharmacology and psychotherapy to the promotion of cellular survival and/or function in the brain and in periphery through the modulation of molecular mediators of ageing. Adapted from [44]

ageing. As summarized in Fig. 14.4, the modulation of intracellular Wnt/b-catenin or PI3K/Akt signalling pathways, the interaction with BDNF and 5-HT, and the antioxidant properties could represent possible mechanisms by which the certain psychiatric medications (mainly SSRIs and lithium) or psychotherapeutic interventions could modulate TA, TL and mtDNAcn [44, 77]. The potential of TA, TL and mtDNAcn in supporting cellular survival and/or function in the brain and in the periphery could, in turn, represent a neurobiological substrate through which these molecules can contribute to mediate the therapeutic effect of such interventions [44, 77].

From a psychotherapeutic perspective, a few pioneering randomized control trials provided information on the effect of mindfulness meditation or mindfulness-based psychotherapy on TA. As reviewed by Schutte and Malouff in 2014, mindfulness is a flexible state of consciousness that consists of non-evaluative awareness [78]. Higher levels of mindfulness are associated with indices of better physical and mental health [78]. Mindfulness meditation consists of practice in processes of attention regulation, body awareness, emotion regulation, and changes in views of the self and others; preliminary evidence suggests that regular practice of mindfulness mindfulness, reduces anxiety, depression and stress, and results in immune-function improvements [78]. In their meta-analysis on 190 subjects,

Schutte and Malouff found (effect size $d = 0.46$) that mindfulness meditation led to significantly increased TA (possible underlying mechanisms are summarized in Fig. 14.4) in peripheral blood mononuclear cells, suggesting therefore that mindfulness-based approaches may be beneficial in a range of somatic, in addition to psychiatric, conditions [78].

14.5 Conclusion

There is accumulating evidence indicating that integrated bio-psycho-social interventions play a crucial role in all areas of medicine and especially in psychosomatic diseases. From a research perspective, in order to better understand the mechanistic underpinnings of psychosomatics it is important to develop translational skills and to integrate findings from neuroscience, experimental psychology, physiology, genetics, pharmacology and molecular biology [3]. From a clinical perspective, psychosomatic medicine integrates interdisciplinary evaluation and management involving diverse specialties ranging from psychiatry to internal medicine. It is therefore important for psychiatrists to undergo specific training to be able to treat psychosomatic conditions with an integrated approach, and it is important for health institutions to set up specific clinical services of consultation-liaison psychiatry.

As reviewed by Kornfeld, in 1937 Billings et al. reported that their psychiatric consultation-liaison service at Denver General Hospital reduced the overall length of patients' stays from 28 to 16 days, with subsequent substantial reduction of costs [79]. Since then, similar findings have been obtained in several other studies, indicating that the presence of consultation-liaison psychiatrists, i.e. health professionals specifically trained in psychosomatic medicine, can lead to relevant cost–benefit advantages [79].

Now and in the future, "*the psychiatric needs of patients will always exist, astute clinical observations remain to be made and studied, and new effective interventions will need to be instituted*" [79]. Trained consultation-liaison psychiatrists or psychosomatic medicine specialists should therefore be increasingly included in all aspects of medicine in order to successfully face the complexity of the bio-psycho-social aspects of health and disease.

References

1. American Psychiatric Association. Diagnostic and statistical manual of mental disorders. 5th ed. Washington, DC: American Psychiatric Association; 2013.
2. Biondi M, Bersani FS, Valentini M. The Italian edition of DSM-5Riv Psichiatr. 2014;49(2):57–60.
3. Levenson JL. Essentials of psychosomatic medicine. Arlington, VA: American Psychiatric Press; 2006.
4. Prince M, et al. No health without mental health. Lancet. 2007;370(9590):859–77.
5. Biondi M. Beyond the brain-mind dichotomy and toward a common organizing principle of pharmacological and psychological treatments. Psychother Psychosom. 1995;64(1):1–8.

6. World Health Organization. Mental health: new understanding, new hope. 2001.
7. Helzer JE, et al. Dimensional approaches in diagnostic classification. Refining the research agenda for DSM-V. Arlington, VA: American Psychiatric Association; 2008.
8. Biondi M, Pasquini M. Dimensional psychopharmacology in somatising patients. Adv Psychosom Med. 2015;34:24–35.
9. Biondi M, et al. Dimensional psychopathology of depression: detection of an 'activation' dimension in unipolar depressed outpatients. J Affect Disord. 2005;84(2–3):133–9.
10. Dazzi F, et al. Predictors of inpatient psychiatric admission in patients presenting to the emergency department: the role of dimensional assessment. Gen Hosp Psychiatry. 2015;37(6):587–94.
11. Pancheri P, et al. Validazione della scala per la valutazione rapida dimensionale "SVARAD". Riv Psichiatr. 1999;34:84–93.
12. Pasquini M, et al. Detection and treatment of depressive and anxiety disorders among cancer patients: feasibility and preliminary findings from a liaison service in an oncology division. Depress Anxiety. 2006;23(7):441–8.
13. Pasquini M, et al. Relevance of anger and irritability in outpatients with major depressive disorder. Psychopathology. 2004;37(4):155–60.
14. Pasquini M, et al. Combining an SSRI with an anticonvulsant in depressed patients with dysphoric mood: an open study. Clin Pract Epidemiol Ment Health. 2007;3:3.
15. Pancheri P, et al. Costruzione della "SVARAD", una scala per la valutazione rapida dimensionale. Riv Psichiatr. 1999;34:72–83.
16. McEwen BS. The neurobiology of stress: from serendipity to clinical relevance. Brain Res. 2000;886(1–2):172–89.
17. Olff M, et al. Changes in cortisol and DHEA plasma levels after psychotherapy for PTSD. Psychoneuroendocrinology. 2007;32(6):619–26.
18. Fischer S, Cleare AJ. Cortisol as a predictor of psychological therapy response in anxiety disorders-systematic review and meta-analysis. J Anxiety Disord. 2017;47:60–8.
19. Epel E, et al. Can meditation slow rate of cellular aging? Cognitive stress, mindfulness, and telomeres. Ann N Y Acad Sci. 2009;1172:34–53.
20. O'Donovan A, et al. Stress appraisals and cellular aging: a key role for anticipatory threat in the relationship between psychological stress and telomere length. Brain Behav Immun. 2012;26(4):573–9.
21. Kessler TA. The cognitive appraisal of health scale: development of psychometric evaluation. Res Nurs Health. 1998;21(1):73–82.
22. Levine AB, Levine LM, Levine TB. Posttraumatic stress disorder and cardiometabolic disease. Cardiology. 2014;127(1):1–19.
23. Lazarus RS, Folkman S. Stress, appraisal, and coping. Berlin: Springer; 1984.
24. Bigatti SM, Steiner JL, Miller KD. Cognitive appraisals, coping and depressive symptoms in breast cancer patients. Stress Health. 2012;28(5):355–61.
25. Lin FY, Rong JR, Lee TY. Resilience among caregivers of children with chronic conditions: a concept analysis. J Multidiscip Healthc. 2013;6:323–33.
26. Harmell AL, et al. A review of the psychobiology of dementia caregiving: a focus on resilience factors. Curr Psychiatry Rep. 2011;13(3):219–24.
27. Schulz R, Beach SR. Caregiving as a risk factor for mortality: the caregiver health effects study. JAMA. 1999;282(23):2215–9.
28. McCombie AM, Mulder RT, Gearry RB. Psychotherapy for inflammatory bowel disease: a review and update. J Crohns Colitis. 2013;7(12):935–49.
29. Gearry RB, et al. Population-based cases control study of inflammatory bowel disease risk factors. J Gastroenterol Hepatol. 2010;25(2):325–33.
30. Bouma G, Strober W. The immunological and genetic basis of inflammatory bowel disease. Nat Rev Immunol. 2003;3(7):521–33.
31. Nicholson RA. Chronic headache: the role of the psychologist. Curr Pain Headache Rep. 2010;14(1):47–54.
32. Lumley MA. Beyond cognitive-behavioral therapy for fibromyalgia: addressing stress by emotional exposure, processing, and resolution. Arthritis Res Ther. 2011;13(6):136.

33. Salviati M, et al. A brain centred view of psychiatric comorbidity in tinnitus: from otology to hodology. Neural Plast. 2014;2014:817852.
34. Salviati M, et al. Tinnitus: clinical experience of the psychosomatic connection. Neuropsychiatr Dis Treat. 2014;10:267–75.
35. Hanifin JM, et al. Guidelines of care for atopic dermatitis, developed in accordance with the American Academy of Dermatology (AAD)/American Academy of Dermatology Association "Administrative Regulations for Evidence-Based Clinical Practice Guidelines". J Am Acad Dermatol. 2004;50(3):391–404.
36. Colom F. The evolution of psychoeducation for bipolar disorder: from lithium clinics to integrative psychoeducation. World Psychiatry. 2014;13(1):90–2.
37. Adams RJ. Improving health outcomes with better patient understanding and education. Risk Manag Healthc Policy. 2010;3:61–72.
38. Bersani FS, et al. Psychoeducational intervention focused on healthy living improves psychopathological severity and lifestyle quality in psychiatric patients: preliminary findings from a controlled study. J Ment Health. 2017;26(3):271–5.
39. Chochinov HM, et al. Dignity therapy: a novel psychotherapeutic intervention for patients near the end of life. J Clin Oncol. 2005;23(24):5520–5.
40. Costantini A, Levenson JA, Bersani FS. In: Wise TN, Biondi M, Costantini A, editors. The crisis of discovery—psychological and psychopathological reaction to the disease, in psycho-oncology. Washington, DC: American Psychiatric Association; 2013.
41. Blackburn EH. Telomere states and cell fates. Nature. 2000;408(6808):53–6.
42. Blackburn EH. Telomeres and telomerase: the means to the end (Nobel lecture). Angew Chem Int Ed Engl. 2010;49(41):7405–21.
43. Blackburn EH, Greider CW, Szostak JW. Telomeres and telomerase: the path from maize, Tetrahymena and yeast to human cancer and aging. Nat Med. 2006;12(10):1133–8.
44. Bersani FS, et al. Telomerase activation as a possible mechanism of action for psychopharmacological interventions. Drug Discov Today. 2015;20(11):1305–9.
45. Starkweather AR, et al. An integrative review of factors associated with telomere length and implications for biobehavioral research. Nurs Res. 2014;63(1):36–50.
46. Bersani FS, et al. Association of dimensional psychological health measures with telomere length in male war veterans. J Affect Disord. 2016;190:537–42.
47. Lindqvist D, et al. Psychiatric disorders and leukocyte telomere length: underlying mechanisms linking mental illness with cellular aging. Neurosci Biobehav Rev. 2015;55:333–64.
48. Martin-Ruiz C, et al. Telomere length predicts poststroke mortality, dementia, and cognitive decline. Ann Neurol. 2006;60(2):174–80.
49. Cawthon RM, et al. Association between telomere length in blood and mortality in people aged 60 years or older. Lancet. 2003;361(9355):393–5.
50. Fitzpatrick AL, et al. Leukocyte telomere length and cardiovascular disease in the cardiovascular health study. Am J Epidemiol. 2007;165(1):14–21.
51. Gorbunova V, Seluanov A. Telomerase as a growth-promoting factor. Cell Cycle. 2003;2(6):534–7.
52. Saretzki G. Extra-telomeric functions of human telomerase: cancer, mitochondria and oxidative stress. Curr Pharm Des. 2014;20(41):6386–403.
53. Scheffler IE. Mitochondria make a come back. Adv Drug Deliv Rev. 2001;49(1–2):3–26.
54. Johannsen DL, Ravussin E. The role of mitochondria in health and disease. Curr Opin Pharmacol. 2009;9(6):780–6.
55. Kasahara A, Scorrano L. Mitochondria: from cell death executioners to regulators of cell differentiation. Trends Cell Biol. 2014;24(12):761–70.
56. Campbell CT, Kolesar JE, Kaufman BA. Mitochondrial transcription factor a regulates mitochondrial transcription initiation, DNA packaging, and genome copy number. Biochim Biophys Acta. 2012;1819(9–10):921–9.
57. Clay Montier LL, Deng JJ, Bai Y. Number matters: control of mammalian mitochondrial DNA copy number. J Genet Genomics. 2009;36(3):125–31.

58. Bersani FS, et al. Mitochondrial DNA copy number is reduced in male combat veterans with PTSD. Prog Neuro-Psychopharmacol Biol Psychiatry. 2016;64:10–7.
59. Lee HC, Wei YH. Mitochondrial biogenesis and mitochondrial DNA maintenance of mammalian cells under oxidative stress. Int J Biochem Cell Biol. 2005;37(4):822–34.
60. Moyes C, Battersby B. Regulation of muscle mitochondrial design. J Exp Biol. 1998;201(3):299–307.
61. Laderman KA, et al. Aging-dependent functional alterations of mitochondrial DNA (mtDNA) from human fibroblasts transferred into mtDNA-less cells. J Biol Chem. 1996;271(27):15891–7.
62. Bratic A, Larsson NG. The role of mitochondria in aging. J Clin Invest. 2013;123(3):951–7.
63. Blokhin A, et al. Variations in mitochondrial DNA copy numbers in MS brains. J Mol Neurosci. 2008;35(3):283–7.
64. Choi YS, Kim S, Pak YK. Mitochondrial transcription factor A (mtTFA) and diabetes. Diabetes Res Clin Pract. 2001;54(Suppl 2):S3–9.
65. Kim JH, Im JA, Lee DC. The relationship between leukocyte mitochondrial DNA contents and metabolic syndrome in postmenopausal women. Menopause. 2012;19(5):582–7.
66. Lee HK, et al. Decreased mitochondrial DNA content in peripheral blood precedes the development of non-insulin-dependent diabetes mellitus. Diabetes Res Clin Pract. 1998;42(3):161–7.
67. Macmillan CJ, Shoubridge EA. Mitochondrial DNA depletion: prevalence in a pediatric population referred for neurologic evaluation. Pediatr Neurol. 1996;14(3):203–10.
68. Morten KJ, et al. Liver mtDNA content increases during development: a comparison of methods and the importance of age- and tissue-specific controls for the diagnosis of mtDNA depletion. Mitochondrion. 2007;7(6):386–95.
69. Tiao MM, et al. Early stage of biliary atresia is associated with significant changes in 8-hydroxydeoxyguanosine and mitochondrial copy number. J Pediatr Gastroenterol Nutr. 2007;45(3):329–34.
70. Xing J, et al. Mitochondrial DNA content: its genetic heritability and association with renal cell carcinoma. J Natl Cancer Inst. 2008;100(15):1104–12.
71. Yu M, et al. Reduced mitochondrial DNA copy number is correlated with tumor progression and prognosis in Chinese breast cancer patients. IUBMB Life. 2007;59(7):450–7.
72. Saretzki G. Telomerase, mitochondria and oxidative stress. Exp Gerontol. 2009;44(8):485–92.
73. Kim JH, et al. The relationship between leukocyte mitochondrial DNA copy number and telomere length in community-dwelling elderly women. PLoS One. 2013;8(6):e67227.
74. Tyrka AR, et al. Association of telomere length and mitochondrial DNA copy number in a community sample of healthy adults. Exp Gerontol. 2015;66:17–20.
75. Pieters N, et al. Molecular responses in the telomere-mitochondrial axis of ageing in the elderly: a candidate gene approach. Mech Ageing Dev. 2015;145:51–7.
76. Tyrka AR, et al. Alterations of mitochondrial DNA copy number and telomere length with early adversity and psychopathology. Biol Psychiatry. 2016;79(2):78–86.
77. Hough CM, et al. Leukocyte telomere length predicts SSRI response in major depressive disorder: a preliminary report. Mol Neuropsychiatry. 2016;2(2):88–96.
78. Schutte NS, Malouff JM. A meta-analytic review of the effects of mindfulness meditation on telomerase activity. Psychoneuroendocrinology. 2014;42:45–8.
79. Kornfeld DS. Consultation-liaison psychiatry: contributions to medical practice. Am J Psychiatry. 2002;159(12):1964–72.

Ethical Counselling for a Patient-Centred Approach in the Context of Psychosomatic Medicine

15

Giovanni Boniolo

> *Even if one manages to comprehend biological, psychological, and social findings and to describe them in their respective languages, even if a method for the analysis of their mutual relationship has been created, there is still no answer to the pertinent question: Why did this person fall ill at this moment? (Langewitz [1], p. 434; for detailed information on psychosomatic medicine, see also von Uexküll [2])*

Abstract

There is an increasing demand for help whenever ethical problems intersect clinical decisions, in particular decisions within psychosomatic medicine. In this chapter, we show how an ethical counselling centred on the needs and on the biographies of the patients could ameliorate their decisional process concerning which clinical option should be pursued. And, of course, the ethical counselling approach we propose does not diminish patient autonomy but, actually, increases patient empowerment.

G. Boniolo
Dipartimento di Scienze Biomediche e Chirurgico Specialistiche, Università di Ferrara, Ferrara, Italy
e-mail: bnlgnn@unife.it

L. Grassi et al. (eds.), *Person Centered Approach to Recovery in Medicine*, Integrating Psychiatry and Primary Care, https://doi.org/10.1007/978-3-319-74736-1_15

15.1 Ethical Counselling and Ethical Problems in Psychosomatic Medicine

An increasing number of physicians, health-care providers, patients and their families are turning to ethics consultants as they increasingly face moral questions that require professional appraisal.[1] As few physicians have been trained to help solve clinical ethical problems, a movement towards providing ethics consultation has grown in the past decades.[2] Consultants can help health-care teams with complex matters that often accompany cases involving issues like patient autonomy or informed consent. According to the American Society for Bioethics and Humanities (ASBH), ethics consultation can be defined as "the identification, analysis and resolution of ethical issues as they emerge in clinical cases in healthcare institutions".[3]

Especially in the context of psychosomatic patients, it seems to be necessary to develop an appropriate ethic dimension to sufficiently deal with the patient and his/her problems and causes.[4]

Psychosomatic medicine, as a subspecialty of psychiatry, deals with the interface of psychological, ethical, social and legal issues arising in clinical medicine.[5] One of its primary goals is "the incorporation of its operational strategies into clinical practice. […] Only recently, there has been increasing awareness of the limitations of disease as the primary focus of medical care. It is not that certain disorders lack an organic explanation; it is our assessment that is inadequate in most clinical encounters."[6]

Therefore and due to the complex nature of this area, it is necessary to provide both clinicians and patients with suitable approaches for ethical counselling.

But what would be a suitable approach? First of all, the ethical counselling should be seen not as "an imposition but a disposition of values".[7]

This leads us to a second question: What is an ethical problem? According to Salloch et al., the identification of ethical problems in medicine "is a theoretically and methodologically demanding enterprise which should not be exclusively dominated by the perspective of ethical theory but develops methods for integrating lay and expert perspectives."[8] The problems that medical ethics take care of stand out due to the fact that they confront the players with actual and practically relevant challenges. Ethical problems don't necessarily exist in an objective way but are named by persons affected or by researchers or physicians involved. At times, patients experience a treatment situation as ethically problematic, while the practitioner, who is captivated in his routines, does not perceive any deficiency. The ethical counsellor who is approaching the situation from an external perspective brings

[1] Arnold et al. [3], pp. 69–69.

[2] La Puma [4], p. 633.

[3] Gaucher et al. [5], p. 75.

[4] Ponesicky [6], p. 16.

[5] Patel et al. [7], p. 63. For a detailed analysis of the challenges psychosomatic medicine can possess see: Ibid., pp. 63ff.

[6] Fava et al. [8], p. 333.

[7] Thomasma [9], p. 138.

[8] Salloch et al. [10], p. 268.

in an additional perspective. He/she can be aware of ethical deficits which are not perceived as such by other participants.[9]

Psychosomatic medicine has specialized in understanding not only the rational elements of ethical reasoning but also the irrational elements, as ethical conflicts in this context arise in situations of emotional stress and conflict. Therefore reflecting on ethical problems in the practice of psychosomatic medicine will "improve the patient's functioning, improve the care of his family and community"[10] and lead to a better assessing of the patient's and the practitioner's interests and problems.

In what follows, we present a particular approach to the *ethical counselling* developed over the years[11] and intended as *a dialogic activity implementable in the cases in which clinical decisions involve ethical issues. It always involves the presence of two actors—the ethical counsellor and the counselee—and it has two different purposes. On the one hand, by clarifying and investigating patients' point of view, it assists them (with or without their relatives) to break through their ethical decisional paralysis in clinical settings and to choose the option more in line with their ethical sensitivity. On the other hand, it trains clinicians to properly examine the ethical problematic situation that their patients are facing, in order to go beyond their commonsensical and intuitive moral understanding and to avoid the dangerous conviction that their own point of view is better than patients' one.*

Moreover in our conception, ethical counselling should not be thought of as a form of psychological support, even if, being directed towards patients beliefs, it might cross with some psychological aspects. It is not aimed at providing solutions. Rather, it is conceived as a "way of cleaning the windows" in order to look deeper through ethical problems. This, in turn, is done to allow patients to be more aware of their choices and clinicians of the situation they are addressing. It should be considered as a tool by means of which the counsellor serves the patient or the clinician (according to two different methodologies, as we will see) to reflect and thus to tame the first intuitive answer. Note that this *reflection slot* between the rising of the problem and the proposal of the possible solution allows also for a critical examination of the representation of the clinical event the patient is living. Usually, human beings have a starting representation of the event at issue, and they proceed to make a moral evaluation based on it. Thus, if an ethical counsellor introduces time to discuss such a representation, this could be better considered or reconsidered, and, probably, a better moral evaluation and solution could come out.

15.2 Ethical Counselling for Patients

Philosophy has derogatorily been considered as a purely theoretical discipline without any impact on real life: mere words and thoughts without any effect on the practice, very far from the empirical results found in biology, or the treatments offered in the clinics. In contrast, the idea lying behind the proposal of ethical

[9] Ibid., p. 273.

[10] Barbosa [11], pp. 224, 226, 234.

[11] See Boniolo and Sanchini [12].

counselling for patients is precisely inspired by the opposite conviction, namely, that philosophy is a life-changing enterprise having a relevant bearing on human relations. This idea has a long-standing tradition within the history of philosophy.

If we are willing to accept what Pierre Hadot (*Exercices Spirituels Et Philosophie Antique*) or Martha Nussbaum (*The Therapy of Desire*)—to name just a few—suggested, philosophy ceases to be considered as a mere theoretical enterprise and starts to acquire a pivotal role in orienteering our choices and life. This is precisely the line of thought upon which our approach to ethical counselling is grounded. Indeed, philosophical reasoning can play a very important role in the improvement of human decision-making. This occurs in particular when some philosophical issues are involved, as it happens when clinical decisions intersect ethical questions.

By taking into consideration this point, we propose a methodology grounded upon the history of philosophy, which could be applied whenever clinical decision-making crosses with ethical decision-making. This methodology is directed *towards the patient* who finds himself/herself confronted with a difficult ethical decision or an ethical dilemma and voluntarily asks for a consultation. We distinguish it from another methodology that we are going to present in a while, which is addressed *to clinicians*. Notably, these two methodologies differ, not just because they are directed towards two different kinds of stakeholders but also because their respective aims are different. The methodology presented in this section aims at helping patients in making decisions that are consonant with their values and beliefs. The next methodological section aims at providing clinicians with a tool to support a patient's decision-making on the ethical issues he/she has to cope with.

15.2.1 Aristotelian Practical Philosophy

The Aristotelian approach of practical philosophy is at the basis of our view on ethical counselling for patients. Very briefly, the term "practical philosophy" appears for the first time in *Metaphysics* (II, 1, 993 b 19–23), where Aristotle distinguishes it from metaphysics (the first philosophy or theoretical philosophy). The latter has as its main purpose the investigation of truth, whereas the former deals with human action (*praxis*) in order to ameliorate it (*eupraxia*) and, thus, to improve human agency.

The place in which Aristotle better develops his account of practical philosophy is, however, the *Nicomachean Ethics*. At the end of *Book I*, he distinguishes between the intellectual and the ethical virtues. The former have to do with reason (*dianoia*) and the latter (the moral excellences, *areté*) with characters, customs and behaviours (*ethos*). In the central *Book VI*, he claims that philosophical wisdom (*sophia*) is the virtue of theoretical philosophy, while practical wisdom (*phronesis*) is the virtue of practical philosophy. By *practical wisdom* Aristotle means man's capacity to deliberate well, that is, the ability to ponder our goals in life and the most effective means to reach them. Practical philosophy consists in the *examination* of the different opinions that are on the stage in order to find out the best one/s through practical wisdom.

A last point is necessary in order to complete the picture. A good decision-maker is someone who necessarily possesses another ethical virtue: temperance (*sophrosyne*). This is the virtue that prevents passions from ruining a proper deliberation.

Summing up, in order to bring about a good decision, one should (1) *control* the irrational part with the help of temperance; (2) *examine* the situation from a rational standpoint, therefore evaluating the epistemological plausibility and the logical tenability of the pros and the cons of each option; and (3) *deliberate* with the help of one's practical wisdom, in favour of what constitutes the best option for him/her.

These three conditions are of extreme importance for us since we consider them the peculiar features of our own account of ethical counselling. Indeed, whenever a patient finds himself/herself in the condition to have to opt for an ethical decision or to solve an ethical dilemma concerning a diagnostic or therapeutic path, the ethical counsellor should exercise an advisory role and, in particular, help the patient to tame his/her emotions and examine, in the Aristotelian sense, his/her possible moral options and their consequences and finally assist the patient to use his/her practical wisdom and thus to individuate what constitutes for him/her the best decision and course of action.

15.2.2 Methodology

Ethical counselling for patients is therefore a service aimed at unlocking a patient's decisional paralysis when addressing clinical choices, imbued with ethical beliefs. Ethical counselling for patients is articulated in an ordered succession of four well-defined phases: (1) *relational phase*, (2) *medical assessment phase*, (3) *ethical analysis phase* and (4) *wrap-up phase*.

1. *Relational phase*. The ethical counsellor starts creating a cooperative relationship by explaining the goals of this service and individuating the aim of the colloquium with the patient. In particular, in this first phase the ethical counsellor presents the ethical counselling as a discretionary service at the patient's disposal. This, in turn, means briefly explaining to the patient that ethical counselling focuses on ethical dilemmas arising in the clinical setting. Moreover, the ethical counsellor tells the patient that the very general aim of this consultation is to identify and assess his/her ethical problematic situation.
2. *Medical assessment phase*. The ethical counsellor focuses on the patient's knowledge in order to verify if he/she is provided with the relevant medical information to make a properly informed choice. Especially in the context of psychosomatic medicine, this might be a difficult task which requires a lot of empathy and a certain amount of psychiatric specialized knowledge on the part of the counsellor. If the patient is uninformed, the ethical counsellor may ask him/her to obtain permission to consult the physician to clarify any aspect left unclear. Obviously, the patient should not perceive this process as if someone is trying to verify his/her knowledge. By contrast, it is very important that the ethical counsellor sets up this process in a dialogic and sympathetic manner.
3. *Ethical analysis phase*. Once the examination of the medical aspects is concluded, the ethical counsellor supports the patient to analyse his/her ethical dilemma. This is done by helping him/her to investigate all the available options from an ethical standpoint. Fleshing out the values promoted or privileged by any option could help in gaining a different and more complete picture of the decisional scenario.

4. *Wrap-up phase*. The ethical counsellor summarizes what has been found asking the patient whether he/she is satisfied or whether a phase of the counselling process needs to be rerun. It is important to note that even if the aim is to break a decisional paralysis, it is not necessary that the patient makes a decision by the end of the colloquium. In other words, the important feature here is that he/she has fairly clear ideas regarding the options at stake, thus having gained all the relevant elements he/she might need in order to make a choice.

15.3 Ethical Counselling for Physicians

We have just briefly discussed a methodology of ethical counselling directed towards patients. However, ethical counselling—partially modified—appears to have some benefits not only for patients but also for those indirectly affected by ethical problematic situations, i.e. physicians.

There are several reasons why health-care providers ask for ethical counselling: be it assistance in decision-making, assistance in case management or assistance in resolving disagreements—consultants in clinical ethics should be competent in both medicine and ethics and have strong interpersonal and communications abilities to help physicians reach ethical solutions in a broad range of cases.[12]

Indeed, extensive literature exists as to the importance of considering the physician not only as the professional figure that is expected to cure patients but also as a partner for both therapeutic and nontherapeutic decisions in care pathways. Ethical counselling requires ethical assessment skills (to identify and analyse ethical issues emerging in clinical cases), process skills (to resolve uncertainties and conflicts in health-care settings) and interpersonal skills.[13]

In addition to the skills mentioned here, ethical counsellors must have at their disposal knowledge in areas like bioethical concepts, clinical context, relevant policies and health law—to name just a few.[14]

When directed towards clinicians, ethical counselling is rather aimed at elucidating a case also from an ethical standpoint, so as to allow them to deal appropriately with patients' ethical questions. This does not mean that physicians are supposed to be provided with as much ethical knowledge as an ethicist is supposed to have. Rather, they should be given the ethical knowledge that enables them establishing, also very generally, the framework within which a case they are facing is ethically located.

This recognition implies that ethical counselling for physicians has to be structured differently from the one envisaged for patients. More specifically, we propose that ethical counselling for professionals be rooted in the Medieval *disputatio* and, in particular, in its first part: the *status quaestionis*, that is, the presentation of the problem and of its justified solutions. The physician facing a patient's ethical questions should not try to solve them but to be informed about the wider moral context. Since physicians ought just to help the patient deciding according to his/her personal

[12] La Puma [4], p. 636.

[13] Arnold et al. [3], pp. 59–69.

[14] Ibid.

philosophy, it could be useful for the former to understand the dilemma in its entirety and complexity with the guidance of a well-constructed ethical counselling service.

15.3.1 The Medieval Origin

Universities, since their origin in the twelfth century, were the institutional places in which knowledge was both produced and transmitted from mentors to disciples. They have been the cornerstones on which modern and contemporary sciences and humanities have been built. Although each medieval university had its own regulation, there was a certain degree of homogeneity to be discovered in the didactic structure, based on *lectiones* (lectures) and *disputationes* (disputes).

The *disputatio* was structured as a debate between two students of an equal level of education and chaired by a master. This latter introduced a topic (*casus* or *thema*) and posed a question (*problema* or *quaestio*). Then, one of the students, the *opponens* (or *impugnans*), had to offer some arguments to which the other student, the *respondens* (or *defendens*), had to reply with counterarguments. In the end, the master stopped the dispute by proposing his view and his arguments, which were considered as the *determinatio* or *solutio*.

Therefore, the medieval student was first and foremost asked to expose the *status quaestionis*, by going through the following steps:

1. *Outline the relevant context* (situating the problem).
2. *Briefly state the problem to be addressed* (to emphasize the issue and to show that what was under discussion was well-understood).
3. *Define the terms to be used* (to eliminate any possible source of terminological ambiguity or confusion).
4. *Show the relevance of the problem and the impact of its solution* (to underline that no irrelevant issue had to be addressed).
5. *Expose the solutions which are alternative to the one you want to support and argue why they are not acceptable.*
6. Finally, *formulate the solution.*

After the presentation of the *status quaestionis*, the student had to argue in favour of his proposed solution. To sum up, two steps were therefore considered essential for the proper examination of an issue: (1) exposition of the *status quaestionis* and (2) exposition of the justification of the proposed solution.[15]

15.3.2 Methodological Proposal and Conclusion

As already said, ethical counselling—when devised for clinicians—deals much more with problem-conceptualizing rather than with problem-solving. The methodology hereby presented is primarily aimed at guiding clinicians to have the most

[15] On this method and on its pervasiveness and usefulness, see Boniolo [13].

complete picture of the ethical dilemma they are confronted with, so that they can non-paternalistically deal with the patients and/or their relatives. By taking all of this into consideration, the first step of a well-constructed *disputatio*, that is, the presentation of the *status quaestionis*, is exactly what meets our needs. This means that ethical counselling for clinicians should move, in a series of meetings, along the following seven phases:

1. *Presentation of the clinical case.* Here the physician is asked to present the case from a clinical standpoint, to have an overall medical picture of the problem to be addressed and of the possible clinical paths the patient might decide to follow.
2. *Presentation of the consequences for the patient to choose in favour of one medical option over another.* Here the physician is asked to present what the clinical consequences of the possible options are. This is done in order to clarify the data and to ground the following ethical analysis on qualified scientific information.
3. *Presentation of the ethical issues raised by the clinical case.* Here the ethical counsellor helps the physician to examine an ethical dilemma behind the case to map it also from an ethical point of view.
4. *Definition of the ethical terms.* Before analysing the case from an ethical standpoint, the ethical counsellor properly defines the main terms to be used. This step is essential in order to avoid any possible source of semantic ambiguity or lexical confusion.
5. *Presentation of the ethical arguments in favour and against each medical option the patient might decide to follow.* Here the ethical counsellor, in a dialogue with the physician, puts on the table all the ethical pros and cons of each medical alternative the patient might pursue. This is done in order to allow the physician to clarify all the possible ethical standpoints in the specific case and allow him/her to make a preliminary trade-off between both ethical values and medical options for the case under consideration.
6. *Examination of the patient's beliefs.* Here the counsellor helps the physician to understand whether the patient has ideological, philosophical or religious beliefs that could influence his/her decision-making process and shift the balance in favour of one option over another.
7. *Conclusive summary.* In this last step, the ethical counsellor proposes an ethical summary of the case in question to the clinician to be sure that he/she has a complete ethical picture of the case.

Conclusions

According to our point of view, the ethical counselling has not to be a mandatory tool that has to be imposed on patients. Instead, it might be proposed to them and they might use it, in case they feel the necessity for it. Differently, some nudges to undergo an ethical counselling process seem to be necessary for clinicians, since an intuitive moral understanding does not prove to be enough in problematic cases involving patients.

However, it remains to accentuate once more that the strategy of ethical counselling described here needs to comply with the characteristics of psychosomatic medicine, and this could be a new field of empirical and theoretical studies. Do not forget, indeed, that physicians—in whatever domain they work— "constantly have to strike a balance between the realm of the uncertain and of subjective facts, which can at best be articulated on one's own behalf, and the realm of objective facts, which everyone can articulate as long as he[/she] is knowledgeable enough and able to express himself[/herself] sufficiently".[16]

Nevertheless, proposing an ethical counselling structured as the above, one means proposing a patient-centred approach where *patients come first*, i.e., patients' quality of life and the imbricated quality of their decisional processes, especially now in the age of patient empowerment.

References

1. Langewitz W. A theory of psychosomatic medicine: an attempt at an explanatory summary. Semiotica. 2009;173:431–52.
2. von Uexküll T. Lehrbuch der Psychosomatischen Medizin. Munich: Urban and Schwarzenberg; 1979.
3. Arnold R, et al. Health care ethics consultation: nature, goals, and competencies: a position paper from the Society for Health and Human Values-Society for bioethics consultation task force on standards for bioethics consultation. Ann Intern Med. 2000;133:59–69.
4. La Puma J. Consultations in clinical ethics—issues and questions in 27 cases. West J Med. 1987;146:633–7.
5. Gaucher N, et al. How do national guidelines frame clinical ethics practice? A comparative analysis of guidelines from the US, the UK, Canada and France. Soc Sci Med. 2013;85:74–8.
6. Ponesicky J. Psychotherapie und Ethik—Der psychosomatische Patient und sein Arzt. Balint. 2003;4:16–8.
7. Patel K, Weinrieb R. Ethical and legal aspects of psychosomatic medicine. J Psychiatry Law. 2012;40:63–74.
8. Fava G, Sonino N. Psychosomatic assessment. Psychother Psychosom. 2009;78:333–41.
9. Thomasma D. Why philosophers should offer ethics consultations. Theor Med. 1991;12:129–40.
10. Salloch S, et al. Was ist ein ethisches Problem und wie finde ich es? Theoretische, methodologische und forschungspraktische Fragen der Identifikation ethischer Probleme am Beispiel einer empirisch-ethischen Interventionsstudie. Ethik Med. 2016;28:267–81.
11. Barbosa A. Relational ethics and psychosomatic assessment. Adv Psychosom Med. 2012;32:223–39.
12. Boniolo G, Sanchini V, editors. Ethical counselling and medical decision-making in the era of personalized medicine. Heidelberg: Springer; 2016.
13. Boniolo G. The art of deliberating. democracy, deliberation and the life sciences between history and theory. Heidelberg: Springer; 2012.

[16] Langewitz [1], p. 448.

Organization of Psychosomatic Service in Health Systems: The German Perspective

16

Stephan Zipfel, Anne Herrmann-Werner, and Florian Junne

Abstract

Psychosomatic Medicine in Germany is either practiced as an integrated approach in mainly internal medicine or specifically focusses on psychotherapeutic methods. There are stepped levels of training for doctors ranging from basic care as a GP to specialist degrees. Patients are treated in inpatient and day-patient facilities with usually interprofessional multi-modal therapy programs. Additionally there are rehabilitation centers particularly focusing on work-related aspects of disability prevention. Usually, hospitals also host a strong psychosomatic outpatient sector and consultation-liaison service including specific care e.g. in psycho-oncology or transplant psychosomatics.

16.1 Introduction

Psychosomatic medicine in Germany is rooted in two traditions—one of an integrated psychosomatic approach mainly based in internal medicine and a second one focusing on psychotherapeutic and psychiatric methods. As a consequence psychosomatic medicine in Germany is not a synonym for consultation-liaison psychiatry but represents a comprehensive field [1] as well as a specialized medical discipline [2].

This development is reflected by the foundation of the German College of Psychosomatic Medicine (DKPM) founded by internists and psychotherapists [3] in 1974 in close relation to thoughts and activities of the International College of

S. Zipfel (✉) · A. Herrmann-Werner · F. Junne
Department of Psychosomatic Medicine and Psychotherapy, University Medical Hospital, Tuebingen, Germany
e-mail: Stephan.Zipfel@med.uni-tuebingen.de

L. Grassi et al. (eds.), *Person Centered Approach to Recovery in Medicine*, Integrating Psychiatry and Primary Care, https://doi.org/10.1007/978-3-319-74736-1_16

Psychosomatic Medicine [2]. This college (with about 400 members today) was and is an interdisciplinary, integrative scientific professional association with activities in the whole field of medicine for doctors, psychologists and other professions. In this time—as a main aim of DKPM—grew up close co-operations to many psychosomatic societies of other specialties (e.g. general practitioners, gynaecologists, dermatologists, orthopaedists) and with psychological societies (medical and clinical psychology) in the concept of (holistic) integrated psychosomatic care in all fields of medicine. Beside the new development at the universities in training of all medical students, later it runs and promotes post-graduate research-based training and advancement in all areas of psychosomatic medicine.

The most important step was reached with the introduction of a specialty of psychotherapeutic medicine (this was already installed in the former German Democratic Republic some years ago) at the German Physicians Congress in 1992 specially, and heads of the departments of psychosomatic medicine committed themselves to establish psychosomatic medicine as an independent specialty in medicine. They were convinced that only a specialization allows an intensive training in psychotherapy and psychosomatic medicine. In 1992 the German Society for Psychosomatic Medicine and Psychotherapy was founded.

As a consequence psychosomatic medicine in Germany has a larger institutional basis than in any other country and has developed well over the last decades. It benefits from its institutional independence and the progressive changes in health care. The clinical core competency of German psychosomatic medicine is centred on integrated care for the following disorders: somatoform/functional disorders, eating disorders, somatopsychic disorders (including psycho-oncology, psychocardiology, neuropsychosomatics and psychodiabetology) and psychotraumatology. An overlap with psychiatry and psychology exists in the fields of treatment of depressive, anxiety and personality disorders.

16.2 Stages of Training and Specialization

In 1993, the General Assembly of German Physicians voted for a three-level approach and, thus, a differentiated and stepped-care qualification training process for specializing in psychosomatic medicine and psychotherapy, which are as follows:

(a) Psychosomatic basic care includes an 80-h structured training comprising theoretical and clinical instruction with psychosomatic patients and reflection of the doctor-patient relationship. All clinically practicing medical specialists can enrol in this training. Psychosomatic basic care is also an integral part of specialist training in general medicine and gynaecology. About 35,000 general practitioners and 12,000 gynaecologists have obtained this qualification [4].
(b) A post-graduate degree in psychotherapy for those already holding a specialization degree (18,000 medical doctors with an additional qualification in psychotherapy [5]. The training is extra-occupational and conveys basic psychotherapeutic skills (120 h of supervised psychotherapy, 120 h of

theoretical input and personal therapy). There are an additional group of 3180 medical doctors with a post-graduate degree in psychoanalysis.

(c) A 5-year specialization to become a specialist in psychosomatic medicine and psychotherapy (to date: including 1 year each of internal medicine and psychiatry, from 2018 ff. 4 years in psychosomatic medicine and one additional year in a clinical subject). This training comprises 1500 h of supervised psychotherapy, 240 h of theoretical input and personal therapy in both individual and group settings. The main emphasis is on the specialized psychotherapeutic and integrated psychosomatic treatment of patients with mental, psychosomatic, somatopsychic and stress disorders. Among physicians who practise psychotherapy in Germany, a specialist in psychosomatic medicine and psychotherapy has received the most intensive psychotherapeutic training. A specialist in psychiatry and psychotherapy has to provide only 240 h of supervised psychotherapy. Thus, a specialist in psychosomatic medicine and psychotherapy is the most qualified expert within the medical psychotherapeutic and psychosomatic care fields. Up to now, there are $n = 5180$ specialists of psychosomatic medicine and psychotherapy [5].

16.3 Psychosomatic Facilities and Structure

One historical milestone was the establishment of the first psychosomatic inpatient hospital that was opened in Berlin already in 1927. Since then, a significant number of hospitals and departments developed specifically to address psychosomatic issues all across Germany. Data based on a 2015 survey [6, 7] show that there are a total of 223 hospitals covering more than 10,000 inpatient beds. The mean length of stay was around 40 days. These figures demonstrate that the number of inpatient beds in Germany nearly tripled this millennium. There has also been a steep increase of psychosomatic day-patient facilities in recent years.

The following figure illustrates the structure of an academic psychosomatic department in Germany. In 1970, psychosomatic medicine became an obligatory subject in the medical school curriculum at the 37 official medical schools in Germany. Building on this advancement, the majority of the medical schools ($N = 26$) decided to establish independent and entire departments of psychosomatic medicine.

16.4 Inpatient and Day-Patient Facilities

To date there are different types of psychosomatic hospital facilities in Germany:

1. Hospitals for psychosomatic medicine with a superregional coverage area. The hospitals often include specialized subunits (e.g. eating disorders, PTSD, chronic pain) comprising more than 200 beds.
2. Departments of psychosomatic medicine at general hospitals providing regional coverage. The departments administer a consultation/liaison service for the entire hospital but have limited inpatient facilities (9–36 beds).

3. Departments of psychosomatic medicine and psychotherapy as academic institutions at university hospitals. These departments are responsible for patient care (20–70 beds), teaching and research (see Fig. 16.1).
4. Departments of psychosomatic medicine that are part of a psychiatric hospital (20–30 beds).
5. Consultation/liaison services for psychosomatic medicine at general and university hospitals (without own treatment unit).

Health insurance (public or private) covers treatment costs from a budget separate from the one for psychiatry. Costs for psychosomatic care are based on length of treatment rather than on the diagnosis-related group. This refunding system will probably change in the next few years.

Aside from the health insurance-covered hospital sector, there is a separate system of rehabilitation centres in Germany, which target the clinical areas of cardiology, oncology, neurology, orthopaedics and psychosomatic medicine. Their particular focus is on work-related aspects of disability prevention. Pension insurance covers the costs for these centres. There are 141 centres for psychosomatic medicine in this system, which provide about 16,000 additional inpatient beds with average treatment duration of 37 days (for more details see [8]).

Psychosomatic inpatient and day-patient treatment programmes are mostly combined multimodal therapy programmes, combining psychotherapy in individual and group formats, oriented on treatment guidelines and best practice experiences. Very often, psychodynamic and cognitive-behavioural approaches are both used in a coherent overall framework. Based on the leading diagnosis additional therapies, e.g. stress-reduction techniques, physiotherapy, body psychotherapy and creative therapies (art

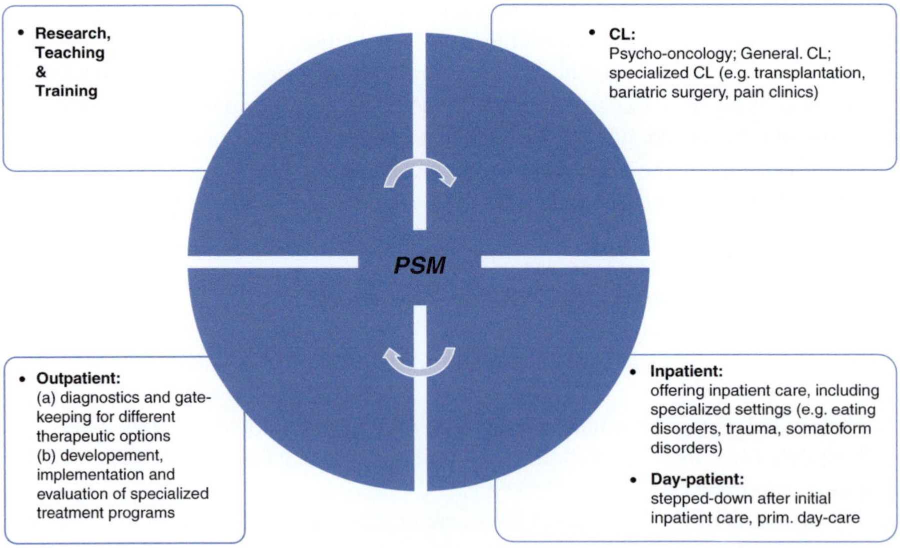

Fig. 16.1 Structure of an academic psychosomatic (PSM) department in Germany

and/or music therapy) are often part of the combined treatment package. Problems in the interpersonal and psychosocial field are in the major focus of family-/partner-oriented treatments often supplemented by a psychosocial skills training. As part of the new reimbursement system, the dosage of psychotherapy is monitored as a key input factor.

16.5 Integrated and Collaborative Care in German Psychosomatic Medicine

The majority of psychosomatic departments and hospitals take part in stringent quality assurance programmes in order to monitor their treatment programme and to provide transparency to the patients. In addition in respective regions and states, registries were introduced to provide outcome data on basic factors, e.g. duration of treatment, leading diagnosis and number of comorbid disorders [9].

Although it is hardly possible to design intervention studies to test such complex interventions such as multimodal in- or day-patient treatments, a recent systematic review and meta-analysis on pre-post studies [10] revealed a medium within group effect size of $g = 0.72$ for symptom change and 0.35 for change of interpersonal problems. However there are first multisite RCTs in Germany, investigating setting effects of day- and inpatient psychosomatic treatment in patients with a depressive disorder [11, 12].

16.6 Models of Psychosomatic Inpatient Services

The predominant model of inpatient psychosomatic services as rooted in the tradition of internal medicine in Germany is based on the "Heidelberg" model of psychosomatic inpatient services. The model was originally founded by Ludolf Krehl (1861–1937) and his scholars Richard Siebeck (1883–1965) und Viktor von Weizsäcker (1886–1957). The model entails a continuum of care where somatic diagnostic and therapeutic services and a focus on internal medicine interventions represent the one end of the spectrum and a focus on psychotherapeutic interventions represents the other end of the continuum. The intensity or setting where a patient is treated thereby depends on the specific needs of the individual. Rooted in this tradition, the Clinic for General Internal Medicine and Psychosomatics in Heidelberg, for example, is organized into three main units, one with a primary focus on internal medicine where the psychosomatic perspective is included, one unit where psychosomatic-psychotherapeutic interventions are equally represented together with somatic services and two units where the focus lies on psychosomatic-psychotherapeutic interventions.

Although other clinical centres for psychosomatic medicine may not differentiate across independent units along this continuum, the model of care with differing dosage of interventions (e.g. within different specialized therapeutic settings) of either diagnostic and therapeutic focus (somatic or psychotherapeutic), depending on the needs of the individual patient, can be seen as the gold standard of psychosomatic inpatient care in Germany.

The treatment components of inpatient services in a multimodal therapy programme in Germany include single and group psychotherapy sessions with dosages varying between one and three single sessions of 25–50 min, respectively, per week and between two and three group therapy sessions with 50–100 min, respectively, per week. In addition, there are usually specialized group therapies in disorder-specific settings, for example, specialized group therapy for patients with chronic pain, depressive disorders, eating disorders, post-traumatic stress disorders or somatoform disorders with 50–100 min per week. In total a typical dosage of psychotherapy may contain 75 min of single psychotherapy sessions, 100 min psychodynamic or cognitive-behavioural group therapy and 75 min disorder-specific group therapy per patient and week. The latter exemplary numbers thereby represent settings with a focus on psychosomatic-psychotherapeutic services. Settings with a primary focus on somatic entities might have less intense dosages of psychotherapy (e.g. one single session and one group session per week).

Besides the psychotherapeutic single and (specialized) group interventions (including family therapy), creative therapies such as art therapy, music therapy, creative writing or land-art therapy (gardening therapy) are offered at most institutions for psychosomatic medicine in Germany. Dosages of creative therapies may vary substantially and may range from 50 to 200 min per week for either of the approaches. Art therapy on the one hand may entail diverse techniques such as painting using different techniques (drawing, painting in oil or watercolours) or pottery and stonecutter. These techniques mainly serve the common aims of expressing and reflecting emotional states and biographic motifs which eventually may then be worked on further in, e.g. single or group therapy sessions.

Music therapy on the other hand may, for example, consist of singing sessions, percussion groups or instrumental groups, where patients may choose from a range of different music instruments (e.g. guitar, harp, xylophone, triangle, pipes, drums and others), for example, to express their (emotional) states, feelings and wishes and to try out other forms of communication among the group of patients to (musically) interact. Music therapy thereby may be a means of expressing one-self as much as improving (empathic) listening skills and to make experiences of new ways of interacting with new mediums (in this case music instruments) with others. In addition to psychotherapy and creative therapies, most centres for psychosomatic medicine in Germany will offer further specialized therapies such as physiotherapy, social interaction training (e.g. exercised by role-plays), social counselling (e.g. on work-related issues), relaxation and meditation techniques, biofeedback, stabilization techniques (especially in settings for patients with post-traumatic stress disorders), diverse approaches of body therapy (especially in settings for patients with eating disorders), activation techniques and sports (walking, swimming, gymnastics, ergometer training).

See Table 16.1 for an exemplary treatment schedule for patients with chronic pain (as practised at the University Medical Hospital Tuebingen, Department for Psychosomatic Medicine and Psychotherapy).

These therapy components in the multimodal therapy process are accompanied by structured team processes where the team members of a psychosomatic inpatient unit exchange their perspectives on the current state of therapy of a given patient

Table 16.1 Exemplary psychosomatic inpatient treatment schedule for patients with chronic pain

Monday	Tuesday	Wednesday	Thursday	Friday
7.15–7.45 Morning activation (physiotherapy)	**7.15–7.45** Morning activation (physiotherapy)	**7.15–7.45** Morning activation (physiotherapy)	**7.15–7.45** Morning activation (physiotherapy)	**7.15–7.45** Morning activation (physiotherapy)
8.00–8.30 Breakfast	**8.00–8.30** Breakfast	**8.00–8.30** Breakfast	**8.00–8.30** Breakfast	**8.00–8.30** Breakfast
08.50–9.40 Music/singing group **8.45–10.00** **Art therapy** **11.00–12.00** **Biofeedback**	**9.00–9.50** **Group psychotherapy** **10.15–10.40** **Physiotherapy** **9.00–9.50** **Individual psychotherapy**	**8.45–10.00** Nordic walking **10.00–11.00** **Body therapy** **11.00–12.00** **Biofeedback**	**8.30–11.00** **Ward round (with consultant physician)** **8.45–9.10** **Physiotherapy** **11:00–11:50** **Individual psychotherapy**	**9.00–9.50** **Group psychotherapy** **10.00–11.00** **Body therapy** **10.45–11.35** **Nordic walking**
10.50 **Educational movie for chronic pain**	**11.10–12.00** Nordic walking			**11.00** **Water gymnastics (physiotherapy)**
12.00–12.20 Meditation	**12.00–12.20** MBT/meditation	**12.00–12.20** MBT/meditation	**12.00–12.20** MBT/meditation	**12.00–12.20** MBT/meditation
12.30–13.00 Lunch	**12.30–13.00** Lunch	**12.30–13.00** Lunch	**12.30–13.00** Lunch	**12.30–13.00** Lunch
15.00–15.25 **Stabilization therapy** **15.45–17.00** **Social therapeutic group Including role-play**	**13.15–15.15** **Art therapy** **15:30–15:55** **Specific group therapy for chronic pain patients**	**15.10–16.00** Progressive muscle relaxation **16.00–16.50** Qigong **17.00–17.25** **Patient assembly**	**15.05–15.55** **Specific group therapy for chronic pain patients** **16.00–17.30** **Gardening therapy**	**13.15–14.05** **Music therapy** **13.15–14.05** **Dance therapy** **15.20–16.10** **Progressive muscle relaxation** **16.15–16.40** **Patient assembly (preparation for weekend)**

and where the focus of the therapy is elaborated and supervised. In weekly ward rounds, the patient is seen by the members of the treatment team including the consultant of the unit. In addition, in a separate weekly team process, the current state and treatment progress of every patient is reflected on by the treatment team of the unit (physicians for psychosomatic medicine, psychologists, nurses, creative therapists, physiotherapists, social counsellors and others). Depending of the predominant school of psychotherapy, the team processes may rely on different structured instruments of diagnostic and assessment such as the operationalized psychodynamic diagnostic system (OPD-2, Arbeitskreis OPD 2006) to plan, conceptualize and operationalize the individual treatment goals.

Among the most specialized disorder-specific treatment settings in psychosomatic clinics and departments are, for example, the settings for patients with chronic pain (see Table 16.1) eating disorders and somatoform/functional disorders. For patients with eating disorders, specialized centres may offer (in addition to the treatment components described above) regular meetings of the patient with a nutritionist, and concepts may entail a weekly specialized group therapy for patients with eating disorders where, for example, the dietitian, eventually together with a specialized nurse or physician/psychologist, reflects on the weekly progresses with the patient concerning eating structure, activity levels and other functional and dysfunctional behaviours and their determinants. Furthermore, settings for patients with eating disorder will contain standardized weightings (e.g. twice a week), single sessions of mirror exposure therapy, body image directed group therapy, guided cooking sessions, guided exposure to natural consumption (shopping) and eating environments, family therapy sessions (diagnostic and therapeutic including the parents of one patient only) and psychoeducational/therapeutic (with parents of multiple patients) in group sessions.

16.7 In the Outpatient Sector

To date [13] there are 3058 specialists in psychosomatic medicine and psychotherapy as well as $n = 4154$ specialists in psychiatry and psychotherapy working in the outpatient sector. In Germany, only medical doctors and certified clinical psychologists are allowed to practise psychotherapy for adults.

In particular, specialists in psychosomatic medicine and psychotherapy are treating 190,000 outpatients per year and those medical doctors with an additional degree in psychotherapy another 170,000 outpatients per year. The majority of these patients are between 35 and 54 years old (mean 43.2 years), and their primarily diagnosis are depressive disorders, anxiety disorders and adjustment disorders [14]. The majority of patients are treated with a psychodynamic approach in short-, intermediate- or long-term treatments. As a consequence a mean outpatient psychosomatic practice is caring for about 170 patients per year. This is roughly the same number than a practice run by a clinical psychologist in Germany. Since 2005 specialists in psychosomatic medicine and psychotherapy in Germany have a distinct catalogue as the basis for refunding by the German health-care system. In this German system until now, there is a clear separation between the inpatient and outpatient sector, provided mainly by hospitals and the separated outpatient sector mainly structured and organized in outpatient practices run by independent specialists.

16.8 Consultation-Liaison Psychosomatic Medicine (CL PSM)

The first psychiatric CL service was established at the University of Colorado General Hospital by E.G. Billings in 1939 [15]. "Consultation" covers the patient-centred aspect, whereas "liaison" refers to a team-based intervention approach. In Germany—as opposed to many other countries worldwide—there are two different specialities providing CL service in the field of psychological comorbidities: psychiatry and psychosomatic medicine. Until the 1960s it was not common to have psychiatric departments in general hospitals, which started to change after the German "psychiatry-enquête" and its demand for more integrated care [16]. With the introduction of the speciality "psychosomatic medicine and psychotherapy" in 2003, the duality of CL service in the field of psychological comorbidities started, and until now there is a wide overlap in service, though psychosomatic doctors usually do not see patients with substance abuse, deliberate self-harm, psychosis and prominent suicidality. Up to one third of patients treated for medical-surgical health problems have clinically relevant psychological comorbidities which is in contrast to CL PSM referral rates of around 3% [17]. CL PSM seems to be cost-effective, and accepted with staff and patients though concordance to CL PSM recommendations varies [17, 18].

In 2008, a task force was created by the board of the European Association of Consultation-Liaison Psychiatry and Psychosomatics (EACLPP) and the Academy of Psychosomatic Medicine (APM) to define core characteristics (roles, competencies, work content) for physicians in the field of consultation-liaison psychosomatics ([19], see also Table 16.2). In general, CL PSM takes care of patients with psychological symptoms or syndromes being treated for other reasons in a

Table 16.2 CanMEDs roles and corresponding competencies for CL PSM doctors [19, 20]

CanMEDs role	Competencies
Medical expert	• Facilitate optimal care through effective diagnostic and evidence-based therapeutic skills including a biopsychosocial approach • Apply or refer to therapeutic interventions (psychoeducation, psychotherapy, pharmacotherapy)
Communicator	• Establish a good doctor-patient relationship regardless of the patient's background (e.g. gender, religion, ethnicity) • Communicate effectively with patients, relatives and other health-care professionals
Collaborator	• Interact effectively with all stakeholders involved (health-care professionals, patients, relatives) while taking into account each person's level of understanding mental health and CL PSM • Help educating other health-care professionals on CL PSM, and clearly explain recommended treatments to enhance adherence • Be part of integrative care teams and/or supply with information on post-inpatient care options in the sector of mental health
Manager	• Provide CL PSM service evidence-based with attention to cost-effectiveness • Supervise and evaluate performance of other CL PSM team members
Health Advocate	• Identify important determinants that affect patients' health and contribute effectively to their improvement • Prevent stigmatization of mental health problems
Scholar	• Engage actively in continuing professional development • Stay up to date with and critically assimilate latest research findings in the field of CL PSM • Engage in teaching of medical students as well as other health-care professionals and the interested public
Professional	• Recognize and acknowledge one's own limitations and act accordingly • Reflect upon one's decisions and actions critically and realize its impact on others • Awareness of relevant legal issues and laws and regulations related to health care

non-mental health setting. Patients might have a medical-surgical condition and mental illness complicating each other's management, medically unexplained symptoms or a mental illness directly due to a general medical condition or its treatment. Additionally, they might show social situations, health beliefs and behaviours or personality traits that hamper successful treatment of the medical-surgical condition [19]. CL PSM doctors thus treat medical-surgical patients with comorbid psychological symptoms as well as actively identifying those at risk to develop mental health problems.

Usually, the CL PSM service is either part of the general psychosomatic outpatients' department or run independently as an own subdepartment. CL PSM doctors should have at least a couple of years work experience to guarantee their firm knowledge of psychosomatic disorders and established treatments. Additionally, there are special training classes preparing doctors for CL PSM challenges [21].

Helpful screening instruments in the context of CL PSM are the Hospital Anxiety and Depression Scale (HADS), the Patient Health Questionnaire-9 (PHQ 9), the 36-Item Short Form Health Survey (*SF-36*) and the State-Trait Anxiety Inventory (STAI). CL PSM service comprises diagnostic evaluation, differential diagnostic referrals (e.g. further lab screening, other CL services) and treatment recommendations (psychological interventions like patient education, behaviour management or counselling, psychotherapy, pharmacotherapy) [18, 19]. An important issue is that usually not the patient initiated the encounter in the first place and the hospital setting as well as underlying medical-surgical conditions might hamper effective psychotherapy even in the willing ones [22]. Thus, brief psychotherapeutic interventions going beyond psychoeducation in the medically ill usually have to be specifically tailored to the patient's condition. For example, medically severely ill patients having difficulties to come to terms with their disease primarily receive resource-oriented, supportive interventions focussed on their main leading-affect and the often severely low self-esteem. Comorbid depression or anxiety in the CL setting can be treated with short psychodynamic or cognitive-behavioural psychotherapy though it will usually still be rather supportive than exploratory or confrontational. For traumatized patients, crisis interventions like stabilizing exercises and supportive relief are often the first choice. However, in general, time within CL PSM service is limited, which makes recommendations for after discharge always a crucial part of the CL PSM service.

16.9 Examples of Special Areas Within CL PSM

16.9.1 Transplant CL PSM

The need for transplant surgery is always a difficult situation asking for a solid evaluation scheme of potential recipients assessing their mental health status as well as their ability to adhere to necessary lifelong treatment. It is well-known that the outcome of the procedure is highly correlated with the recipient's mental health status [23]. With the shortage of post-mortal donations, the concept of living organ donation becomes more popular. This poses a special context with an ethical issue due to the fact that a healthy donor is risking his or her health for the live and health condition of the recipient. Thus, respect for the donor's autonomy is currently the main justification for allowing this risky procedure, and there are usually strict national guidelines on the evaluation process. CL PSM evaluation thus comprises assessment of the donor's motivation, voluntariness, knowledge about the procedure and its possible complications, relation with the potential recipient, mental health history, socio-economic background and long-term outcomes [24]. Within living organ donations, the very recent uterus transplantation is a new field with certain distinctive features compared to other organs: it is classified into the group of "non-vital and quality of life-enhancing types of transplantation" and usually only for the temporary purpose of giving birth to children [25]. Here in particular, a common evaluation of both, potential donor and recipient, together after the individual assessment has been completed successfully is considered crucial although it might also be helpful in other living organ donation situations [26]. In general, donors report satisfactory post-operative outcomes or even positive effects like a boost in self-esteem which has to be balanced against possible failures on the recipients' side and the dangers for the donors [24, 27].

16.9.2 Psychocardiology

It is well accepted that psychosocial stressors play a crucial role in the development, progress and outcome of cardiovascular diseases [28]. The negative impact seems to come from the risk factors themselves via enduring, dysfunctional activation of the autonomous nervous system, the endocrine and inflammatory system as well as the factor's influence on patient behaviour (e.g. the risk factor "low socio-economic status" is associated with increased smoking rates which in turn are risk factors for cardiovascular events) [29]. Particularly depressive and anxious symptoms are far more present in patients with cardiovascular diseases than in the normal population with negative impact on patient outcome [30]. Several meta-analyses could show that psychosocial interventions—as offered by CL PSM—could provide a positive effect on quality of life, health-related behaviour and somatic risk factors as well as partially on cardiovascular morbidity and mortality [31, 32]. There is also strong recommendation that psychological comorbidities like depression or anxiety disorders need further psychotherapeutic treatment [28].

16.9.3 Chronic Pain

Patients with medically unexplained pain are often first admitted to medical-surgical departments and show negative associations like longer hospital stays, greater overall costs and more frequent usage of health-care systems [33]. CL PSM offers support in assessing if these symptoms presented are truly functional and can be explained as representatives of a mental illness addressing the patient's health beliefs and trying to link psychosocial issues to physical symptoms whenever possible [33]. Additionally, patients with chronic pain explained by underlying medical-surgical reasons have a higher comorbidity of mental illnesses such as major depression or PTSD and need to be assessed for substance abuse [34, 35]. Aside from this traditional CL PSM service, more collaborative care programmes are also dealing with chronic pain patients. Pain-related somatic disciplines like neurology or orthopaedics can offer complex chronic pain treatment for 1–2 weeks on the condition that they include other specialities like psychosomatic medicine into their treatment programme. Here, patients get psychosocial evaluation and basic psychoeducation as well as special recommendations for further treatment options if necessary. Also, CL PSM doctors offer clinics within the anaesthesiological pain clinic. Anaesthesiologists can refer patients they consider suitable for evaluation, and patients don't even have to change location or go through the sometimes subjectively embarrassing task of entering a mental health clinic. The climax in this chain of constellations are interdisciplinary pain-specific day units, where PSM CL doctors work together with anaesthesiologists, neurologists, neurosurgeons or orthopaedic doctors on a constant basis to guarantee best possible health care. These truly collaborative integrated care models have shown to be effective even in long-term follow-ups [36, 37].

16.9.4 Psycho-oncology

The field of psycho-oncology is also closely linked to psychosomatic medicine in Germany. In the majorities of the Comprehensive Cancer Centres, which are linked to academic medicine, psycho-oncology is delivered by departments of psychosomatic medicine. However, also specialists from psychosomatic medicine need some additional extra training and a specific additional certification.

Conclusion

To conclude, combining its two traditions, German psychosomatic medicine has developed well over the last decades, benefitting from its institutional independence. Clinically, disorder-oriented psychotherapy is a core method integrated with other modes of therapy. So the German model of psychosomatic medicine is a strong advocate for psychotherapy in medicine and just celebrating its 25th anniversary of an independent discipline within medicine.

References

1. Fava GA, Belaise C, Sonino N. Psychosomatic medicine is a comprehensive field, not a synonym for consultation liaison psychiatry. Curr Psychiatry Rep. 2010;12:215–21.
2. Deter HC. Psychosomatic medicine and psychotherapy: on the historical development of a special field in Germany. Adv Psychosom Med. 2004;26:181–9.

3. von Uexküll Thure WW. Integrierte Medizin als Gesamtkonzept der Heilkunde: Ein bio-psycho-soziales Modell. In: Adler RWH, Joraschky P, Köhle K, Langewitz W, Söllner W, Wesiak W, editors. Psychosomatische Medizin: Theoretische Modelle und klinische Praxis, vol. 7. München: Elsevier GmbH; 2011. p. 3–40.
4. Kassenärztliche Bundesvereinigung. 2014. http://www.kbv.de/html/. Accessed 6 Oct 2017.
5. Bundesärztekammer. 2014. http://www.bundesaerztekammer.de/weitere-sprachen/english/german-medical-association/. Accessed 6 Oct 2017.
6. Zipfel S, Giel KE, Bulik CM, Hay P, Schmidt U. Anorexia nervosa: aetiology, assessment, and treatment. Lancet Psychiatry. 2015;2:1099–111.
7. Zipfel S, Herzog W, Kruse J, Henningsen P. Psychosomatic medicine in Germany: more timely than ever. Psychother Psychosom. 2016;85:262–9.
8. Linden M. Psychosomatic inpatient rehabilitation: the German model. Psychother Psychosom. 2014;83:205–12.
9. Probst T, von Heymann F, Zaudig M, Konermann J, Lahmann C, Loew T, et al. The effectiveness of psychosomatic inpatient treatment—results of a multicentre follow-up study. Z Psychosom Med Psychother. 2009;55:409–20.
10. Liebherz S, Rabung S. Do patients' symptoms and interpersonal problems improve in psychotherapeutic hospital treatment in Germany? A systematic review and meta-analysis. PLoS One. 2014;9:e105329.
11. Dinger U, Klipsch O, Kohling J, Ehrenthal JC, Nikendei C, Herzog W, et al. Day-clinic and inpatient psychotherapy for depression (dip-d): a randomized controlled pilot study in routine clinical care. Psychother Psychosom. 2014;83:194–5.
12. Zeeck A, von Wietersheim J, Weiss H, Eduard Scheidt C, Volker A, Helesic A, et al. Symptom course in inpatient and day clinic treatment of depression: results from the INDDEP-study. J Affect Disord. 2015;187:35–44.
13. Bundespsychotherapeutenkammer. 2016. http://www.bptk.de/. Accessed 6 Oct 2017.
14. Herzog W, Beutel M, Kruse J. Psychosomatische Medizin und Psychotherapie heute—zur Lage des Fachgebietes in Deutschland. Stuttgart: Schattauer; 2012.
15. Billings EG. Liaison psychiatry and intern instruction. J Assoc Am Med Coll. 1939;14:375–85.
16. Diefenbacher AC. Psychiatry and psychosomatic medicine in Germany: lessons to be learned. Austr N Zeal J Psychiatry. 2005;39:782–94.
17. Laner B, Staufer C, Giesinger JM, Gross R, Kohl C, Malik P, et al. Psychiatric consultation-liaison interventions: recollection, perception and outcome. J Psychosom Res. 2013;75:184–6. https://doi.org/10.1016/j.jpsychores.2013.06.007.
18. Wood R, Wand AP. The effectiveness of consultation-liaison psychiatry in the general hospital setting: a systematic review. J Psychosom Res. 2014;76:175–92. https://doi.org/10.1016/j.jpsychores.2014.01.002.
19. Leentjens AF, Rundell JR, Wolcott DL, Diefenbacher A, Kathol R, Guthrie E. Psychosomatic medicine and consultation-liaison psychiatry: scope of practice, processes, and competencies for psychiatrists or psychosomatic medicine specialists. A consensus statement of the European Association of Consultation-Liaison Psychiatry and the Academy of Psychosomatic Medicine. Psychosomatics. 2011;52:19–25.
20. Frank JR, Danoff D. The CanMEDS initiative: implementing an outcomes-based framework of physician competencies. Med Teach. 2007;29:642–7.
21. Söllner W, Creed F, European Association of Consultation-Liaison Psychiatry and Psychosomatics Workgroup on Training in Consultation-Liaison. European guidelines for training in consultation-liaison psychiatry and psychosomatics: report of the EACLPP workgroup on training in consultation-liaison psychiatry and psychosomatics. J Psychosom Res. 2007;62:501–9.
22. O'Dowd MA, Gomez MF. Psychotherapy in consultation-liaison psychiatry. Am J Psychother. 2001;55:122–32.
23. Olbrisch ME, Benedict SM, Ashe K, Levenson JL. Psychological assessment and care of organ transplant patients. J Consult Clin Psychol. 2002;70:771–83.

24. Jowsey SG, Schneekloth TD. Psychosocial factors in living organ donation: clinical and ethical challenges. Transplant Rev (Orlando). 2008;22:192–5. https://doi.org/10.1016/j.trre.2008.04.008.
25. Järvholm S, Johannesson L, Clarke A, Brännström M. Uterus transplantation trial: psychological evaluation of recipients and partners during the post-transplantation year. Fertil Steril. 2015;104:1010–5. https://doi.org/10.1016/j.fertnstert.2015.06.038.
26. Erim Y, Beckmann M, Valentin-Gamazo C, Malago M, Frilling A, Schlaak J, et al. Selection of donors for adult living-donor liver donation: results of the assessment of the first 205 donor candidates. Psychosomatics. 2008;49:143–51. https://doi.org/10.1176/appi.psy.49.2.143.
27. Potts M, Evans DW. Is solid organ donation by living donors ethical? The case of kidney donation. In: Weimar W, Bos MA, Busschbach JJ, editors. Organ transplantation: ethical, legal and psychosocial aspects. Towards a common European policy. Lengerich: Pabst Sci Publ; 2008.
28. Ladwig KH, Lederbogen F, Albus C, et al. Position paper on the importance of psychosocial factors in cardiology: update 2013. Ger Med Sci. 2014;12:Doc09. https://doi.org/10.3205/000194.
29. Rozanski A, Blumenthal JA, Davidson KW, et al. The epidemiology, pathophysiology, and management of psychosocial risk factors in cardiac practice: the emerging field of behavioral cardiology. J Am Coll Cardiol. 2005;45:637–51.
30. Albus C, Ladwig KH, Herrmann-Lingen C. Psychocardiology. Clinically relevant recommendations regarding selected cardiovascular diseases. Dtsch Med Wochenschr. 2014;139:596–601.
31. Rutledge T, Redwine LS, Linke SE, et al. A meta-analysis of mental health treatments and cardiac rehabilitation for improving clinical outcomes and depression among patients with coronary heart disease. Psychosom Med. 2013;75:335–49.
32. Whalley B, Rees K, Davies P. Psychological interventions for coronary heart disease. Cochrane Database Syst Rev. 2011; CD002902.
33. Grover S, Kate N. Somatic symptoms in consultation-liaison psychiatry. Int Rev Psychiatry. 2013;25:52–64.
34. Elman I, Zubieta JK, Borsook D. The missing p in psychiatric training: why it is important to teach pain to psychiatrists. Arch Gen Psychiatry. 2011;68(1):12–20. https://doi.org/10.1001/archgenpsychiatry.2010;174.
35. Voon P, Karamouzian M, Kerr T. Chronic pain and opioid misuse: a review of reviews. Subst Abuse Treat Prev Policy. 2017;12:36. https://doi.org/10.1186/s13011-017-0120-7.
36. Turk DC. Clinical effectiveness and cost-effectiveness of treatments for patients with chronic pain. Clin J Pain. 2002;18:355–65.
37. Zeeberg P, Olesen J, Jensen R. Efficacy of multidisciplinary treatment in a tertiary referral headache centre. Cephalalgia. 2005;25:1159–67.

17 Training in Consultation-Liaison Psychiatry and Psychosomatic Medicine

Wolfgang Söllner, Else Guthrie, and Alexandre Berney

Abstract

Training is a central issue for consultation-liaison (C-L) psychiatrists and specialists in psychosomatic medicine (PM), firstly for their own education. There is a wide variety of training of residents and fellows in different countries. Guidelines for training were developed and agreed in the USA, in Australia and New Zealand, and in Europe.

Secondly, C-L and PM specialists have an important role as teachers. They educate medical students and give courses in communication skills and psychosomatic competencies for general practitioners, residents and specialists of other medical specialties, and other health-care professionals like nurses or case managers. Such training courses proved effective to improve communication with and treatment of patients with comorbid medical and mental health problems.

In this chapter, we review training modalities (a) for residents and fellows in C-L psychiatry and PM and (b) for nonpsychiatric health-care professionals in different countries. In this review, we mainly focus on the situation in the USA, Europe, and Australia and New Zealand.

W. Söllner (✉)
Department of Psychosomatic Medicine and Psychotherapy, Paracelsus Medical School, General Hospital Nuremberg, Nuremberg, Germany
e-mail: wolfgang.soellner@klinikum-nuernberg.de

E. Guthrie
Leeds Institute of Health Sciences, University of Leeds, Leeds, UK

A. Berney
Department of Psychiatry, Lausanne University Hospital, Lausanne, Switzerland

L. Grassi et al. (eds.), *Person Centered Approach to Recovery in Medicine*, Integrating Psychiatry and Primary Care, https://doi.org/10.1007/978-3-319-74736-1_17

17.1 Introduction

Consultation-liaison psychiatry (CLP) and psychosomatic medicine (PM) are overlapping fields of health care (HC), research, and education at the interface between "general" and mental health. CLP emerged with the establishment of psychiatric departments in general hospitals in the middle of the last century. It is based on a psychiatric service for the "somatic" departments—organized either on demand (consultation) or in a more integrated way with a consultant embedded in the somatic department (liaison). In some countries, special competencies (e.g., "liaison psychiatry" in the UK) or subspecializations ("psychosomatic medicine" in the USA, "consultation-liaison psychiatry" in Switzerland) were established.

While CLP is a well-defined form of HC intervention, psychosomatic medicine (PM) is based on a broader concept. On the one hand, it espouses a general approach to medicine which integrates psychological and social aspects of disease; on the other hand, it describes—similar to liaison psychiatry—integrated forms of interventions of PM specialists in general health care. In most countries, PM is seen and performed as a "holistic" biopsychosocial approach to medicine, including an important educational role for medical students and primary care physicians. In some European countries (Germany, Latvia, Czech Republic), medical specializations in PM were established separately and alongside general psychiatry.

Depending on the view of CLP and PM as a more general "holistic" concept in medicine or a more specialized field of medical intervention, the requirements for training are very different. Medical students and residents in general medicine and medical specializations should be educated to consider psychological and socioeconomic factors as well as physical factors in the diagnosis and treatment of diseases, and they should be trained in adequate communication skills to meet the needs of their patients. Psychiatrists and psychosomatic doctors involved in CLP and PM services need special knowledge, skills, and attitudes. The knowledge must include both somatic aspects of disease and psychological and social aspects. Skills must include biological as well as psychological treatment methods and specific communication skills to perform clinical work at the borderline between general and mental health care, collaborating with different professions and health-care teams. Approaches must be based on a biopsychosocial theoretical framework and a humanistic view of the world (*Weltanschauung*). As a consequence, in this chapter, we will first discuss essential training in psychosomatic competencies for medical students and general practitioners, followed by specialized training for psychiatrists and specialists in PM.

So far, different examples of training have been established, evaluated, and published, and there is a wide variety of education and training methods. The principles of the biopsychosocial paradigm and basic psychosomatic knowledge and skills have been included in many medical curricula. In some countries (e.g., Austria, Germany, Switzerland), curricula in "basic psychosomatic competencies" were developed for residents in general medicine and for GPs [1, 2]. Recently such programs have been established in China, Laos, and Vietnam [3]. Courses in communication skills seem to be well accepted by internists [2, 4] and particularly by oncologists [5]. A meta-analysis has shown the benefit of such training [6]. In some countries, such courses became mandatory for oncologists (e.g., the UK and Switzerland).

The CanMEDS framework for postgraduate education (PGME), which was originally developed in Canada and first published in 1996, has now been adopted by many countries to shape training and practice for doctors [7]. Although the CanMEDS framework does not specifically refer to psychosomatic aspects of disease in its broad themes, it does place great significance on the role of doctor as a communicator and a collaborator.

Regarding specialized training in CLP and PM, the Manchester courses in liaison psychiatry [8] were considered the "gold standard" for training of psychiatric and psychosomatic residents in C-L. They were a melting pot of ideas and enhanced the spread of C-L services throughout Europe. Similar courses emerged in other countries (Austria, Germany, Italy).

In the USA, the Academy of Psychosomatic Medicine (APM) published consensus papers on the training of psychiatric residents in CLP [9] and on the core competencies for the fellowship "psychosomatic medicine" [10]. The European Association of Consultation-Liaison Psychiatry and Psychosomatics (EACLPP), the precursor of the European Association of Psychosomatic Medicine (EAPM), established a working group which elaborated and agreed guidelines for training in C-L psychiatry and psychosomatics [11]. Surveys on the organization and practice of training in C-L were undertaken and published in Western Europe [11], in Eastern Europe [12], and in the USA [13].

Finally, APM and EACLPP published a joint consensus paper on the scope of practice, processes, and competencies for CLP and psychosomatics [14]. In the section on competencies and skills, the CanMEDS framework [7] was adopted with specific psychosomatic competencies described for each of the CanMEDS areas: medical expert, communicator, collaborator, manager, health advocate, scholar, and professional.

17.2 Undergraduate Education of Medical Students

The biopsychosocial theoretical concept of diseases and medical care [15–17] replaced the biomechanical paradigm and became the predominant paradigm in Western medicine. However, it is not unanimously accepted [18], and its implementation in the practice of medical training has been patchy and inadequate in most medical faculties. There is wide variation in how the biopsychosocial approach is taught, both in theoretical and in clinical aspects of the medical curriculum. The formats include clinical courses, communication skills training courses, and clinical clerkship.

- Small-group clinical courses in which students practice conducting medical interviews with real patients or with simulated patients, using trained actors, have been shown to improve students' interviewing skills and patient-centered attitudes and are positively evaluated by medical students [19–22].

- In some medical schools, psychosomatic/C-L faculty members are engaged in interprofessional courses and seminars together with nursing schools teaching team communication and difficult topic areas of communication with patients (e.g., breaking bad news, medical error communication) [23].
- Clinical clerkship rotations in psychosomatic/C-L departments strengthen a biopsychosocial understanding of illness [24–26]. Unfortunately, most of these clerkship rotations are voluntarily. In the evaluation of these programs students as well as faculty report a high practical value of such education and recommend that it should be mandatory in the undergraduate curriculum.

17.3 Postgraduate Training of Residents in General Medicine, Primary Care Physicians (PCPs) and Nonpsychiatric Specialists

In the USA, only about 50% of patients with mental illness are primarily seen only in primary care settings. Only a minority of patients receive effective treatment. This results in under treatment of patients with mental health problems but also in social problems and increased costs because treatment of mental illness in the medical health sector produce much more costs than in the mental health sector [27]. This is not only an American problem but to a larger or smaller degree a worldwide problem. In a White Paper on the Integration of Psychiatry and Primary Care the American Psychiatric Association [28] strongly recommended the development and implementation of mental health services integrated in primary care. Another urgent task is to train GPs and physicians of other medical specialties to better understand, diagnose, and treat mental health disorders and to more effectively cooperate with mental health specialists.

In some countries (e.g., Germany), residents in general medicine are obliged to perform courses in "basic psychosomatic competencies" ; in other countries (e.g., Austria, Switzerland, Denmark), such courses are voluntary and, on completion, involve receipt of a Diploma of the Medical Association. The extent and the content of these courses is very different in different countries. Frequently taught subjects are the diagnosis and treatment of somatoform/somatic symptom disorders, psychosocial aspects of chronic pain, as well as anxiety, depression, and substance abuse in the medically ill. Usually the leaders and teachers of these courses are specialists in psychosomatic medicine or C-L psychiatrists. As an example, we show in Table 17.1 the number of hours of training and the types of training experience for courses in "basic psychosomatic competencies" in Austria, Germany, and Switzerland. In some countries, physicians who have completed these courses receive higher fees for medical consultations from the health insurance companies. In Germany, more than 60.000 of the 360.000 German PCPs have attended such courses [29].

Some university hospitals (Aarhus, Denmark; Freiburg, GE; Manchester, UK) offer special trainings for the diagnosis and treatment of somatoform/somatic symptom disorders for primary care physicians and other nonpsychiatric specialists. A very specific example is the "reattribution model" developed by Goldberg and coworkers [30] in Manchester, England, for use by GPs in their everyday practice.

Table 17.1 Number of hours of training in courses in basic psychosomatic competency in Austria, Germany, and Switzerland

	Austria		Germany	Switzerland
	Voluntary		Mandatory for PCPs and gynecologists, voluntary for other specialists	Mandatory for gynecologists and oncologists, voluntary for other specialists
Mandatory/voluntary	Step 1	Step 2		
Course size in hours	80	240	80	40
Contents (hours)				
– Theory	40	80	20	10
– Communication skills training			30	10
– Case conference/ Balint group	40	80	30	
– Relaxation training				20
– Self-experience in groups		80		
Examination	Case report	Written case report	Case report	Case report

This program was further refined by the Aarhus Research Unit on Functional Disorders ("The Extended Reattribution and Management (TERM) model" [31] and by the Psychosomatic Department of Freiburg University [1]. These programs aim to increase knowledge about somatoform/somatic symptom disorders, change GPs' attitude toward these disorders, and train them in interview techniques and specific treatment techniques for these disorders. The training programs last between 24 and 30 h (usually 2 full days and several evenings). They are based on micro skills training in small groups including role-playing and feedback and take into account the very limited available time that GPs have for the treatment of these patients. The programs proved to be suitable for improving communication with patients with functional disorders. After the training doctors and their patients were more satisfied with the interaction and the treatment and patients' somatoform symptoms were more reduced than in patients treated by GPs without such training [32, 33], although outcome is variable [34]. The TERM model is now mandatory for the training of GPs in some regions in Denmark. In Germany, 35,000 GPs and 12,000 gynecologists performed such training.

An interesting project to train and supervise primary care providers in rural areas, the ECHO project, was developed and evaluated in Ontario, Canada. In the framework of a video-based collaborative care approach, GPs, nurses, social workers, and other community health workers participated in the program. Using weekly video conferences, an interdisciplinary team including C-L psychiatrists offered case discussion and didactic lectures to the participants. Evaluation of the program showed high satisfaction of 131 participants in 26 rural sites. They reported increased knowledge of mental health issues, a reduced professional isolation, and a trend toward higher self-efficacy. Moreover, they reported to have implemented 76% of the experts' recommendations from cases in practice [35].

In some sectors of health care and particularly in specialties where a high number of severely ill and chronically ill patients are treated (like oncology, cardiology, transplantation medicine, treatment of chronic pain patients, and palliative care), physicians are in need of intensive further education and training in psychosocial aspects of illness and communication skills. In many countries, C-L psychiatrists and specialists in psychosomatic medicine offer communication skills training (CST) and contribute to specialized courses in psychosocial oncology, psychocardiology, palliative care, and chronic pain treatment for physicians, nurses, and other health-care professionals. CST courses are effective to improve the communication with severely ill patients and their caregivers and their satisfaction with medical treatment [4, 6]. As a consequence CST became mandatory for the training of oncologists in some countries (e.g., Switzerland, UK).

17.4 Training of Psychiatric Residents

Training of psychiatric residents in psychosomatics is variable. Most trainings focus on traditional mental disorders such as schizophrenia, bipolar disorder, and anxiety/depressive states. There is relatively little emphasis on psychological aspects of physical disease or psychosomatic conditions. In the UK, the first 3 years of psychiatric training focuses upon the development of core competencies, and there is virtually no reference to liaison psychiatry skills in the learning outcomes that early career doctors have to achieve. Some psychiatry training schemes offer 6 month placements in liaison psychiatry, but these are not mandatory and are only available to a small number of trainees.

Training in CLP is mandatory in other European countries, e.g., in Austria, Germany, Portugal, and Spain. However, training and rotation to C-L departments are very heterogeneous in different countries. Rotation to C-L departments ranges from 2 to 6 months.

In Australia and New Zealand, trainees do a basic first 12-month training in general psychiatry and then have to spend a 6-month attachment in a C-L post during the next 24 months of their training (Stage 2). This training experience is mandatory, as is a training experience in child psychiatry.

The Academy of Psychosomatic Medicine (APM) published a consensus paper on the training of psychiatric residents in PM [9]. The working group on training in C-L of the European Association of Consultation-Liaison Psychiatry and Psychosomatics (EACLPP), the precursor of the European Association of Psychosomatic Medicine (EAPM), agreed guidelines for training in C-L psychiatry and psychosomatics [11]. The European guidelines recommend a larger timeframe for the rotation to a C-L department and a similar number of performed consultations (see Table 17.2). Both guidelines recommend similar contents of training including the acquirement of attitudes, knowledge, and skills such as:

- The assessment and management of psychiatric and psychosomatic disorders, e.g., suicide/self-harm, somatic symptom disorder/somatization, chronic pain, and mental disorders and problematic illness behavior in the medically ill

Table 17.2 Recommendations of the APM and EACLPP guidelines for the organization of training in C-L for psychiatry residents

	APM	EACLPP
Model of rotation	Block model	Block model
Duration of the rotation to a C-L department:		
– Minimum	3 months FTE	6 months FTE
– Ideal	4–6 months	
Numbers of new consultations performed by the trainee		
– Minimum	50	100
– Ideal	100	
Ideal year of rotation during residency	3 or 4	Second half of residency
Rotation to outpatient C-L experience	Recommended	
Liaison activities	Encouraged	Recommended
Specialty areas	Recommended (e.g., oncology, transplantation, ICU, geriatrics)	Recommended
Supervision	Clearly defined frequency and duration of supervision sessions by an experienced C-L expert	Clearly defined frequency and duration of supervision sessions; named supervisor

- Quickly forming a therapeutic alliance under a variety of clinical settings
- Crisis intervention and supportive psychotherapy appropriate for the medically ill
- Psychopharmacology in the medically ill
- Appropriate communication with the severely ill and dying patient and his or her caregivers
- Appropriate communication with the consultees and the medical staff
- Promoting coordination of care for the complex patient across several disciplines

In addition, the APA Ad Hoc Work Group Report on the Integration of Psychiatry and Primary Care [28] recommends to include exposure to integrated care models into psychiatric residency.

17.5 Advanced Training (Special Competence, Fellowship, Subspecialization, Specialization)

The treatment of severely and chronically ill patients suffering from somatoform/somatic symptom disorders, eating disorders, and complex comorbid medical and psychiatric conditions and the research in these areas of health care and the undergraduate and postgraduate education of primary care physicians and specialists need specialized physicians. In most countries these are psychiatrists with a special training or a subspecialization in C-L psychiatry; in some countries (Germany,

Austria, Latvia, Czech Republic), own specialization in psychosomatic medicine was established. In the UK, psychiatric trainees in their 3 years of higher training can spend 1 year in liaison psychiatry and obtain a subspecialty endorsement in liaison psychiatry, which equips them to apply for a consultant post in liaison psychiatry at the end of their training.

17.5.1 Special Competence

For many years, such competence was acquired in an ad hoc manner or by learning from an expert in psychosomatic medicine/CLP in a hospital with an excellent reputation in C-L. Formal courses and trainings in C-L psychiatry were organized locally:

- In the USA, fellowship programs appeared in several academic hospitals supported by NIMH training grants in the 1970s [36].
- In Europe, the course for liaison psychiatry in Manchester, England, was the first attempt to offering some training to psychiatrists in C-L [8]. This was a week-long intensive course that set up in 1992. The course was attended by many psychiatrists from other countries, too. This spread knowledge and competence throughout Europe and enhanced the building of a network. Similar courses were organized in Austria and Germany [37, 38].

Since the middle of the 1950s of the last century, researchers in the field of PM met for a biannual scientific meeting, the European Conference of Psychosomatic Research. In the mid-1990s, several multicenter research projects funded by the European Union brought together experts in the field who formed the European C-L Workgroup [39]. This was the core group for the foundation of the European Association of C-L Psychiatry and Psychosomatics (EACLPP) in 1999 [40]. The EACLPP found that there were serious shortcomings and unacceptable variation of the expertise and standard of training in C-L psychiatry and psychosomatics throughout Europe. For this reason, EACLPP founded a working group on training in C-L that agreed and published guidelines for training in C-L based on formal consensus procedures [11]. These guidelines stated that advanced training in C-L psychiatry and psychosomatics should enable the trainees to [11]:

- *"identify and assess complex patients with increased care needs and to formulate an appropriate treatment plan and care co-ordination for these patients;*
- *provide comprehensive psychological and pharmacological treatment for medically ill patients with psychiatric co-morbidity;*
- *work effectively in a liaison role;*
- *sensitise physicians and nurses to the psychosocial aspects of patient care, to the prevention of the development of psychosocial problems in the physically ill, and the early detection and treatment of psychiatric co-morbidity;*

- *provide support to medical staff and mediate conflicts between patients and medical staff*
- *educate other specialties' physicians and staff;*
- *participate in the training of residents in C-L psychiatry and psychosomatics*
- *plan and/or conduct research in C-L psychiatry and psychosomatics;*
- *conduct quality management in a C-L service;*
- *organise and implement a new C-L service in a particular medical department".*

The guidelines recommended that advanced training should:

- Cover a minimum of 12-month full-time rotation to a C-L department and/or a PsychMed unit or a psychosomatic unit (2-year training is preferable):
    - Trainees should gain practical experience in several clinical fields including intensive care and palliative care where they have clinical responsibility throughout their training under the direct supervision of an experienced C-L psychiatrist.
    - Practical experience should include classical consultation services as well as more intensive and integrated cooperation with a somatic ward or department (liaison).
    - The increase in knowledge should not only include knowledge about diagnostic and screening methods and treatment modalities but also knowledge about the development and organization of C-L services, research methods in C-L, as well as economic aspects and ethical dilemmas in this clinical field.
    - The trainees should acquire specific communication skills at the interface of medicine and psychiatry including a comprehensive understanding of the systemic and scenic aspects of the referral and issues of transference/countertransference in the relationship between physicians, staff, and patients. They should learn to effectively communicate with a multidisciplinary team.
    - Trainees should learn to coordinate care for the complex patient across several disciplines in secondary and primary care.
    - Trainees should be supervised by a named attending physician with experience in C-L psychiatry/psychosomatics. They should attend weekly case conferences, theoretical seminars, and journal clubs.
    - Assessment of competency should include feedback of tutors and be based upon trainees' performance at clinical supervision. It should be concluded with a formal examination.

So far, formal advanced training in C-L psychiatry which is accredited by the National Board of Physicians is rare. In Finland, a 2-year approved training leads to the recognition of "special competence" in General Hospital Psychiatry. In the UK 1 year of full-time training in a C-L unit leads to a "special endorsement" in C-L psychiatry as part of specialist training and is linked to the attainment of specific competencies outlined by the Royal College of Psychiatrists [41].

In Australia and New Zealand, advanced training in CLP has been well developed. In the third stage (advanced stage) of the psychiatry training program which lasts for 24 months, trainees can spend 6 months in CLP [42]. This is in addition to a mandatory 6 months in CLP which has to be completed during their second stage of training. As trainees enter their advanced stage of training, they can choose to undertake a Certificate in Advanced Training in various areas of practice, one of which is CLP.

17.5.2 Subspecialization in Psychosomatic Medicine/C-L Psychiatry (Fellowship)

In the USA, "psychosomatic medicine" received approval as a subspecialty field of psychiatry in 2003. Earlier this field was better known as consultation-liaison (C-L) psychiatry, and recently the name of the subspecialty was changed into "consultation-liaison psychiatry." Most physicians who are active in this field are members of the Academy of Psychosomatic Medicine (APM). Training in this subspecialty provides special competencies in the diagnosis and treatment of patients with complex medical conditions and psychiatric comorbidities. Fellowship training is based on a 1-year full-time rotation (or a longer-lasting part-time rotation, at least half-time) to a PM clinical and teaching unit after completion of a residency in general psychiatry. It must meet the minimum faculty standard of two specialists who are board certified in psychiatry and psychosomatic medicine. Board certification of the subspecialty requires reexamination every 10 years.

In a consensus procedure, directors of training programs agreed core competencies for such training [10]. The American Accreditation Council for Graduate Medical Education (ACGME) has established a set of six core competencies for residency and fellowship certifications: clinical care, medical knowledge, professionalism, interpersonal and communication skills, system-based learning, and practice-based learning. These core competencies were agreed for the fellowship programs in CLP, too. The training is focused on the evaluation and treatment of (a) complex medically ill patients suffering from medical and psychiatric conditions and (b) patients with somatic symptom disorder/somatoform disorder or chronic pain in acute hospital settings. Fellows are trained to perform diagnostic evaluation and the development and implementation of treatment and care plans for such patients in inpatient and outpatient settings. In addition, they are expected to develop skills to professionally communicate with other HC providers, to implement liaison activities, and to develop multiprofessional care for complex patients. Trainees are supervised on a day-to-day basis. Fellowship programs include seminars, literature clubs, rounds, and bedside teaching, and—at least in academic hospitals—participation in research activities. Trainees and supervisors have to undergo a formal evaluation twice a year.

In Switzerland, a significant step was achieved about 10 years ago (in 2008) with the recognition of C-L psychiatry as a subspecialty of adult psychiatry by the Swiss Medical Chamber. The Swiss Society of Consultation-Liaison Psychiatry was established in 2001 and developed C-L training requirements, influenced by the official recognition of the subspecialty in the USA (described above), as well as the recommendations made by the EACLPP [11].

The C-L subspecialty training program consists of a minimum of 2-year full-time work (or equivalent part-time) at an accredited C-L training center. Centers can be accredited for 2 years (academic and large centers entailing a multidisciplinary C-L team as well as specialized consultations, e.g., psycho-oncology, transplantation, bariatric surgery) or for 1 year (smaller centers). At least 1 year has to be performed after the specialization in psychiatry. In addition to tutorials, supervision, journal clubs, and case conferences directly offered by the C-L units, candidates for the subspecialty have to attend theoretical training. The theoretical course (60 h) covers modules in C-L psychiatry, psychopharmacology, and psychotherapy in the C-L context, as well as topics related to specific areas (e.g., neuropsychiatry, oncology, transplantation, pain patients, eating disorders, and substance abuse). The course is provided both in German- and French-speaking areas. During their training candidates must perform a minimum of 300 written and supervised referrals as well as 10 interdisciplinary team-counseling sessions. A minimum of 120 hours of individual or group supervision offered by at least two certified C-L psychiatrists—one of them not serving in the department where the training is carried out—is required. Outcome and competency assessments include a learning objective-based evaluation by the tutors and an examination consisting of a thesis (or a first author peer-reviewed paper) and an oral examination focusing on clinical cases (for details see [43] and www.ssclp.ch).

17.5.3 Specialization in Psychosomatic Medicine

In Germany, psychosomatic medicine became a mandatory subject in the education of medical students in 1970. Consequently, departments of PM emerged in most university hospitals. They were built on a long-standing tradition of "holistic" bio-psychosocial approaches in internal medicine and neurology. Some of these departments belonged to centers of internal medicine, others to centers of psychosocial medicine. In addition to education of medical students, they conducted research and provided clinical care for patients with medical and mental comorbidity. In 1992, PM became a separate medical specialization alongside general psychiatry and child psychiatry.

The main emphasis of the new specialty is the diagnosis and treatment of patients with comorbid somatic and mental conditions and disorders (e.g., anxiety and depression in the medically ill, somatoform disorders, adjustment disorders accompanying physical diseases, chronic pain syndromes, eating disorders). Training of specialists lasts 5 years including 1 year in internal medicine, 1 year in psychiatry, and 3 years of specialized training in psychosomatic medicine (at least 2 years in a psychosomatic department; 1 year can be performed in a certified psychosomatic practice). The residents must undergo a training involving attachment to psychosomatic wards (med-psych units), outpatient services, and consultation-liaison services. Compared to subspecialty training, residents in PM have much more intensive training in psychotherapeutic methods for the treatment of medically ill patients with psychological problems or mental comorbidities. Short-term and long-term psychotherapy sessions are supervised closely by faculty experts. Residents have to undergo a psychotherapeutic experience themselves outside the training facility. At the end of the training, residents perform an oral examination.

To date, about 5000 physicians have completed such specialization in Germany, 3000 of them working in outpatient facilities and 2000 in departments of PM [28]. Psychosomatic departments are an established part of most tertiary care and many secondary care centers.

Outside Germany, a specialization in psychosomatic medicine exists in Austria, Latvia and in the Czech Republic.

17.6 Education of Other Health-Care Professionals

17.6.1 Training of Nurses

In many countries, the biopsychosocial approach to illness and medical treatment is a theoretical basis of the training for nurses. Nurse trainees receive training in communication skills with patients, their relatives, and within teams. In most German federal states, training in psychosomatic medicine is integrated in the education of psychiatry nurses, e.g., in Nuremberg psychiatry nurses undergo a 1-week theoretical training in PM and a 6-month rotation to a PM ward. In Saxonia there is a 2-year formal education of specialized PM nurses.

There is no specific training in liaison psychiatry in the UK for nurses, but a nurse competence framework has been developed for mental health liaison nursing by Eales and colleagues [44]. It consists of 19 competencies, one of which is working with people with psychosomatic disorders. Liaison nurses also deliver psychological treatments in the UK including cognitive behavioral therapy and psychodynamic interpersonal therapy. To carry out this work, nurses undergo the relevant training with supervision.

17.6.2 Training of Care/Case Managers

Case managers who take care of complex, multimorbid patients work at the intersection of medical and mental health care. They are a core element in the provision and coordination of care for patients with medical and mental comorbidity and their caregivers. However, depending on their professional background and experience care managers often focus solely on the physical aspects of care or solely on the mental aspects of care. This hinders an effective coordination of the care patients need. Uncoordinated care may lead to treatment errors, miscommunication, waste of resources, and patient dissatisfaction. Integrated medical and mental health care has proven more effective than fragmented care [45]. For this reason, the Case Management Society of America (CMSA) has implemented a project to train case managers in an integrated evaluation and care of complex patients with medical and psychiatric comorbidity. Based on the INTERMED method [46, 47], Latour and co-workers [48] developed a manual for the biopsychosocial evaluation and care planning for complex patients, the IM-CAG. The CMSA have included this tool and related communication skills in their training for care managers to provide integrated multiprofessional care for complex patients.

17.7 Future Tasks and Developments

Experts agree that a more intensive training of all physicians and other HC providers who treat complex patients with medical and mental comorbidity in general medical settings is necessary. Such training should include knowledge about the evaluation and treatment of complex medically ill and specific communication skills to address the needs of these patients. Training courses for the evaluation and treatment of patients with somatoform disorders and to improve communication skills with cancer patients have been shown effective [1, 6, 32]. To achieve this goal, we need more physicians who are specialized in PM to train general practitioners, residents, and specialists in different medical specialties, nurses, care managers, and other health-care professionals.

In many countries, training of psychiatric residents in PM/C-L has been implemented or improved during the last decade. However, surveys on the organization and practice of such training programs [11–13, 49] identified a couple of problems and shortcomings:

- In most countries, there is a lack of clear objectives and of guidelines.
- There are not enough PM/C-L specialties to teach residents and fellows.
- The time of rotation of residents to C-L units is not sufficiently long.
- Often the rotation is not organized as a "block," and obligations in other departments or sectors of psychiatry had to be performed.
- Training in supportive psychotherapy and other psychological interventions is not sufficient.
- Systemic and psychodynamic aspects of the consultation and the trainees' attitudes and countertransference reactions are not adequately addressed.
- The evaluation and treatment of complex patients is not sufficient, and practical experience with collaborative care programs is missing in most trainings.
- Costs for such training are not sufficiently covered.

So far, formal subspecialty and specialty training in PM exists only in a few countries. There are attempts in Canada and in some European countries (the Netherlands, Spain, Portugal) to obtain a board certification for a subspecialty. In some countries this may be called psychosomatic medicine, in others C-L psychiatry.

References

1. Fritzsche K, Larisch A. Treating patients with functional somatic symptoms. A treatment guide for use in general practice. Scand J Primary Health Care. 2003;21(3):132–5.
2. Fritzsche K, Scheib P, Ko N, Wirsching M, Kuhnert A, Hick J, et al. Results of a psychosomatic training program in China, Vietnam and Laos: successful cross-cultural transfer of a postgraduate training program for medical doctors. Biopsychosoc Med. 2012;6(1):17. https://doi.org/10.1186/1751-0759-6-17.
3. Smith RC, Lyles JS, Mettler J, Stoffelmayr BE, Van Egeren LF, Marshall AA, et al. The effectiveness of intensive training for residents in interviewing—a randomized, controlled study. Ann Intern Med. 1998;128:118–26.
4. Langewitz WA, Eich P, Kiss A, Wössmer B. Improving communication skills—a randomized controlled behaviorally oriented intervention study for residents in internal medicine. Psychosom Med. 1998;60(3):268–76.
5. Stiefel F, Barth J, Bensing J, Fallowfield L, Jost L, Razavi D, et al. Communication skills training in oncology: a position paper based on a consensus meeting among European experts in 2009. Ann Oncol. 2010;21(2):204–7. https://doi.org/10.1093/annonc/mdp564.
6. Barth J, Lannen P. Efficacy of communication skills training courses in oncology: a systematic review and meta-analysis. Ann Oncol. 2011;22(5):1030–40. https://doi.org/10.1093/annonc/mdq441.
7. Royal College of Physicians and Surgeons of Canada. 2005. http://rcpsc.medical.org/canmeds/CanMEDS2005/index.php. Accessed 2 Nov 2017.
8. Guthrie E, Creed F. Postgraduate training. In: Benjamin S, House A, Jenkins P, editors. Liaison psychiatry. Defining needs and planning services, vol. 1994. London: Gaskell; 1994. p. 99–103.
9. Gitlin DF, Schindler BA, Stern TA, Epstein SA, Lamdan RM, McCarty TA, et al. Recommended guidelines for consultation-liaison psychiatric training in psychiatry residency programs. A report from the Academy of Psychosomatic Medicine Task Force on Psychiatric Resident Training in Consultation-Liaison Psychiatry. Psychosomatics. 1996;37(1):3–11.
10. Worley LL, Levenson JL, Stern TA, Epstein SA, Rundell JR, Crone CC, et al. Core competencies for fellowship training in psychosomatic medicine: a collaborative effort by the APA Council on Psychosomatic Medicine, the ABPN Psychosomatic Committee, and the Academy of Psychosomatic Medicine. Psychosomatics. 2009;50(6):557–62. https://doi.org/10.1176/appi.psy.50.6.557.
11. Söllner W, Creed F, European Association of Consultation-Liaison Psychiatry and Psychosomatics Workgroup on Training in Consultation-Liaison Psychiatry and Psychosomatics. European guidelines for training in consultation-liaison psychiatry and psychosomatics: report of the EACLPP Workgroup on Training in Consultation-Liaison Psychiatry and Psychosomatics. J Psychosom Res. 2007;62(4):505–6.
12. Rymaszewska J, Söllner W. Training in consultation-liaison psychiatry in Eastern Europe. J Psychosom Res. 2012;72(6):460–2. https://doi.org/10.1016/j.jpsychores.2012.02.006.
13. Heinrich TW, Schwartz AC, Zimbrean PC, Wright MT, Academy of Psychosomatic Medicine's Residency Education Subcommittee. The state of the service: a survey of psychiatry resident education in psychosomatic medicine. Psychosomatics. 2013;54(6):560–6. https://doi.org/10.1016/j.psym.2013.07.005.
14. Leentjens AF, Rundell JR, Diefenbacher A, Kathol R, Guthrie E. Psychosomatic medicine and consultation-liaison psychiatry: scope of practice, processes, and competencies for psychiatrists working in the field of CL psychiatry or psychosomatics. A consensus statement of the European Association of Consultation-Liaison Psychiatry and Psychosomatics (EACLPP) and the Academy of Psychosomatic Medicine (APM). Psychosomatics. 2011;52(1):19–25. https://doi.org/10.1016/j.psym.2010.11.022.
15. Engel GL. The clinical application of the biopsychosocial model. Am J Psychiatry. 1980;137:535–44.

16. Adler RH. Engel's biopsychosocial model is still relevant today. J Psychosom Res. 2009;67(6):607–11.
17. Fava GA, Sonino N. From the lesson of George Engel to current knowledge: the biopsychosocial model 40 years later. Psychother Psychosom. 2017;86(5):257–9. https://doi.org/10.1159/000478808.
18. Benning TB. Limitations of the biopsychosocial model in psychiatry. Adv Med Educ Pract. 2015;6:347–52. https://doi.org/10.2147/AMEP.S82937.
19. Nestel D, Kidd J. Peer assisted learning in patient-centred interviewing: the impact on student tutors. Med Teach. 2005;27(5):439–44.
20. Doering S, Schneider G, Burgmer M, Sensmeier J, Schrewe FB, Friederichs H, Heuft G. Evaluation of the clinical course psychosomatics and psychotherapy employing standardized patients. Z Psychosom Med Psychother. 2010;56(4):385–98.
21. Keifenheim KE, Teufel M, Ip J, Speiser N, Leehr EJ, Zipfel S, et al. Teaching history taking to medical students: a systematic review. BMC Med Educ. 2015;15:159. https://doi.org/10.1186/s12909-015-0443-x.
22. Keifenheim KE, Petzold ER, Junne F, Erschens RS, Speiser N, Herrmann-Werner A, et al. Peer-assisted history-taking groups: a subjective assessment of their impact upon medical students' interview skills. GMS J Med Educ. 2017;34(3):Doc35. https://doi.org/10.3205/zma001112.
23. Berger S, Goetz K, Leowardi-Bauer C, Schultz JH, Szecsenyi J, Mahler C. Anchoring interprofessional education in undergraduate curricula: the Heidelberg story. J Interprof Care. 2017;31(2):175–9. Epub 2016 Nov 23. https://doi.org/10.1080/13561820.2016.1240156.
24. Shulman R. Psychosomatic education: who teaches what and where at the University of British Columbia. J Psychosom Res. 1983;27(1):17–20.
25. Voineskos G, Hsu K, Hunter RC. The teaching of consultation-liaison psychiatry in the undergraduate curriculum of Canadian medical schools. Gen Hosp Psychiatry. 1984;6(2):117–22.
26. Lobo A, Campayo A, de-la-Cámara C, Saz P, Salvador H, Lobo-Escolar L, et al. The teaching of liaison psychiatry. J Psychosom Res. 2012;72(6):457–9. https://doi.org/10.1016/j.jpsychores.2012.01.012.
27. Kathol RG, Melek S, Bair B, Sargent S. Financing mental health and substance use disorder care within physical health: a look to the future. Pschiatr Clin North Am. 2008;31(1):11–25.
28. American Psychiatric Association Ad Hoc Work Group on the Integration of Psychiatry and Primary Care. https://www.psychiatry.org/psychiatrists/practice/professional-interests/integrated-care/
29. Zipfel S, Herzog W, Kruse J, Henningsen P. Psychosomatic medicine in Germany: more timely than ever. Psychother Psychosom. 2016;85(5):262–9. https://doi.org/10.1159/000447701.
30. Goldberg D, Gask L, O'Dowd T. The treatment of somatization: teaching techniques of reattribution. J Psychosom Res. 1989;33:689–95.
31. Fink P, Rosendal M, Toft T. Assessment and treatment of functional disorders in general practice: the extended reattribution and management model—an advanced educational program for nonpsychiatric doctors. Psychosomatics. 2002;43(2):93–131.
32. Toft T, Rosendal M, Ørnbøl E, Olesen F, Frostholm L, Fink P. Training general practitioners in the treatment of functional somatic symptoms: effects on patient health in a cluster-randomised controlled trial (the Functional Illness in Primary Care study). Psychother Psychosom. 2010;79(4):227–37. https://doi.org/10.1159/000313691.
33. Larisch A, Schweickhardt A, Wirsching M, Fritzsche K. Psychosocial interventions for somatizing patients by the general practitioner. A randomized controlled trial. J Psychosom Res. 2004;57:507–14.
34. Morriss R, Dowrick C, Salmon P, Peters S, Dunn G, Rogers A, et al. Cluster randomised controlled trial of training practices in reattribution for medically unexplained symptoms. Br J Psychiatry. 2007;191:536–42.
35. Sockalingam S, Arena A, Serhal E, Mohri L, Alloo J, Crawford A. Building provincial mental health capacity in primary care: an evaluation of a project ECHO mental health program. Acad Psychiatry. 2017. https://doi.org/10.1007/s40596-017-0735-z.

36. Houpt JL, Weinstein HM, Russell ML. The application of competency-based education to consultation-liaison psychiatry: II. Intervention knowledge and skills. Int J Psychiatry Med. 1976–1977;7(4):309–20.
37. Maislinger S, Rumpold G, Kantner-Rumplmair W, Stelzig M, Riessland-Seifert A. Curriculum for a course in C-L psychiatry, psychology, and psychosomatics in Austria. J Psychosom Res. 2007;62(5):599–600.
38. Fritzsche K, Stein B, Larisch A, Weidner K, Diefenbacher A, Burian R, Söllner W. First curriculum for care of patients with mental and psychosomatic disorders in the context of a consultation-liaison service. Psychother Psychosom Med Psychol. 2009;59:246–7.
39. Huyse FJ, Herzog T, Lobo A, Malt UF, Opmeer BC, Stein B, et al. Consultation-liaison psychiatric service delivery: results from a European study. Gen Hosp Psychiatry. 2001;23:124–32.
40. Leentjens A, Lobo A. On the history of the European Association of Consultation-Liaison Psychiatry and Psychosomatics (EACLPP). J Psychosom Res. 2011;70(6):575–7.
41. Royal College of Psychiatrists. https://www.rcpsych.ac.uk/pdf/Liaison_Psychiatry_Curriculum_August_2016.pdf
42. Royal Australian and New Zealand College of Psychiatrists. Curriculum for fellowship. https://www.ranzcp.org/Pre-Fellowship/About-the-training-program.aspx
43. Georgescu D, Berney A. Consultation–liaison psychiatry: a new psychiatric subspecialty in Switzerland. J Psychosom Res. 2011;71(6):429–30.
44. Eales S, Wilson N, Waghorn J. A competence framework for liaison. Mental Health Nursing. 2014;1–31. https://www.rcpsych.ac.uk/pdf/A Competence Framework for Liaison. Mental Health Nursing 2014.pdf
45. Kathol RG, Butler M, McAlpine DD, Kane RL. Barriers to physical and mental condition integrated service delivery. Psychosom Med. 2010;72(6):511–8. https://doi.org/10.1097/PSY.0b013e3181e2c4a0.
46. Huyse FJ, Lyons JS, Stiefel F, Slaets J, de Jonge P, Latour C. Operationalizing the biopsychosocial model: the intermed. Psychosomatics. 2001;42(1):5–13.
47. Stiefel FC, Huyse FJ, Söllner W, Slaets JP, Lyons JS, Latour CH, et al. Operationalizing integrated care on a clinical level: the INTERMED project. Med Clin North Am. 2006;90(4):713–58.
48. Latour C, Perez R, Kathol RG, Huyse F, Cohen JS. The integrated case management manual: assisting complex patients regain physical and mental health. New York: Springer; 2010.
49. Jiménez X, Thorkelson G. Medical countertransference and the trainee: identifying a training gap. J Psychiatr Pract. 2012;18(2):109–17. https://doi.org/10.1097/01.pra.0000413276.03467.49.

Wolfgang Söllner, MD, is Professor of Psychosomatic Medicine and Psychotherapy at Paracelsus Medical University in Nuremberg, Germany. He is director of the Department of Psychosomatic Medicine and Psychotherapy at the Nuremberg General Hospital. He is Fellow of the Academy of Psychosomatic Medicine and from 2002 to 2018 he was president of the European Association of Psychosomatic Medicine. He conducted research mainly in the areas of psycho-oncology, psychosocial aspects of chronic pain, and psychotherapy with the medically ill. He was active in the training of GPs, oncologists, and residents in psychiatry and psychosomatic medicine. He is co-editor of the German Textbook of Psychosomatic Medicine.

Else Guthrie, MD, is Professor of Psychological Medicine in the Leeds Institute of Health Sciences, University of Leeds. She is co-author of Psychodynamic-Interpersonal Therapy: A conversational Model, Sage 2016 (with M Barkham, G Hardy and F Margsion) and Psychiatry Master Medicine: Churchill Livingstone; 2002 (with S Lewis). She is co-editor of The Handbook of Liaison Psychiatry, Cambridge 2007 (with G Lloyd) and Seminars in Liaison Psychiatry Gaskell 1996 and Seminars in Liaison Psychiatry Second Edition Gaskell 2007 (with S Rao and M Temple). She is former Chair of the Faculty of Liaison Psychiatry, Royal College of Psychiatrists and has published widely on psychological treatments in liaison psychiatry and psychosomatic medicine.

Alexandre Berney, MD, is Associate Professor at the Lausanne University Hospital, Switzerland. He is both psychiatrist and psychotherapist, specialized in C-L psychiatry and psychosomatics, and leads a C-L Unit at Lausanne University Hospital. His research interests and publications focus on neuropsychiatry, functional disorders, and physician–patient communication. He served several years as President of the Swiss Society for Consultation-Liaison Psychiatry and contributed to the recognition in 2008 of C–L psychiatry as a subspecialty of adult psychiatry by the Swiss Medical Chamber.

MIX
Papier aus verantwortungsvollen Quellen
Paper from responsible sources
FSC® C105338

If you have any concerns about our products,
you can contact us on
ProductSafety@springernature.com

In case Publisher is established outside the EU,
the EU authorized representative is:
Springer Nature Customer Service Center GmbH
Europaplatz 3, 69115 Heidelberg, Germany

Printed by Libri Plureos GmbH
in Hamburg, Germany